D1068626

ITI Treatment Guide
Volume 10

ITI
Treatment
Guide

Editors:
D. Buser, S. Chen, D. Wismeijer

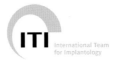

ITI International Team
for Implantology

Authors:
V. Chappuis, W. Martin

Volume 10

Implant Therapy in the Esthetic Zone:

Current Treatment Modalities
and Materials
for Single-tooth Replacements

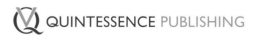
QUINTESSENCE PUBLISHING

Berlin, Barcelona, Chicago, Istanbul, London,
Milan, Moscow, New Delhi, Paris, Prague,
São Paulo, Seoul, Singapore, Tokyo, Warsaw

German National Library CIP Data

The German National Library has listed this publication in the German National Bibliography. Detailed bibliographical data are available at http://dnb.ddb.de.

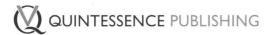

© 2017 Quintessenz Verlags-GmbH
Ifenpfad 2 – 4, 12107 Berlin, Germany
www.quintessenz.de

Illustrations:	Ute Drewes, Basel (CH), www.drewes.ch
Copyediting:	Triacom Dental, Barendorf (DE), www.dental.triacom.com
Graphic concept:	Wirz Corporate AG, Zürich (CH)
Production:	Juliane Richter, Berlin (DE)
Printing:	Bosch-Druck GmbH, Landshut (DE), www.bosch-druck.de

Printed in Germany
ISBN: 978-3-86867-343-2

The ITI Mission is ...

"... to serve the dental profession
by providing a growing global
network for life-long learning
in implant dentistry through
comprehensive quality education
and innovative research to the benefit
of the patient."

Preface

It has been ten years since the publication of the first volume of the Treatment Guide series that addressed single-tooth replacements in the esthetic zone. Today, a decade later, many more practitioners are routinely involved in providing patients with implant therapy, and the field has seen many advances.

Progress and developments in implant design, surgical techniques, and materials, abutment design and restorative materials, as well as patient evaluation add up to make this a timely moment to revisit single-tooth replacements in the esthetic zone. From the first consultation to follow-up and maintenance, volume 10 focuses on the treatment modalities and materials that implant dentistry has to offer today.

The Consensus Statements and clinical recommendations from the 5th ITI Consensus Conference are the starting point of this volume. They are followed by a detailed protocol for evaluation and treatment planning and execution for patients with esthetic needs who require single-tooth replacement with a dental implant.

Fourteen complex clinical case presentations form the core of this volume with step-by-step descriptions of procedures for achieving stable long-term esthetic outcomes. The aim is to support clinicians in their decision-making processes and in preventing complications.

D. Buser   S. Chen   D. Wismeijer

Acknowledgment

The authors would like to express their gratitude to Dr. Kati Benthaus for her excellent support in the preparation and coordination of this Treatment Guide. We would also like to thank Ms. Ute Drewes for the professional illustrations, Ms. Juliane Richter (Quintessence Publishing) for the typesetting and for the coordination of the production workflow and Mr. Per N. Döhler (Triacom Dental) for the language editing. We also acknowledge Institut Straumann AG, the corporate partner of the ITI, for its continuing support.

Editors and Authors

Editors:

Daniel Buser
   DDS, Dr med dent, Professor
   Chair, Department of Oral Surgery and Stomatology
   School of Dental Medicine
   University of Bern
   Freiburgstrasse 7
   3010 Bern
   Switzerland
   E-mail: daniel.buser@zmk.unibe.ch

Stephen Chen
   MDSc, PhD, FRACDS
   Clinical Associate Professor
   School of Dental Science
   University of Melbourne
   720 Swanston Street
   Melbourne, VIC 3010
   Australia
   E-mail: schen@periomelbourne.com.au

Daniel Wismeijer
   DMD, Professor
   Head of the Department of Oral Implantology and
   Prosthetic Dentistry
   Section of Implantology and Prosthetic Dentistry
   Academic Center for Dentistry Amsterdam (ACTA)
   Free University
   Gustav Mahlerlaan 3004
   1081 LA Amsterdam
   Netherlands
   E-mail: d.wismeijer@acta.nl

Authors:

Vivanne Chappuis
   DDS, Dr med dent, PD, Assistant Professor
   Department of Oral Surgery and Stomatology
   School of Dental Medicine
   University of Bern
   Freiburgstrasse 7
   3010 Bern
   Switzerland
   E-mail: vivianne.chappuis@zmk.unibe.ch

William Martin
   DMD, MS, Clinical Professor
   The University of Florida
   Center for Implant Dentistry
   1395 Center Drive, Room D7-6
   Gainesville, FL 32610-3003
   United States of America
   E-mail: wmartin@dental.ufl.edu

Contributors

Urs Belser
  DMD, Dr med dent
  Professor emeritus, University of Geneva
  Guest Professor, University of Bern
  Freiburgstrasse 7
  3010 Bern
  Switzerland
  E-mail: urs.belser@unige.ch

Dieter Bosshardt
  PhD, Associate Professor
  University of Bern
  Head, Robert K. Schenk Laboratory of Oral Histology
  School of Dental Medicine
  Freiburgstrasse 7
  3010 Bern
  Switzerland
  E-mail: dieter.bosshardt@zmk.unibe.ch

Allen Russell Burgoyne
  BSc, DDS, MSD, Cert Prostho
  966 King Street West
  Suite 101
  Kitchener, ON N2G 1G4
  Canada
  E-mail: dr.burgoyne@sympatico.ca

Daniel Buser
  DDS, Dr med dent, Professor
  Chair, Department of Oral Surgery and Stomatology
  School of Dental Medicine
  University of Bern
  Freiburgstrasse 7
  3010 Bern
  Switzerland
  E-mail: daniel.buser@zmk.unibe.ch

Paolo Casentini
  DDS, Dr med dent
  Via Anco Marzio 2
  20123 Milano
  Italy
  E-mail: paolocasentini@fastwebnet.it

Stephen Chen
  MDSc, PhD, FRACDS
  Clinical Associate Professor
  School of Dental Science
  University of Melbourne
  720 Swanston Street
  Melbourne, VIC 3010
  Australia
  E-mail: schen@periomelbourne.com.au

Wagner Duarte
  DDS, PhD
  University of Brasilia
  SCN Quadra 2 Bloco D Sala 516/517
  Edificio Liberty Mall, Asa Norte
  Brasília, DF
  70712-903
  Brazil
  E-mail: duartew@yahoo.com

Michael Gahlert
  Dr med dent
  High Tech Research Center
  University Hospital Basel
  Spitalstrasse 21
  4031 Basel
  Switzerland
  E-mail: mgahlert@uhbs.ch, m.gahlert@knihagahlert.de

Jason Gillespie
DDS, PA
4118 McCullough Ave
San Antonio, TX 78212-1905
United States of America
E-mail: jrgillespiedds@sbcglobal.net

Adam Hamilton
BDSc, FRACDS, DCD
Harvard School of Dental Medicine
Restorative Dentistry and Biomaterials Sciences
Division of Regenerative and Implant Sciences
188 Longwood Avenue
Boston, MA 02115-5819
United States of America
E-mail: adam_hamilton@hsdm.harvard.edu

Alessandro Januario
DDS, MS, PhD
Aria Institute
Centro Médico Lúcio Costa
SGAS 610 Lote 74 Bloco II Sala 307
Brasília, DF
70200-700
Brazil
E-mail: januarioal@gmail.com

Scott Keith
DDS, MS
1111 Civic Drive
Suite 320
Walnut Creek, CA 94596-3894
United States of America
E-mail: skeithdds@hotmail.com

Chatchai Kunavisarut
DDS, MS, Assistant Professor
Mahidol University
School of Dentistry
Advanced General Dentistry Department
6 Yothee Road
Bangkok 10400
Thailand
E-mail: drjub@hotmail.com

Eduardo R. Lorenzana
DDS, MS
3519 Paesano's Parkway
Suite 103
San Antonio, TX 78231-1266
United States of America
E-mail: drlorenzana@yahoo.com

Dean Morton
BDS, MS, Professor
Professor and Chair, Department of Prosthodontics
Assistant Dean for Strategic Partnerships and
Innovation
Director, Center for Implant, Esthetic and
Innovative Dentistry
Indiana University School of Dentistry —
Prosthodontics
1121 W Michigan Street, DS-S316
Indianapolis, IN 46202-5186
E-mail: deamorto@iu.edu

Paulo Eduardo Pittas do Canto
DDS
Prosthodontics
Contento – Odontologica Especializada
Rua Marcelo Gama, 1148
Porto Alegre, RS
90540-041
Brazil
E-mail: pittasdocanto@gmail.com

Waldemar D. Polido
DDS, MS, PhD
Clinical Professor and Program Director,
Predoctoral Oral and Maxillofacial Surgery
Co-Director, Center for Implant, Esthetic and
Innovative Dentistry, Indiana University
School of Dentistry
1050 Wishard Boulevard, Room 2200
Indianapolis, IN 46202-2872
United States of America
E-mail: cirurgia.implantes@polido.com.br

Simon Storgård Jensen
DDS
Department of Oral and Maxillofacial Surgery
Copenhagen University Hospital
Blegdamsvej 9
2100 København Ø
Denmark
E-mail: simon.storgaard@jensen.mail.dk

Daniel S. Thoma
PD, Dr med dent, Head of Academic Unit
Clinic of Fixed and Removable Prosthodontics and
Dental Material Science
Center for Dental Medicine, University of Zürich
Plattenstrasse 11
8032 Zürich
Switzerland
E-mail: daniel.thoma@zzm.uzh.ch

Table of Contents

1   Introduction 1
        W. Martin, V. Chappuis

2   Consensus Statements: Statements and Recommendations Obtained
    from the 5th ITI Consensus Conference 3
        V. Chappuis, W. Martin

2.1   Contemporary Surgical and Radiographic Techniques in Implant Dentistry 4

2.2   Restorative Materials and Techniques for Implant Dentistry 8

2.3   Optimizing Esthetic Outcomes in Implant Dentistry 11

2.4   Implant-loading Protocols 15

2.5   Prevention and Management of Biological and Technical Implant Complications 18

3   Preoperative Risk Assessment and Treatment Planning
    for Optimal Esthetic Outcomes 23
        W. Martin, V. Chappuis, D. Morton, D. Buser

3.1   Patient Selection 26
3.1.1   SAC Classification for Single-tooth Replacement 28

3.2   Esthetic Risk Assessment 29
3.2.1   Medical Status 31
3.2.2   Smoking Habit 31
3.2.3   Gingival Display at Full Smile 32
3.2.4   Width of the Edentulous Span 33
3.2.5   Shape of Tooth Crowns 35
3.2.6   Restorative Status of Adjacent Teeth 37
3.2.7   Gingival Phenotype 38
3.2.8   Infection at the Implant Site 40
3.2.9   Soft-tissue Anatomy 41
3.2.10   Bone Level at the Adjacent Teeth 42

3.2.11 Facial Bone-wall Phenotype 42

3.2.12 Anatomy of the Alveolar Crest 44

3.2.13 Patients' Esthetic Expectations 46

3.3 Treatment Planning 47

3.3.1 Anatomical Considerations 49

3.3.2 Indications for CBCT in the Esthetic Zone 50

3.3.3 Digital or Conventional Planning 52

3.3.4 Surgical Templates for Implant Placement 54

4 Selecting Biomaterials for Implant Procedures 57

  V. Chappuis, S. S. Jensen, D. D. Bosshardt, D. Buser

4.1 Ceramic vs. Titanium Implant Materials 58

4.1.1 Commercially Pure Titanium Implants 58

4.1.2 Titanium-alloy Implants 61

4.1.3 Ceramic Implants 62

4.2 Bone Grafts and Bone Substitute Materials 64

4.2.1 Autologous Bone Grafts 66

4.2.2 Allografts 72

4.2.3 Xenografts 76

4.2.4 Alloplastic Bone Substitutes 76

4.3 Biologics 77

4.3.1 Growth Factors 77

4.3.2 Enamel Matrix Derivative 77

4.3.3 Autologous Platelet Concentrates 78

4.4 Membranes 79

4.4.1 Non-resorbable Membranes 80

4.4.2 Resorbable Membranes 80

4.4.3 New Development in Membranes with a Functionally Graded Structure 81

5 Surgical Considerations for Optimal Esthetic Outcomes 83

  V. Chappuis, S. Chen, D. Buser

5.1 Post-extraction Dimensional Ridge Alterations in the Esthetic Zone 85

5.1.1 Flapless Low-trauma Tooth Extraction to Reduce Dimensional Alterations 85

5.1.2 Post-extraction Dimensional Alterations of the Hard Tissues 89

5.1.3 Post-extraction Dimensional Alterations of the Soft Tissues 90

5.2 Indications for Post-extraction Ridge Preservation 92

5.2.1 Ridge Preservation by Root Maintenance 92

5.2.2 Ridge Preservation by Socket Grafting 94

5.3 Indications for Soft-tissue Grafting 97

5.3.1 Increasing the Band of Keratinized Mucosa 97

5.3.2 Improving the Soft-tissue Volume 99

5.4	Flap Design and Suture Techniques	101
5.4.1	Flapless Approach	101
5.4.2	Elevation of a Mucoperiosteal Flap	103

5.5	Implant Selection	105
5.5.1	Selection Criteria for Soft-tissue-level (STL) vs. Bone-level (BL) Implants in the Anterior Maxilla	106
5.5.2	Implant Diameters in the Anterior Maxilla	108
5.5.3	Implant Lengths in the Anterior Maxilla	110

5.6	Correct Three-dimensional Implant Positioning	111
5.6.1	Mesiodistal Dimensions	113
5.6.2	Orofacial Dimensions	113
5.6.3	Coronoapical Dimensions	113
5.6.4	Implant Angulation	113

5.7	Surgical Approach: Simultaneous vs. Staged GBR	114
5.7.1	Simultaneous GBR	114
5.7.2	Staged GBR	115

5.8	Surgical Approach: Immediate vs. Early vs. Late Implant Placement	116
5.8.1	Immediate Implant Placement (Type 1)	116
5.8.2	Early Implant Placement (Type 2 and 3)	120
5.8.3	Late Implant Placement (Type 4)	123

6	Prosthetic Management for Optimal Esthetic Outcomes	133
	W. Martin, A. Hamilton	

6.1	Evaluation of Esthetic Outcomes in Single-tooth Replacement	134

6.2	Interim Prostheses	137
6.2.1	Before Implant Placement	137
6.2.2	After Implant Placement	140

6.3	Management of Peri-implant Tissue	144
6.3.1	Shaping the Transition Zone	144
6.3.2	Capturing the Transition Zone	145

6.4	Laboratory Communication	149
6.4.1	Photography	149
6.4.2	Records	151
6.4.3	Prescription	151

6.5	Screw-retained vs. Cemented Restorations	152

6.6	Material Selection for Abutments and Crowns	154
6.6.1	Prefabricated Abutments	154
6.6.2	Cast Custom Abutments	156
6.6.3	CAD/CAM Custom Abutments	157
6.6.4	Original vs. Non-original	160

6.6.5   Abutment Materials 160

6.6.6   Biocompatibility 161

6.6.7   Influence on Esthetics 161

6.6.8   Physical Properties 161

6.7   Prosthetic Design 163

6.7.1   Crown/Veneer Materials 163

6.8   Handling of Abutments and Restorations 167

7   Clinical Case Presentations 169

7.1   Replacement of a Failing Upper Left Central Incisor: Immediate Placement
      of an RC Bone Level Implant and Provisionalization 170
      E. R. Lorenzana, J. Gillespie

7.2   Replacement of a Perforated Upper Left Central Incisor: Early Placement
      of an RC Bone Level Implant 181
      A. Januário, W. Duarte

7.3   Replacement of an Upper Right Central Incisor with a Root Fracture:
      Early Placement of an RC Bone Level Implant, Variobase Abutment 192
      C. Kunavisarut

7.4   Replacement of a Failing Upper Right Central Incisor: Ridge Preservation
      and Late Placement of a NC Bone Level Implant 202
      W. D. Polido, P. E. Pittas do Canto

7.5   Replacement of an Upper Right Central Incisor with Root Resorption:
      Ridge Preservation, Delayed Placement of an NC Bone Level Roxolid Implant 222
      P. Casentini

7.6   Replacement of an Upper Right Central Incisor with Root Resorption:
      Ridge Preservation, Early Placement of an RC Bone Level Implant 234
      S. Chen

7.7   Replacement of an Ankylosed Central Incisor with a Gingival Recession:
      Tooth Extraction with Socket Grafting and Late Implant Placement with
      Simultaneous Contour Augmentation 244
      D. Buser, U. Belser

7.8   Replacement of a Compromised Upper Right Central Incisor: Hard- and
      Soft-tissue Augmentation, Late Placement of an RC Bone Level Implant 258
      P. Casentini

7.9   Replacement of a Failing Restored Upper Right Central Incisor:
      Ridge Preservation and Early Placement of an RC Bone Level Implant 273
      D. Thoma

7.10 Replacement of a Fractured Upper Left Central Incisor: Delayed Placement
      of a Bone Level Tapered Implant Using a Staged Approach 288
      S. Keith

7.11 Replacement of an Ankylosed Upper Left Central Incisor: Bone Augmentation and Socket Grafting, Late Placement of an RC Bone Level Implant 300
    A. Burgoyne

7.12 Replacement of a Missing Upper Left Central Incisor: Late Placement of an RC Bone Level Implant, CAD/CAM Zirconia Abutment... 318
    E. R. Lorenzana, J. Gillespie

7.13 Replacement of a Missing Upper Left Central Incisor: Late Placement of an RC Bone Level Implant and Adjacent Tooth Restoration 330
    A. Hamilton

7.14 Replacement of a Fractured Upper Left Central Incisor: Early Placement of a Monotype Zirconia Implant, Semi-submerged Transmucosal Healing 340
    M. Gahlert

8   Esthetic Complications 351
    V. Chappuis, W. Martin, D. Buser

8.1 Causes of Esthetic Complications 352

8.1.1 Incorrect 3D Implant Position.. 353
8.1.2 Implant Selection 358
8.1.3 Insufficient Facial Bone Wall... 360
8.1.4 Esthetic Failure Due to Late Facial Growth... 361
8.1.5 Esthetic Failure Due to Implants and Third-party Implant Components Lacking Scientific Validation......... 362

8.2 Management of Esthetic Complications 364

8.2.1 Decision Criteria for Salvaging Esthetic Implants.................................... 364
8.2.2 Criteria for Implant Removal 375

9   Conclusions.. 389
    W. Martin, V. Chappuis

10   References 393

1 Introduction

W. Martin, V. Chappuis

The history of successful dental implant treatment has led to its large-scale use in today's clinical practice, providing patients with solutions for the treatment of all forms of edentulism. Clinicians and patients alike benefit from the possibility to use these implants to retain prostheses in a variety of situations, ranging from anterior to posterior tooth replacement to fully edentulous situations. Several authors have reported long-term survival rates of > 90%, leading to a higher acceptance of the dental implant as a primary option for tooth replacement (Adell and coworkers 1990; Lindquist and coworkers 1996; Wennström and coworkers 2005; Buser and coworkers 2012; Chappuis and coworkers 2013a). Of critical note, implant survival does not necessarily correlate with successful esthetic rehabilitation, since success criteria have varied over time. For esthetically sensitive areas, success criteria must include measurements of the peri-implant mucosa as well as the restoration and its relationship to the surrounding dentition (Belser and coworkers 2004; Smith and Zarb 1989).

Patients with failing or missing teeth in the esthetic zone present with their own set of clinical challenges for the clinician to achieve a natural-looking outcome. Any esthetic rehabilitation has to be predictable, which requires a reproducible and stable outcome in the short and long term. The ability to achieve this depends on the interaction between clinicians and technicians (experience) as well as biologic (anatomic factors, host response), surgical (procedures, materials, techniques), implant (dimensions, compositions, surface characteristics, designs), and prosthetic factors (techniques and materials).

The ITI has recognized the challenge of treating patients with esthetic needs and focused attention on them in its numerous publications (SAC Classification, ITI Treatment Guides) and the Proceedings of the 1st through 5th ITI Consensus Conferences over the past sixteen years. The SAC Classification provides information on the degree of restorative and surgical difficulty in the treatment of patients with dental implants and incorporates the use of the Esthetic Risk Assessment (ERA) in determining the risks to achieving an esthetic outcome based upon clinical factors associated with individualized treatment situations. Several ITI Treatment Guides have described the influence of treatment protocols on esthetic outcomes, beginning with Volume 1, Implant Therapy in the Esthetic Zone: Single-tooth Replacements and continuing with volumes 2 through 8. The Proceedings of the (1st to 5th) Consensus Conferences with its consensus statements and clinical recommendations have focused on the treatment of patients with high esthetic needs through treatment guidelines focusing on patient evaluation and treatment, timing of implant placement, loading protocols, and complications related to restorative materials.

In 2007, the ITI published the first volume of the ITI Treatment Guide series, focusing on single-tooth replacement in the esthetic zone. Since then there have been many advances in patient evaluation, implant design, surgical techniques and materials, abutment design and restorative materials, necessitating a revisit to this timely topic.

This volume of the ITI Treatment Guide series begins with the most recent consensus statements and clinical recommendations of the 5th ITI Consensus Conference, followed by a detailed protocol for evaluation and treatment planning for patients with esthetic needs requiring single-tooth replacement with a dental implant and restoration. The ERA table will be reviewed, and an updated version will be presented that is in line with current evaluation procedures and techniques incorporating digital technology.

Implant therapy performed in the esthetic zone requires careful attention to surgical procedures and materials utilized to regain lost tissue support for placing implants in ideal three-dimensional positions based upon the restorative plan. Implant materials, bone grafts, bone substitutes, biologics, and membranes will be presented and indications and techniques for their use outlined. Various surgical situations commonly encountered in the esthetic zone will be presented and treatment recommendations provided.

Prosthetic treatment in the esthetic zone requires advanced knowledge of clinical techniques and materials that can contribute to creating predictable and long-term esthetic outcomes. This volume will highlight the clinical management of the proposed implant site before and after implant placement through the use of interim prostheses, laboratory communication, abutment design, restorative material selection, and prosthesis delivery.

A unique characteristic of all ITI Treatment Guides has been the incorporation of clinical case presentations contributed by clinicians from all over the world that embrace the ITI's philosophy of an evidence-based approach to treatment and treatment planning. This volume will present several clinical cases highlighting various approaches, both surgical and restorative, in the treatment of patients requiring single teeth to be replaced with a dental implant. In addition, causes and case management approaches related to esthetic implant complications will be reviewed, highlighting surgical and prosthetic options to recover from compromised outcomes.

Our goal with this Treatment Guide has been to present a comprehensive, evidence-based approach to assist practitioners in the successful treatment of their patients who desire esthetic outcomes, from the initial consultation to follow-up.

2 Consensus Statements: Statements and Recommendations Obtained from the 5th ITI Consensus Conference

V. Chappuis, W. Martin

2.1 Contemporary Surgical and Radiographic Techniques in Implant Dentistry

International Journal of Oral and Maxillofacial Implants 2014, Vol. 29 (Supplement): Contemporary Surgical and Radiographic Techniques in Implant Dentistry (Michael M. Bornstein and coworkers 2014)

Introductory remarks

Successful dental implant rehabilitation requires accurate preoperative planning of the surgical intervention based on prosthodontic considerations and validated treatment methods. The introduction and widespread use of cross-sectional imaging in implant dentistry using cone-beam computed tomography (CBCT) over the last decade has enabled clinicians to diagnose and evaluate the jaws in three dimensions before and after insertion of dental implants, thus replacing computed tomography (CT) as the standard of care. Furthermore, computer-guided implant surgery uses data from cross-sectional imaging derived from CBCT scans on a routine basis. Considering rapid changes in science and clinical practice, two systematic reviews in this group, by Bornstein and coworkers (2014 a) and Tahmaseb and coworkers (2014), have centered their focus questions on these topics.

There are two possible surgical interventions for the treatment of the narrow edentulous ridge. The use of narrow-diameter implants has been suggested to avoid augmentation procedures and thus decrease patient morbidity. Nevertheless, this has not been validated in a systematic review of the literature to date. Horizontal augmentation procedures are widely used to increase the bone available for subsequent implant placement. However, knowledge on the efficacy and long-term outcomes of this procedure in the anterior maxilla is still limited. Therefore, the systematic reviews prepared by Klein and coworkers (2014) and by Kuchler and von Arx (2014) evaluated the existing data for these two rather different treatment approaches.

Cone-beam computed tomography (CBCT) in implant dentistry

Consensus statements

With respect to CBCT imaging in dental implant therapy and respective use guidelines, specific indications and contraindications for use, and the associated relative radiation does risk, the following statements can be made:

- Current clinical practice guidelines for CBCT use in implant dentistry provide recommendations that are consensus-based or derived from non-standardized methodological approaches.
- Published indication for CBCT use in implant dentistry vary from preoperative analysis to postoperative evaluation, including complications. However, a clinically significant benefit for CBCT imaging over conventional two-dimensional methods resulting in treatment plan alteration, improved implant success, survival rates, and reduced complications has not been reported to date.
- CBCT imaging exhibits a significantly lower radiation does risk than conventional CT, but higher than that of two-dimension radiographic imaging. Different CBCT devices deliver a wide range of radiation doses. Substantial dose reduction can be achieved by using appropriate exposure parameters and reducing the field of view (FOV) to the actual region of interest (ROI).

Treatment guidelines
- The clinician performing or interpreting CBCT scans for implant dentistry should take into consideration current radiologic guidelines.
- The decision to perform CBCT imaging for treatment planning in implant dentistry should be based on individual patient needs following thorough clinical examination.

- When cross-sectional imaging is indicated, CBCT is preferable over CT.
- CBCT imaging is indicated when information supplemental to the clinical examination and conventional radiographic imaging is considered necessary. CBCT may be an appropriate primary imaging modality in specific circumstances (e.g., when multiple treatment needs are anticipated or when jawbone or sinus pathology is suspected).
- The use of a radiographic template in CBCT imaging is advisable to maximize surgical and prosthetic information.
- The FOV of the CBCT examination should be restricted to the ROI whenever possible.
- Patient- and equipment-specific dose reduction measures should be used at all times.
- To improve image data transfer, clinicians should request radiographic devices and third-party dental implant software applications that offer fully compliant DICOM data export.

For a pdf copy of the full article (free of charge) from the ITI Consensus Paper, please check out the ITI Online Academy's ITI Consensus Database. See what else the Online Academy has to offer (charges may apply) at **academy.iti.org**

Computer-guided implant surgery

Consensus statements
- Implants placed utilizing computer-guided surgery with a follow-up period of at least 12 months demonstrate a mean survival rate of 97.3% (n = 1,941), which is comparable to implants placed following conventional procedures.
- There are significantly more data to support the accuracy of computer-guided implant surgery compared to 2008. Meta-analysis of the accuracy revealed a mean error of 0.9 mm at the entry pint (n = 1,530), 1.3 mm at the implant apex (n = 1,465), and a mean angular deviation of 3.5 degrees (n = 1,854) with a wide range in all measurements.
- Mucosa-, tooth-, and mini-implant-supported templates demonstrated accuracy of implant placement superior to that of bone-supported guides.
- After template osteotomy preparation, the accuracy of template implant insertion was superior to free-hand implant insertion.

Treatment guidelines
- Guided surgery should be viewed as an adjunct to, not a replacement for, appropriate diagnosis and treatment planning.
- Guided surgery should always be prosthetically driven. This includes either a radiographic template generated from a wax-up, or appropriate software application to create a digital wax-up.
- Information to be gathered from the combination of high-quality CBCT images and digital planning should include locations of vital structures, desired implant positions and dimensions, the need for augmentation therapy, and the planned prostheses.
- Due to the reported mean deviations, an additional 2 mm should be taken into consideration when planning implant position with relation to vital structures and adjacent implants in all directions. In borderline cases, an intraoperative periapical radiograph should be taken as a safety measure.
- Guided surgery may be utilized with a flapless or raised flap approach.
- Only mucosal- and/or tooth- or implant-supported surgical templates should be utilized.
- For improved accuracy, implants should be inserted in a fully guided manner (versus guided implant bed preparation alone) whenever possible.
- Guided surgery may be used with different loading protocols, in partially and fully edentulous indications.
- Indications for guided surgery include: to aid in treatment planning, when encountering complex anatomy, to perform minimally invasive surgery, and to improve patient understanding of therapeutic needs and treatment options.

For a pdf copy of the full article (free of charge) from the ITI Consensus Paper, please check out the ITI Online Academy's ITI Consensus Database. See what else the Online Academy has to offer (charges may apply) at **academy.iti.org**

Narrow-diameter implants

Consensus statements
- One-piece titanium mini-implants with a diameter of 1.8 to 2.9 mm demonstrated a mean survival rate of 94.3% (91% to 100%) after a mean follow-up time of 3.9 years (1 to 6 years) for the indications of overdenture treatment in the edentulous mandible (four implants) and for an anterior single tooth (maxillary lateral incisor, mandibular incisor).
- Two-piece titanium implants with a diameter of 3.0 to 3.25 mm demonstrated a mean survival rate of 98.5% (94% to 100%) after a mean follow-up time of 2.8 years (1 to 5 years) in only a single-tooth treatment (maxillary lateral incisor, mandibular incisor).
- Two-piece titanium implants with a diameter of 3.3 to 3.5 mm demonstrated a mean survival rate of 96.9% (89% to 100%) after a mean follow-up time of 4.1 years (1 to 11 years) for all indications including posterior regions.
- There is insufficient evidence on the success rates for all narrow (reduced)-diameter implants (NDIs). Clinical parameters and treatment protocols are often not sufficiently described and no controlled comparative studies are available, resulting in a high risk of bias.

Treatment guidelines
- NDIs might be indicated in situations with reduce mesiodistal space or reduced ridge width, provided that the general positioning rules are followed.
- NDIs have several indications. However, the risk of biomechanical problems (e.g., fracture) after long-term loading and the limited knowledge of their clinical behavior should be taken into account.

- In this respect, implant diameter should be the widest possible in relation to the emergence profile and ridge configuration.
- NDIs should have a length of 10 mm or more.
- Clinical indications may include:
  1 Single-tooth replacements in the anterior zones: categories* 1, 2, and 3 (category 1 and 2 only for incisors). One-piece implants often have specific prosthodontic disadvantages.
  2 Edentulous jaws to be rehabilitated with overdentures: categories 2 and 3, and category 1 for mandibles only (4 implants).
  3 Single posterior, multiple-unit fixed dental prostheses (FDP), and edentulous jaws to be rehabilitated with FDP: only category 3; individual informed consent should include the possibility of more technical complications. Alternative treatment options should also be discussed.

---

* Category 1: one-piece, < 3.0 mm (mini-implants)
Category 2: two-piece, 3.00 to 3.25 mm
Category 3: two-piece, 3.30 to 3.50 mm

For a pdf copy of the full article (free of charge) from the ITI Consensus Paper, please check out the ITI Online Academy's ITI Consensus Database. See what else the Online Academy has to offer (charges may apply) at **academy.iti.org**

Horizontal ridge augmentation in the anterior maxilla

Consensus statements

- Horizontal bone augmentation in the anterior maxilla is a reliable treatment option to enable the proper placement of implants.
- Mean horizontal bone gain in the staged approach (measured at the time of implant placement) ranged from 2.2 to 5 mm. The included studies do not provide information about the long-term stability of horizontal ridge augmentation.
- There is not enough data available to indicate superiority of one method or material over another.
- Survival and success rates of implants placed in horizontally augmented bone were not different from those reported for implants placed in native bone with adequate width.

Treatment guidelines

- In sites with inadequate ridge width, horizontal bone augmentation is indicated to enable proper implant placement. Ideally, a bone thickness of 2 mm should be achieved on the facial aspect of the implant.
- The primary aim of horizontal ridge augmentation procedures in the anterior maxilla is to optimize implant positioning in order to improve the functional and esthetic outcome. The position and shape of the augmented bone influence the soft-tissue profile, which should follow the contour of the neighboring teeth.
- Clinicians performing horizontal ridge augmentation in the anterior maxilla may choose from a wide range of treatment options, including particulate bone grafts for simultaneous and bone blocks for staged approaches with or without placement of resorbable and nonresorbable membranes.

- Soft-tissue augmentation may be required as an adjunctive procedure to improve the esthetic outcome.
- Horizontal ridge augmentation with simultaneous implant placement is indicated when adequate soft-tissue conditions are present and correct implant positioning with primary implant stability is achievable.
- If defect morphology is such that successful regeneration is unlikely to be achieved using the simultaneous approach, a staged approach should be used.
- In large defects precluding implant primary stability and proper three-dimensional implant positioning, a staged approach is recommended.
- In general, the choice of augmentation materials should assure the long-term stability of the bone volume created and should be based on solid documentation in the literature.

For a pdf copy of the full article (free of charge) from the ITI Consensus Paper, please check out the ITI Online Academy's ITI Consensus Database. See what else the Online Academy has to offer (charges may apply) at **academy.iti.org**

2.2 Restorative Materials and Techniques for Implant Dentistry

International Journal of Oral and Maxillofacial Implants 2014, Vol. 29 (Supplement): Restorative materials and techniques for implant dentistry (Daniel Wismeijer and coworkers 2014)

Introductory remarks

Computer-assisted design (CAD) and computer-assisted machining (CAM) have been increasingly used in implant dentistry over the past 10 years. The continuous improvement of these newer techniques by their developers has started to challenge traditional techniques of fabricating implant-supported prostheses. The premise that there is an improvement in outcome compared with traditional fabrication techniques is fundamental to the use of CAD/CAM. The systematic review by Kapos and Evans (2014) is focused on the performance of CAD/CAM prostheses when compared to conventionally manufactured prostheses.

Since most patients provided with oral implants are between 40 and 50 years of age, long-term survival rates for implant and prostheses are expected both from the clinician and the patient to ensure the longevity of the reconstruction. "Long-term" has been specified as a follow-up of at least 5 years. Thus, survival rates and the incidence of biologic, technical, and esthetic events should be based on mean observation periods of at least 5 years. However, implant survival rates are not the only essential consideration when advising the patient of different treatment options. Prosthetic and implant/abutment outcomes need to be considered as well. Different kinds of abutments are available with respect to material (metal and ceramic) and shape (prefabricated and customized, both with various internal designs). At this time, metal abutments are classified as the gold standard, although high-strength zirconia abutments are being utilized more widely and may be an adequate alternative to metal abutments for the clinical use. The systematic review by Zembic and coworkers (2014) focuses on the survival rates of metal and ceramic abutments supporting single-implant crowns with a mean observation period of

at least 3 years, as sufficient 5-year data were not available. In addition, the occurrence of negative biologic, technical, and esthetic events was evaluated for metal and ceramic abutments.

One of the important decisions in implant prosthodontics is the choice of the connection type of the final restoration to the implant via the screw-retained abutment. The restorative connection can be either screw- or cement-retained. With screw-retained restorations, an abutment or mesostructure may be separate to the restoration (two-piece) or combined as part of the fabrication procedure (one-piece). In general, both retention types have their advantages and limitations. Clinical and technical issues relevant in making the choice include ease of fabrication, precision, passivity of the framework, retention, occlusion, esthetics, accessibility, retrievability, complications, and costs. The focus of the review by Wittneben and coworkers (2014) is on biologic and technical failures and complication rates observed with cement- and screw-retained fixed implant-supported reconstructions.

CAD/CAM technology for implant abutments, crowns, and superstructures

Consensus statements

With respect to CAD/CAM technology for implant abutments, crowns, and superstructures, the following statements can be made:

- CAD/CAM technology has been successfully incorporated into implant dentistry.
- The clinical performance for implant-supported prostheses produced using CAD/CAM and conventional techniques is similar over the short term (mean: crowns, 1 year [1 to 1.1 years]; abutments, 3.5 years [1 to 5 years]; frameworks, 4 years [1 to 10 years]).
- The variability of CAD/CAM software and hardware used in fabrication implant-supported prostheses makes comparison difficult.

- The variability of outcome measures and material choices in investigations of CAD/CAM implant-supported prostheses makes comparison difficult.
- The short-term (mean, 3.5 years [1 to 5 years] survival rate of individually customized CAD/CAM abutments is similar to that of conventionally fabricated or stock abutments.
- The short-term (mean, 4 years [1 to 10 years]) survival rate of individually customized CAD/CAM frameworks is similar to that of conventionally fabricated frameworks.

Treatment guidelines

- The implementation of CAD/CAM technologies should lead to acceptable clinical outcomes.
- Continuous training for both the restorative dentist and technician is essential to successfully implement CAD/CAM techniques for the restoration of dental implants.
- There is continuous industry-controlled development in CAD/CAM devices, techniques, and materials. The dentist and technician should be aware that product hardware and software, as well as support, will change with generational advances.
- As the dentist remains responsible for treatment outcomes, it is recommended that he/she play an active role, together with the technician, to carefully control CAD/CAM processes and material selection.
- It is recommended that the dentist approve a virtual final prosthesis (virtual diagnostic wax-up) that dictates abutment/framework design.
- It is recognized that digitally derived prostheses can be remanufactured from stored data sets. It is recommended that digital data sets be stored/protected for this eventuality and that digital technology work platforms maintain programming compatibility/transparency.

For a pdf copy of the full article (free of charge) from the ITI Consensus Paper, please check out the ITI Online Academy's ITI Consensus Database. See what else the Online Academy has to offer (charges may apply) at **academy.iti.org**

Survival rate and incidence of complications of single implant-supported fixed reconstructions

Consensus statements

- No differences were found between ceramic and metal abutments in clinical performance based upon esthetic, technical, or biologic outcomes.
- No differences were found between the clinical performance of metal abutments with external or internal connections, based upon esthetic, technical, or biological outcomes (mean, 5 years [3 to 10 years]).
- The reported rate of technical complications is higher than either esthetic or biologic complications (mean, 5 years [3 to 10 years]).

Treatment guidelines

- As many different types of zirconia with differing microstructures and performance are being introduced into implant dentistry, they should be obtained from a reputable/qualified manufacturer.
- For anterior and premolar prostheses, zirconia abutments may be indicated. However, they should not be ground, abraded, or adjusted by the clinician or technician following sintering, unless recommended by the manufacturer.
- Ceramic abutments should not replace metal ones for all indications. Preliminary findings reflect an inherent sensitivity of ceramics to design and processing problems; e.g., stress concentration, thin walls, sintering, and residual machining flaws.
- The design of full ceramic abutments should not be based on metal abutment design to avoid stress concentrations or the development of unfavorable stresses.
- Caution is recommended in the clinical use of ceramic abutments in molar sites, as their behavior in these sites has not been sufficiently described.
- The performance of bonded titanium-zirconia implant abutments is not yet established. Thus, caution is recommended in the clinical use of such abutments due to insufficient data.

For a pdf copy of the full article (free of charge) from the ITI Consensus Paper, please check out the ITI Online Academy's ITI Consensus Database. See what else the Online Academy has to offer (charges may apply) at **academy.iti.org**

Clinical performance of screw- versus cement-retained implant-supported fixed reconstructions

Consensus statements

- High survival rates can be achieved with both cemented and screw-retained fixed implant-supported prostheses. Neither failure nor complication can be avoided by selecting a prosthesis retention type.
- Cemented all-ceramic prostheses have a higher failure rate than cemented metal-ceramic prostheses. However, no difference was found with screw-retained prostheses.
- Based upon the literature reviewed, the type of cement used does not influence the failure rate of cemented prostheses.
- Technical complications occurred (estimated annual event rate of up to 10%) with both cemented and screw-retained prostheses. In the pooled data, the cemented prostheses exhibited a higher rate of technical complications.
- Screw-retained prostheses exhibited a higher rate of ceramic chipping than cemented prostheses.
- Biological complications can be found (estimated annual event rate of up to 7%) with both cemented and screw-retained prostheses. Cemented prostheses exhibit a higher rate of fistula formation and suppuration.

Treatment guidelines

Based on the data in this review, a universal recommendation cannot be made for either cementation or screw retention. However, in a clinical situation that offers a choice of prosthesis retention type, the following recommendations may be made:

Cement retention may be recommended:

- For short-span prostheses with margins at or above tissue level to simplify fabrication procedures
- To enhance esthetics when the screw access passes transocclusally or in cases of malposition of the implant
- When an intact occlusal surface is desirable
- To reduce initial treatment costs
- It is further recommended that the clinician understand that the procedures involved with cement retention for implant-supported crowns are not simple and should be carried out with great caution.

Screw retention may be recommended:

- In situations of minimal interarch space
- To avoid a cement margin and thus the possibility of cement residue (this may be particularly important if the prosthetic margin is placed submucosally, since it has been shown to be more difficult to completely remove cement residue from margins placed > 1.5 mm submucosally)
- When retrievability is of importance
- In the esthetic zone, to facilitate tissue contouring and conditioning in the transition zone (emergence profile)
- To facilitate screw retention, it is recommended that the implant be placed in a prosthetically driven position.

For a pdf copy of the full article (free of charge) from the ITI Consensus Paper, please check out the ITI Online Academy's ITI Consensus Database. See what else the Online Academy has to offer (charges may apply) at **academy.iti.org**

2.3 Optimizing Esthetic Outcomes in Implant Dentistry

International Journal of Oral and Maxillofacial Implants 2014, Vol. 29 (Supplement): Optimizing Esthetic Outcomes in Implant Dentistry (D. Morton and coworkers 2014)

Introductory remarks

In the anterior maxilla, dental implant-supported prostheses need to replicate the dental hard and soft tissues in order to be esthetically acceptable. Three systematic reviews were prepared to address the topic of optimizing esthetic outcomes.

Following tooth extraction, the clinician has the choice of various time points to place implants. Implant placement post extraction is often accompanied by bone augmentation procedures to manage residual bone defects and enhance esthetic results. Thus, the first systematic review by Chen and Buser (2014) analyzed the influence of the timing of implant placement and bone augmentation procedures in relation to their effect on esthetic outcomes.

Unfortunately, complications with implant treatment can occur. In the esthetic zone, these complications often lead to adverse esthetic results due to recession and deficiencies associated with the peri-implant soft tissues. The second paper by Levine and coworkers (2014) therefore reviewed the literature on procedures to treat mucosa defects following the placement and restoration of implants in the esthetic zone. In order to achieve acceptable esthetic outcomes, a number of restorative procedures have been developed with the aim of optimizing esthetic outcomes with implant-supported prostheses. However, these procedures have not been evaluated in a systematic way to determine their efficacy in relation to esthetics. The aim of the third systematic review by Martin and coworkers (2014) was therefore to assess the influence of various restorative procedures on esthetic outcomes.

From these three systematic reviews, a general observation was made that the available data on esthetic outcomes were predominantly represented by case series studies. Relatively few randomized controlled trials (RCTs) and cohort studies were identified, and a minority of these was judged to be at low risk of bias. Nevertheless, the case series studies provided invaluable information in establishing the current clinical trends in techniques and materials related to esthetic outcomes. Indeed, well-designed prospective case series studies of consecutively enrolled subjects with clearly defined inclusion and exclusion criteria can provide important information to validate clinical procedures and materials.

The group recognized that RCTs are not always feasible or ethical when clinical conditions that are known to increase the risk of adverse esthetic outcomes are under investigation. Implant treatment in the esthetic zone is a challenging procedure and classified as advanced or complex according to the SAC classification (Dawson and coworkers 2009). Most patients present with multiple esthetic risk factors and often have high expectations. If esthetic complications occur, they are usually difficult or impossible to manage. As a consequence, the prevention of esthetic complications should be a primary objective. Therefore, a conservative treatment approach is recommended to facilitate successful outcomes with high predictability and a low risk of complications.

Esthetic outcomes following immediate and early implant placement in the anterior maxilla

Consensus statement

The included studies reported on single-tooth implants in post-extraction sites adjacent to natural teeth. For post-extraction implant placement, esthetic outcomes determined by objective indices and positional changes of the peri-implant mucosa can be achieved in the majority of cases. However, adverse esthetic outcomes may occur.

Regarding the position of the soft tissue following immediate implant (type 1) placement, there is considerable variety. Following immediate implant placement, midfacial mucosal recession of 1 mm or more occurs in 9% to 41% (median, 26%) of sites between 1 and 3 years after implant placement.

The factors associated with midfacial recession for immediate implant placement are (1) thin facial bone plate, (2) lack of intact facial bone plate, (3) facial malposition of the implant, and (4) thin soft-tissue phenotype. Following immediate implant placement, the lack of a facial bone wall associated with increased mucosal recession is a frequent observation, based on two retrospective studies with small sample sizes.

Based on a small number of studies (one RCT and one case series), early implant placement (type 2 or 3) demonstrates no midfacial mucosal recession of 1 mm or more. Two studies of early implant placement (type 2) combined with simultaneous bone augmentation with guided bone regeneration (GBR) (contour augmentation) demonstrate a high frequency (above 90%) of a facial bone wall visible on cone-beam computed tomography.

Treatment guidelines

Esthetic outcomes can be achieved at post-extraction sites irrespective of the timing of implant placement. Different placement times, however, present with specific treatment challenges and variable predictability of esthetic outcomes.

With immediate placement, a high level of clinical competence and experience in performing the treatment is needed. Careful case selection is required to achieve satisfactory esthetic outcomes. The following clinical conditions should be satisfied:

- Intact socket walls
- Facial bone wall at least 1 mm in thickness
- Thick soft tissue
- No acute infection at the site
- Availability of bone apical and palatal to the socket to provide primary stability

For immediate placement, a preoperative three-dimensional (3D) radiographic examination may be considered in determining the above-mentioned bony anatomical conditions and to assist in treatment planning.

For predictable esthetic outcomes with immediate placement with or without flap elevation, the following treatment requirements should be met:

- Correct 3D position of the implant platform (according to previous ITI recommendations).
- If that position falls within the extraction socket, a minimum distance of 2 mm between the implant platform and the inner surface of the facial socket wall should be present. A technique should be used to compensate for post-extraction resorption, such as bone filler with a low substitution rate.

If these conditions are not met, immediate implant placement is not recommended.

The above-mentioned preconditions for immediate placement are rarely present. Thus, early implant placement (type 2) is the option of choice in most instances. If, however, it is anticipated that primary stability cannot be achieved, the post-extraction healing period should be extended. Ridge preservation/augmentation procedures may be considered when implant placement needs to be delayed for patient- or site-related reasons.

To optimize the esthetic outcomes of early implant placement (type 2 and 3), the implant platform should be placed in the correct prosthetically driven 3D position. Implant placement is combined with GBR using a low-substitution bone filler to overcontour the facial aspect of the ridge. This is followed by coverage of the augmentation material with a barrier membrane and submergence of the biomaterials.

For a pdf copy of the full article (free of charge) from the ITI Consensus Paper, please check out the ITI Online Academy's ITI Consensus Database. See what else the Online Academy has to offer (charges may apply) at **academy.iti.org**

Soft-tissue augmentation procedures for mucosal defects in the esthetic zone

Consensus statements
The included studies consisted predominantly of case reports and case series of small numbers and short duration. The studies did not always identify the etiology and timing of the facial soft-tissue recession around single implants.

Periodontal soft-tissue surgical procedures were applied to treat facial soft-tissue recession. There is no consensus on how to treat a facial soft-tissue defect in esthetic sites. In some of the papers, the implant restoration was removed and/or facially altered (crown, abutment, and/or implant) in order to facilitate the treatment.

Limited improvement of the soft-tissue (including increase in soft-tissue thickness, keratinized tissue width, and facial marginal soft-tissue level) can be achieved following soft-tissue augmentation procedures.

Following soft-tissue augmentation procedures, complete restoration of the soft-tissue defect ranged from 0% to 75% (3 studies; 32 patients).

Treatment guidelines
A team approach and Esthetic Risk Assessment should be utilized to improve predictability of an esthetic outcome and to reduce risk when managing soft-tissue defects in the esthetic zone.

When soft-tissue recession is found around a single-tooth implant, the clinician needs to diagnose the etiology based on evaluation of 3D implant position, restoration, existing hard and soft-tissue support, as well as factitious (self-inflicted) injury such as tooth brushing and flossing trauma.

The surgical procedures to correct soft-tissue facial recession around a single implant are complex. A systematic assessment and treatment protocol are required. The assessment should include the following:

- Patient's expectations
- Medical status
- Smoking habit
- Visibility of defect upon smiling
- Width of keratinized tissue remaining at the defect site
- Restoration contour
- Infection at the implant site
- Contributing patient-related factors
- 3D implant position
- Proximity of implant to adjacent teeth
- Interproximal radiographic bone loss
- Scarring of soft tissue at implant site

When the above-mentioned factors are favorable, hard- and/or soft-tissue augmentation procedures can be effective. The patient should be made aware of the high variability of the outcome. When the above-mentioned factors are unfavorable, hard- and/or soft-tissue augmentation procedures are less effective. Restorative modifications (abutment/crown replacement and/or reshaping) combined with a surgical approach may be indicated. Implant removal should also be considered as an option. When an implant needs to be removed, techniques that minimize bone loss are preferred. Specialized implant removal kits are available and preferred to trephines.

For a pdf copy of the full article (free of charge) from the ITI Consensus Paper, please check out the ITI Online Academy's ITI Consensus Database. See what else the Online Academy has to offer (charges may apply) at **academy.iti.org**

The influence of restorative procedures on esthetic outcomes in implant dentistry

Consensus statements

The available literature does not demonstrate that esthetic outcomes can be improved by:

- The use of surgical templates (surgical guides)
- The utilization of implant-retained provisional prostheses
- The timing of provisional implant-retained prostheses
- The mode of prosthesis retention (cement- or screw-retained)

There is limited evidence (one study) reporting improved esthetic outcomes (color matching) in implant dentistry associated with ceramic abutment/prosthesis combination.

Esthetic outcomes can be improved (mean, 0.3 mm on the midfacial mucosal margin) by the presence of a horizontal offset, or platform switching (smaller abutment diameter).

Treatment guidelines

The use of surgical templates, development from a prosthetically driven approach that communicates the optimal implant position in 3D respecting the comfort zones as reported in previous ITI publications, is recommended.

The use of provisional implant-retained restorations in the esthetic zone is recommended. Provisional restorations enhance communication between all members of the treatment team and the patient. They should be anatomically and functionally correct, and respect the emergence profile of the restoration apical to the planned mucosal margin (highest convexity) to allow for maximum tissue volume. Screw retention of the interim restoration is considered advantageous for multiple reasons (retrievability, tissue shaping, tissue health and maturation, ease of modification).

Immediate loading or restoration of an implant cannot be recommended as a routine procedure because risks are elevated and esthetic outcomes are variable. In agreement with previously published ITI documents, early loading of dental implants in the esthetic zone is recommended.

In sites of elevated esthetic risk, a horizontally offset (platform switched) implant/abutment design is advantageous for single-tooth replacements. Further, an oversized implant platform and prosthetic components must be avoided to respect the interproximal and facial regions of the site.

The abutment and prosthesis material are a patient- and site-specific choice for the clinician. Provided that the material chosen is of high quality and documented, the design of the abutment and/or prosthesis is more critical than the material chosen, for reasons including:

- Controlling emergence profile
- Material properties and strength
- Access to finish lines
- Retrievability

In patients with thin tissues, a tooth-colored abutment and/or final prosthesis emerging through the tissues can offer esthetic advantages. When the implant angulation allows, screw retention of the prosthesis offers clinical advantages.

For a pdf copy of the full article (free of charge) from the ITI Consensus Paper, please check out the ITI Online Academy's ITI Consensus Database. See what else the Online Academy has to offer (charges may apply) at **academy.iti.org**

2.4 Implant-loading Protocols

International Journal of Oral and Maxillofacial Implants 2014, Vol. 29 (Supplement): Optimizing Esthetic Outcomes in Implant Dentistry (G. O. Gallucci and coworkers 2014)

Introductory remarks

This report summarizes the statements and clinical recommendations for implant loading protocols as per consensus agreement among the participants at the 5th ITI Consensus Conference.

Group 4 was composed of participants from 13 different countries and of variuos specialties in dental medicine. Prior to the conference, scientific evidence on conventional, early, and immediate implant loading protocols was evaluated by four systematic reviews according to well-differentiated clinical situations: single implant crowns, extended edentulous spaces in partially edentulous patients, edentulous jaws with fixed prostheses, and edentulous jaws with overdenture prostheses. The primary outcome was implant survival. In addition, number of implants, prosthetic design, marginal bone loss, stability of peri-implant soft tissue, prosthetic failures, treatment modifiers, esthetics, and patient satisfaction were considered as secondary outcomes.

Reports from previous consensus conferences (Cochran and coworkers 2004; Weber and coworkers 2009) stated that conventional and early implant loading are well-established protocols and should be considered routine. In particular, several clinical studies (Cochran and coworkers 2011; Bornstein and coworkers 2010; Morton and coworkers 2010) demonstrated the high predictability of early loading protocols when compared to conventional healing times, showing no differences in regard to implant survival rates. In this context, the design of the systematic reviews presented at the 5th ITI Consensus Conference aimed to assess whether immediate loading showed similar clinical outcomes to early and conventional loading.

At the conference, the authors presented their methodology, results, and conclusions for the four systematic reviews to all participants in the loading protocols group. These manuscripts provided substance for a comprehensive and methodical discussion leading to the unbiased formulation of consensus statemens, clinical recommendations, and directions for future research on implant loading protocols. The group's determinations were then presented to the plenum, where additional input was collected for the preparation of this final report.

Definition of terms

The definitions of loading protocols presented by Weber and coworkers (2009) were used for the calibration of the systematic reviews and endorsed without modifications by the group as follows:

- *Conventional loading* of dental implants is defined as being greater than 2 months subsequent to implant placement.
- *Early loading* of dental implants is defined as being between 1 week and 2 months subsequent to implant placement.
- *Immediate loading* of dental implants is defined as eing earlier than 1 week subsequent to implant placement.

Loading protocols for single implants in partially edentulous patients

Consensus statements

1. In general, there is a high level of comparative evidence supporting te use of both immediate and conventional loading of single-implant crowns in terms of implant survivial and marginal bone level stability.
2. A minimal insertion torque in the range of 20 to 45 N·cm, a minimal implant stability quotient (ISQ) in the range of 60 to 65, and the need for simultaneous bone augmentation were the most common inclusion/exclusion criteria.

3. There are limited data comparing immediate and conventional loading in terms of stability of the papilla height and of the facial mucosal margin.
4. Esthetics and patient satisfaction were measured only in a few trials that compared immediate and conventional loading, rendering insufficient data to draw conclusions.

Treatment guidelines

The recommendations for immediate and early loading of single-implant crowns are limited to situations fulfilling the following prerequisites:

1. Primary implant stability (insertion torque ≥ 20 to 45 N·cm and/or implant stability quotient (ISQ) ≥ 60 to 65
2. Absence of systematic or local contraindications (eg, parafunctional activities, large bone defects, need for sinus floor elevation)
3. When the clinical benefits exceed the risks
4. For the anterior and premolar regions, immediate and early loading of single-implant crowns are predictable procedures in terms of implant survival and stability of the marginal bone. However, data regarding soft-tissue aspects are not conclusive enough to recommend immediate or early loading of single-tooth crowns in esthetically demanding sites as a routine procedure. Immediate loading in such sites should be approached with caution and by experienced clinicians.
5. For the mandibular molar region, immediate and early loading of single-implant crowns is a predicable procedure and can generally be recommended in cases where clincial benefits are identified.
6. The low amount of data on immediate and early loading of single-implant crowns in the maxillary molar region does not allow general recommendation of these loading procedures. In these sites, conventional loading should be the procedure of choice.

Loading protocols for partially edentulous patients in extended edentulous sites

Consensus statements

1. Based on limited scientific evidence and under strict selection criteria, immediate implant loading in partially edentulous patients with healed posterior extended edentulous sites presents similar implant survival rates compared to early or conventional loading.
2. Insufficient evidence exists to support immediate implant loading in anterior maxillary or mandibular extended edentulous sites.
3. Insertion torque, ISQ values, implant lengths, the need for bone augmentation procedures, the timing of implant placement, smoking, and the presence of parafunctional habits were common criteria in selecting a loading protocol.

Treatment guidelines

1. In the absence of modifying factors, early loading of solid-screw-type implants with a microtextured surface after 4 to 8 weeks in extended edentulous sites of partially edentulous patients is a predictable treatment approach.
2. Immediate loading of posterior implants in healed extended edentulous sites seems to be predictable. However, in such cases immediate implant loading is of limited clinical benefit.
3. Immediate loading of anterior implants in extended edentulous sites of partially edentulous patients should be approached with caution and by experienced clinicians, since insufficient evidence exists to support such treatment.
4. When immediate implant loading is intended, the following criteria should be considered: primary implant stability, need for substantial bone augmentation, implant design and dimension, occlusal factors, patient habits, systemic health, and clinician experience.

 For a pdf copy of the full article (free of charge) from the ITI Consensus Paper, please check out the ITI Online Academy's ITI Consensus Database. See what else the Online Academy has to offer (charges may apply) at **academy.iti.org**

 For a pdf copy of the full article (free of charge) from the ITI Consensus Paper, please check out the ITI Online Academy's ITI Consensus Database. See what else the Online Academy has to offer (charges may apply) at **academy.iti.org**

Loading protocols for fixed prostheses in edentulous jaws

Consensus statements

1. The existing literature provides high evidence that immediate loading of microtextured dental implants with one-piece fixed interim prostheses in both the edentulous mandible and maxilla is as predictable as early and conventional loading.
2. Inclusion criteria, such as insertion torque ≥ 30 N·cm, ISQ ≥ 60, and minimal implant length ≥ 10 mm, have been used in the majority of the included studies.
3. The number of implants used to support a fixed prosthesis varied from 2 to 10 in the mandible and 4 to 12 in the maxilla.

Treatment guidelines

1. The treatment of edentulism with fixed implant-supported prostheses is complex according to the ITI SAC criteria. Therefore, careful case selection and treatment planning, as well as adequate knowledge, skill, and experience of the clinician(s) performing the procedures are key. Immediate, early, or conventional loading with one-piece fixed interim prostheses have demonstrated high implant and prosthesis survival rates and can be recommended for the mandible and maxilla.
2. Patient-centered benefits of immediate loading include the immediate fixed restoration of function, the reduction of postoperative discomfort caused by a removable interim prosthesis, as well as the reduction of overall treatment time.
3. The number, size, and distribution of implants for a full-arch fixed prosthesis needs to be based on the implant-prosthodontic plan, arch form, and bone volume, regardless of the loading protocol.
4. Primary implant stability is critical for predictable osseointegration regardless of the loading protocol. It is suggested that prior to immediate loading in the edentulous arch, the primary stability of each implant must be confirmed.
5. The need for simultaneous procedures such as bone augmentation or sinus floor elevation is considered a relative contraindication for immediate loading.

Loading protocols for implant-supported overdentures in edentulous jaws

Consensus statements

1. Current clinical research supports high survival with the use of threaded, microtextured implants with a minimum diameter of 3 mm for the support of overdenture prostheses when used with immediate, early, or conventional loading protocols. Limited evidence exists for immediate loading of implants supporting overdentures in the maxilla.
2. Descriptive material from the review in this group for immediate loading by Schimmel and coworkers (2014) lists inclusion criteria of: insertion torque (≥ 30 N·cm), ISQ value (≥ 60), two or more implants in the mandible, or four or more implants in the maxilla.
3. Splinting of implants and the type of attachment system had no effect on 1-year survival rate compared to freestanding implants.

Treatment guidelines

1. The intended loading protocol should be selected considering implant-prosthodontic parameters as well as functional, psychosocial, and financial aspects and patient preference.
2. Early loading represents a satisfactory treatment modality in the management of the edentulous jaw, when using implants to support/retain an overdenture prosthesis, and can be recommended as routine in the absence of modifying factors.
3. Immediate loading protocols in implant-supported/retained overdentures appear predictable. The available research arbitrarily uses an insertion torque of 30 N·cm or greater and/or an ISQ value of 60 or greater. The evidence for immediate implant loading in the maxilla is less compelling. However, there is no reliable pretreatment predictor that has determined conclusively that the clinician can perform an immediate loading procedure.
4. Given the lack of research, the use of a single implant in an immediately loaded fashion may not be indicated for support/retention of overdenture prostheses.

For a pdf copy of the full article (free of charge) from the ITI Consensus Paper, please check out the ITI Online Academy's ITI Consensus Database. See what else the Online Academy has to offer (charges may apply) at **academy.iti.org**

For a pdf copy of the full article (free of charge) from the ITI Consensus Paper, please check out the ITI Online Academy's ITI Consensus Database. See what else the Online Academy has to offer (charges may apply) at **academy.iti.org**

2.5 Prevention and Management of Biological and Technical Implant Complications

International Journal of Oral and Maxillofacial Implants 2014, Vol. 29 (Supplement): Optimizing Esthetic Outcomes in Implant Dentistry (L. J. A. Heitz-Mayfield and coworkers 2014)

Introductory remarks

Implant treatment is highly successful, as documented in a wealth of scientific literature. However, patients and clinicians should expect to see complications within their daily practice. The aim of the papers presented by this group was to address the prevention and management of technical and biologic complications in order to make recommendations both for clinical practice and future research. Three topics were chosen within the field of complications of implant treatment, and these addressed prevention and therapy of peri-implant disease and prevention of technical complications.

Three systematic reviews were conducted and formed the basis for discussion of working group 5. The discussions led to the development of statements and recommendations determined by group consensus based on the findings of the systematic reviews. These were then presented and accepted following modifications as necessary at plenary sessions.

Effects of anti-infective preventive measures on biologic implant complications and implant loss

Consensus statements

The aim of the review by Salvi and Zitzmann was to systematically appraise whether anti-infective protocols are effective in preventing biologic implant complications and implant loss after a mean observation period of at least 10 years following delivery of the prosthesis. Out of 15 included studies, only one comparative study assessed the effects of adherence to supportive periodontal therapy (SPT) on the occurrence of biological complications and implant loss. In view of the lack of randomized trials, observational studies including adherence and lack of adherence to SPT were considered valuable in order to estimate the effects of SPT on implant longevity and the occurrence of biological complications.

- Overall, the outcomes of this systematic review indicated that high long-term survival and success rates of dental implants can be achieved in partially and fully edentulous patients adhering to SPT.
- Long-term implant survival and success rates are lower in patients with a history of periodontal disease adhering to SPT compared with those without a history of periodontal disease.
- The findings of this systematic review indicate that pre-existing peri-implant mucositis in conjunction with lack of adherence to SPT was associated with a higher incidence of peri-implantitis.

Treatment guidelines

Preventive measures before implant placement
- Residual periodontal pockets are a risk for peri-implant disease and implant loss. Therefore, completion of active periodontal therapy aiming for elimination of residual pockets with bleeding on probing should precede implant placement in periodontally compromised patients.
- In cases of residual probing depths (PD) ≥ 5 mm with concomitant bleeding on probing, full-mouth plaque scores > 20%, and associated risk factors, retreatment and periodontal reevaluation are recommended before implant placement.
- In subjects diagnosed with aggressive periodontitis, an SPT program with shorter intervals is a prerequisite.
- During implant treatment planning, factors to be considered that may result in biological complications include: insufficient keratinized mucosa and bone volume at the implant recipient site, implant proximity, three-dimensional implant position, and design and cleansability of the prosthesis. Alternative restorative solutions should be considered according to a patient's individual circumstances.

Preventive measures after implant placement

- All oral health care providers, including undergraduate students, should be trained to recognize clinical signs of peri-implant pathology and maintain or reestablish peri-implant health.
- After delivery of the definitive implant-supported prosthesis, clinical and radiographic baseline measurements should be established.
- During SPT, an update of medical and dental history and a clinical inspection of the implant-supported prosthesis including the evaluation of iatrogenic factors (e.g., cement remnants, misfit of prostheses, implant proximity with insufficient access for interproximal oral hygiene) should constitute the basis of a proper diagnostic process.
- Regular diagnostic monitoring of the peri-implant tissues includes assessment of presence of plaque, PD, bleeding on gentle probing (approx. 0.25 N), and/or suppuration.
- Changes in PD from a fixed landmark should be assessed regularly and compared to previous examinations.
- In the presence of clinical signs of disease, an appropriate radiograph is indicated in order to detect radiographic bone-level changes compared to previous examinations.
- A diagnosis of *peri-implant health* is given in the absence of clinical signs of inflammation. A recall frequency of at least once per year is recommended unless systemic and/or local conditions require more frequent intervals. In cases of peri-implant health, professional cleaning including reinforcement of self-performed oral hygiene is recommended as a preventive measure.
- A diagnosis of *peri-implant mucositis* is given in the presence of individual clinical signs of soft-tissue inflammation (e.g., redness, edema, suppuration) and bleeding on gentle probing. If mucositis is diagnosed, in addition to reinforcement of self-performed oral hygiene, mechanical debridement with or without antiseptics (e.g., chlorhexidine) is delivered. The use of systemic antibiotics for the treatment of peri-implant mucositis is not justified. Therapy of peri-implant mucositis should be considered as a preventive measure for the onset of peri-implantitis.
- A diagnosis of *peri-implantitis* is given in the presence of mucositis in conjunction with progressive crestal bone loss. When peri-implantitis is diagnosed, early implementation of appropriate therapy is recommended to prevent further progression of the disease.

Therapy of peri-implantitis

Consensus statements

The focus question for the review by Heitz-Mayfield and Mombelli (2014) was: In patients with osseointegrated implants diagnosed with peri-implantitis, how successful is treatment aimed at resolution of the disease?

Currently, there is no standard of care for treating peri-implantitis. Various clinical protocols for treating peri-implantitis have been proposed, including mechanical debridement, the use of antiseptics and local and systemic antibiotics, as well as surgical and regenerative procedures. In view of the lack of comparable randomized controlled trials (RCTs) this review has taken a broader approach to capture as many relevant studies as possible, including randomized and observational studies, but with consideration to the strengths and limitations of the included research.

The ideal goal of the treatment of peri-implantitis would be the resolution of disease, i.e., no suppuration or bleeding on probing, no further bone loss, and the reestablishment and maintenance of healthy peri-implant tissues. A composite outcome to reflect this would include absence of peri-implant PD ≥ 5 mm with concomitant bleeding on probing and no suppuration, in addition to no further bone loss. If these criteria are met, it can be assumed that no further intervention other than nonsurgical maintenance care would be required, and the treatment outcome would therefore be regarded as successful. Unfortunately, these data were rarely reported in the literature and therefore a compromise composite criterion for successful treatment outcome was employed, ie, implant survival with mean PD < 5 mm and no further bone loss. Although there is no consensus in the literature on whether a 5-mm peri-implant PD alone represents health or disease, this threshold was adopted for the purposes of the review.

This review was based on 33 studies reported in 43 papers including case series of at least 5 patients treated with the same protocol and comparative studies. No studies were found comparing surgical and nonsurgical protocols. Based on this literature, the following conclusions were drawn:

For a pdf copy of the full article (free of charge) from the ITI Consensus Paper, please check out the ITI Online Academy's ITI Consensus Database. See what else the Online Academy has to offer (charges may apply) at **academy.iti.org**

1. The case definition of peri-implantitis remains unclear and varies substantially between studies.
2. There is a great variety of treatment protocols for both nonsurgical and surgical treatment.
   a. Nonsurgical therapy included: debridement with hand and powered instruments, air powder abrasive devices, laser treatment, and local and systemic antimicrobial agents.
   b. Surgical therapy included: elevation of a mucoperiosteal flap and removal of granulation tissue to gain access to the implant and defect surfaces, decontamination of the implant surface (various techniques) with or without implant surface modification. Some studies also evaluated respective therapy or a variety of regenerative procedures. The majority of the studies employed systemic antimicrobial administration.
3. The following elements are common to most protocols for peri-implantitis therapy:
   a. Pretreatment phase including establishment of good oral hygiene
   b. Anti-infective treatment including implant surface cleaning achieved by nonsurgical/surgical access
   c. Supportive maintenance care
4. The available evidence does not allow recommendation of specific treatment options for peri-implantitis. However, improvement of clinical parameters was reported for the majority of patients, although complete resolution according to a composite success criterion was not usually achieved for all patients. Favorable short-term outcomes were reported in many studies; however, lack of disease resolution as well as progression or recurrence of disease and implant loss, despite treatment, were also reported.
5. Interpretation of the results of studies is complicated by unclear or high risk of bias, heterogeneity of study design, and difficulty of generalizing outcomes to practice settings due to frequent exclusion of patients who smoke, those with poorly controlled diabetes, and other conditions that may affect clinical outcomes.
6. There are no data investigating patient-reported outcomes and economic analysis of therapy.
7. Peri-implantitis therapy was associated with soft-tissue recession, which was most evident following surgical treatment. Post-surgery complications including membrane exposure and infection were also reported.

Treatment guidelines

1. As peri-implantitis is an infection associated with the presence of a submucosal bacterial biofilm around implants, the primary goal of therapy must be the resolution of the infection, which is achieved by the disruption of the biofilm, the removal of calculus and/or overhanging restoration margins, and the prevention of recurrence of the disease.
2. It is important to try to establish if iatrogenic or other factors have contributed to the infection, for example, ill-fitting or non-cleansable overcontoured prostheses, malpositioned implants, or foreign bodies such as impression material or excess luting cement. Non-iatrogenic factors may include impacted dental floss.
3. The following sequence of treatment of peri-implantitis is normally recommended.
   a. Pretreatment phase including:
      i. Thorough assessment and diagnosis
      ii. Reduction of risk factors for peri-implantitis; in particular, poor oral hygiene, prostheses that prevent adequate access for plaque control, tobacco use, presence of periodontal diseases, and systemic diseases that may predispose to peri-implant disease
      iii. If required, prosthesis removal and adjustment/replacement
   b. Nonsurgical debridement focused on maximal removal of biofilm, with or without antimicrobials
   c. Early reassessment of peri-implant health; normally within 1 to 2 months
   d. Surgical access if resolution of peri-implantitis has not been achieved. This should include:
      i. Full-thickness mucoperiosteal flaps and removal of granulation tissue to allow thorough cleaning of the implant surface.
      ii. Thorough surface decontamination of the implant and restorative components. The following techniques have been proposed: locally applied chemicals, gauze soaked with saline or antiseptics, hand-powered instruments, air-powder abrasives, Er-YAG lasers, photodynamic therapy, and implant surface modification. There is no evidence for the superiority of any one approach.
      iii. Surgical therapy might also include regenerative or resective approaches
         1. Regenerative approaches include filling of the intraosseous peri-implant defect with a bone substitute/graft/bioactive substance with or without a resorbable barrier membrane. Defect morphology for regeneration would normally require a contained defect. Submerged healing might reduce the risk of membrane exposure. Reestablishment of osseointegration

following treatment has not been demonstrated in humans.

2. Resective approaches include osseous recontouring with apical positioning of the flap.

iv. Immediate postoperative anti-infective protocol should include daily chlorhexidine rinsing during the healing period until mechanical oral hygiene can be resumed. In the absence of evidence comparing surgical treatment with or without antibiotics, peri- or postoperative systemic antibiotics are recommended in view of the aggressive nature of disease. Professional support of healing and plaque control will be needed during this phase.

e. Clinical monitoring should be performed on a regular basis and supplemented by appropriate radiographic evaluation as required. Supportive maintenance therapy including reinforcement of effective oral hygiene and professional biofilm removal should be provided on a frequency determined by oral health and the risk profile, likely to be between every 3 to 6 months.

4. Surgical access is likely to be needed for the majority of deep lesions due to the difficulty of accessing the threads and surfaces of the implant.

5. The patient should be advised that:
   a. Recession of the peri-implant mucosa should be expected following peri-implantitis treatment, in particular after surgical therapy.
   b. Progression or recurrence of disease might require additional therapy or implant removal.

6. The clinician should consider implant removal as a treatment option. Factors influencing this decision may include the severity of the peri-implantitis lesion, the position of the implant, the surrounding tissues, or when the treatment outcomes are likely to be unsatisfactory.

7. Referral to specialist care for nonresponding peri-implantitis should be considered.

8. Regular assessment of peri-implant health is recommended during SPT to identify disease at an early stage.

9. Training of dental team professionals should include diagnosis and management of peri-implant disease.

For a pdf copy of the full article (free of charge) from the ITI Consensus Paper, please check out the ITI Online Academy's ITI Consensus Database. See what else the Online Academy has to offer (charges may apply) at **academy.iti.org**

Survival rates of implant-supported fixed prostheses over the last decades

Consensus statements

The systematic review by Pjetursson and coworkers (2014) was conducted to compare the survival and complication rates of implant supported prostheses published up to the year 2000 with those reported in studies published after the year 2000. An association between period of publication and fixed implant-supported prosthesis outcomes were found with higher survival rates and overall lower rates of mechanical and technical complications reported in more recent clinical studies. However, the incidence of reported technical complications is still high. The difference in survival rates was most evident for screw-retained prostheses, where the reported survival rate of 77.6% in the older publications was increased to 96.8% in the more recent ones.

Treatment guidelines

Risk of fracture—implants

1. Implant fracture is a rare complication. To avoid implant fracture, it is recommended that clinicians consider the use of appropriately designed and manufactured implants with properly investigated and documented low fracture rates. Similarly, the clinician should use implants manufactured from materials that have been thoroughly investigated.

2. The risk of implant fracture can be considered extremely low when:
   a. The appropriate distribution, number, and diameter of implants are used
   b. Implants are placed using a prosthetically driven protocol
   c. Implants are combined with an adequately fitting prosthesis

Risk of fracture and/or loosening—prosthetic screws

Fracture of manufacturer screws made to specified tolerances can be influenced by three factors: mishandling, misfit, and occlusal forces.

1. Mishandling: To reduce the risk of fracture of prosthetic screws, it is recommended that a clinician follow the manufacturer's instructions for use.

2. Misfit: An inadequately fitting framework may be a predisposing factor to prosthetic screw fracture or loosening. It is recommended to prioritize evaluation of the accuracy of the interface between the machined head of the screw and its seating surface over the entire area of contact to reduce the risk of loosening and fracture.

3. Occlusal forces, usually in the presence of other predisposing factors, misfit, and mishandling, may lead to prosthetic screw fracture or loosening.

Risk of fracture and/or loosening—abutments

1. It is recommended that the clinician carefully evaluate the differential etiology of screw loosening, as the literature does not differentiate between abutment or prosthetic screw loosening sufficiently to conclude which type of screw is more likely to loosen.
2. Metal abutment fracture is a rare complication. Greater caution is advised with ceramic abutments. It is recommended that the specific material-based requirements of ceramics should be respected when choosing, designing, and handling these abutments.

Risk of fracture of framework and/or veneering materials

1. Currently framework fracture is a rare complication. The choice of material, appropriate design, and method of fabrication are all factors in reducing the risk of framework fracture.
2. To reduce the risk of fracturing the veneering materials, the framework must provide adequate support for the veneering ceramic or resin in order to avoid excessive thickness of the veneering material.
3. When choosing the material and determining framework design, it is recommended that the final contour of the definitive prosthesis be visualized prior to framework fabrication.
4. Scheduled regular maintenance appointments should include a careful occlusal review. It is recommended that clinicians undertake any required adjustments to the prosthesis, inclusive of meticulous polishing of worn ceramic surfaces, to reduce the risk of fracturing of the veneer material.

Quality assurance

It is recommended that clinicians, technicians, and manufacturers employ a tracking system for implants and restorative components. Clinicians should be aware that not all implant systems have the same level of documentation. The clinician should be aware of the origin of the components used.

 For a pdf copy of the full article (free of charge) from the ITI Consensus Paper, please check out the ITI Online Academy's ITI Consensus Database. See what else the Online Academy has to offer (charges may apply) at **academy.iti.org**

A literature review is not provided at this point, as the relevant literature relating to this volume of the Treatment Guide series is covered extensively in the following chapters.

3 Preoperative Risk Assessment and Treatment Planning for Optimal Esthetic Outcomes

W. Martin, V. Chappuis, D. Morton, D. Buser

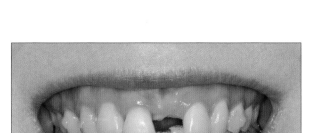

Fig 1   Pre-treatment high lip-line at smile, fully exposing the posterior teeth and gingiva.

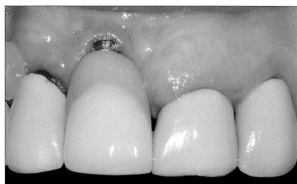

Fig 2   An unfavorable esthetic result with implant 11.

The *esthetic zone* can be defined objectively as any dentoalveolar segment that is visible at full smile, while subjectively it is defined as any dentoalveolar area of esthetic importance to the patient (Fig 1) (Belser and coworkers 2004). Smiles are as unique to individuals as the treatment necessary to maintain their natural appearance. Implant therapy in the esthetic zone is a challenging process, as patient demands on esthetics coupled with pre-existing deficiencies in the anatomy can present obstacles to achieving ideal results. The rehabilitation of missing teeth in the esthetic zone needs to be a predictable process, implying reproducibility and stability of the outcome in the short and long term (Elian and coworkers 2007a). Failure to achieve esthetic and functional results with dental implants could lead to disastrous situations that would require additional surgical and restorative procedures in an attempt to correct the compromise (Fig 2) (Buser and coworkers 2004; Levine and coworkers 2014).

It is therefore important for clinicians to understand their patient's desires and to perform a thorough initial clinical examination to highlight any potential obstacles that may present as a challenge in achieving an ideal esthetic outcome. Clinicians performing a rehabilitation must have a thorough understanding of tissue biology, and a knowledge of all treatment modalities for a given clinical situation, as dental implants may not always be the primary choice.

In an effort to properly diagnose a clinical situation and provide viable treatment options, the clinician should be able to visualize an ideal outcome for both the hard and soft tissues (Magne and Belser 2002). This visualization can then be used to isolate the clinical deficiencies that would require attention during the implant rehabilitation. The treatment endpoint can be defined in the form of an analog wax-up or a digital mock-up that captures the final contours of the planned restoration and supporting tissues (Figs 3a-c). This treatment endpoint will act as a blueprint and can be used to generate the treatment plan and procedures necessary for an esthetic result. Understanding the standards for an ideal esthetic implant restoration can aid in this process. The Proceedings of the 4th ITI Consensus Conference (Belser and coworkers 2004) highlighted these standards for an esthetic fixed implant restoration:

- An esthetic implant-supported prosthesis was defined as one that is in harmony with the perioral facial structures of the patient.
- The health, height, volume, color, and contours of the esthetic peri-implant tissues must be in harmony with the healthy surrounding dentition.
- The restoration should imitate the natural appearance of the missing dental unit(s) in terms of color, form, texture, size, and optical properties.

Applying these parameters during the pre-treatment phase can assist the clinician in determining the overall treatment risk related to the desired treatment outcome. The present chapter will highlight key factors associated with diagnosis and treatment planning for patients requiring single-tooth implants in the esthetic zone.

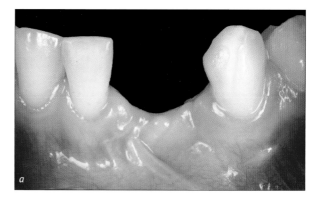

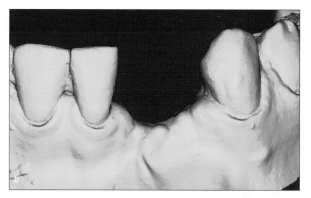

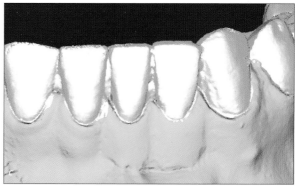

Figs 3a-c   Digital mock-up of hard- and soft-tissue areas.

3.1 Patient Selection

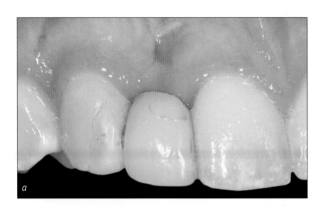

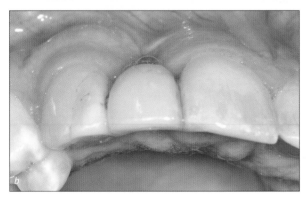

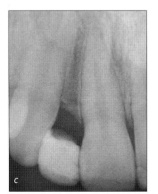

Dental patients present at our offices with the hope that we will address and satisfy their chief complaints, and it is our responsibility as clinicians to properly diagnose, inform and offer treatment recommendations and/or alternatives where available. While dental implants are a viable long-term treatment option for tooth replacement, not all patients are ideal implant candidates (Giannopoulou and coworkers 2003; Esposito and coworkers 2009a; Grütter and Belser 2009). We should make sure to present all treatment alternatives when necessary. In areas of esthetic importance, patients present with a wide variety of clinical situations that can influence our ability to achieve ideal results (Figs 4 to 6). While these situations present several clinical challenges, it is also important to evaluate the patient's general health risk factors that could negatively influence the success of surgical procedures, as reported by Buser and coworkers (2004) (Table 1).

Figs 4a-c   Congenitally missing tooth with limited inter-root space and in-adequate hard-tissue support for a dental implant.

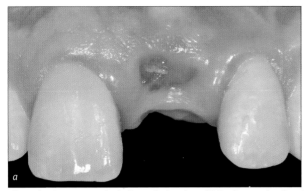
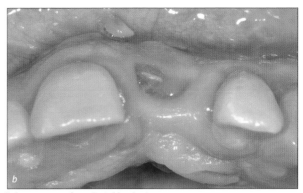

Figs 5a-b   Post-traumatic single-tooth situation with inadequate hard- and soft-tissue support for a dental implant.

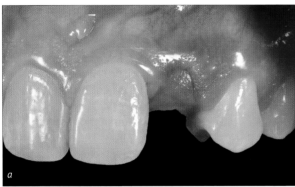
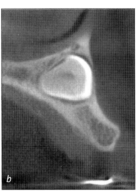

Figs 6a-b   Impacted canine preventing placement of a dental implant to replace tooth 22.

Table 1   General risk factors in candidates for implant therapy (Buser and coworkers 2004).

Risk factor	Remarks
Medical	• Severe bone disease causing impaired bone healing • Immunological disease • Medication with steroids • Uncontrolled diabetes mellitus • Irradiated bone • Others
Periodontal	• Active periodontal disease • History of refractive periodontitis • Genetic predisposition
Oral hygiene/compliance	• Home care measured by gingival indices • Personality, intellectual aspects
Occlusion	• Bruxism

Evaluating our patients using a systematic approach will reduce the possibility of overlooking potential pitfalls in treatment. Several assessment tools have been developed to aid in this process by isolating each clinical factor in an effort to obtain an overall risk of treatment (SAC Classification in Implant Dentistry, Dawson and Chen 2009). Once the overall treatment risk is established, clinicians must determine if their knowledge and skills are adequate for initiating care or if they necessitate a referral. These assessment tools will be introduced throughout the course of this text.

3.1.1 SAC Classification for Single-tooth Replacement

All clinical treatments require proper diagnosis, planning and execution during the surgical and restorative phases. In 2009, the International Team for Implantology (ITI) published a textbook based on a 2007 Consensus Conference to assist in this process called the SAC Classification in Implant Dentistry, focusing on classifying treatment difficulty in the surgical and restorative phases of treatment. This SAC Classification has been adopted by clinicians, teaching institutions, and dental organizations to aid in the diagnosis and planning for patients, based upon clinician experience and treatment difficulty. This classification system is highlighted in the ITI Online Academy as a free virtual tool to assist in examining the overall treatment risk and also to provide a foundation for clinician online education. (More information on the ITI Online Academy can found at www.academy.iti.org.)

The objective of the SAC Classification is to define the degree of treatment difficulty in a given patient, using a rating system of Straightforward (low difficulty and low risk), Advanced (moderate difficulty and moderate risk) and Complex (high difficulty and high risk). The majority of all clinical situations will fit the standard criteria of the SAC Classification and will be considered normative.

What makes the SAC Classification unique is that it also assumes that not all clinical situations are the same and that patients often present with modifying clinical factors that could positively or negatively influence the overall normative classification.

As an example, a patient with esthetic demands requiring a single-tooth central incisor implant would be considered normatively to have an Advanced surgical and restorative classification. But, if the patient presents with a surgical modifying factor, such as vertical bone loss or restorative modifying factor, such as planned immediate restoration, the overall treatment risk would be elevated to Complex. One clinical modifier of importance is the Esthetic Risk Assessment (ERA), first published in 2006 in Volume 1 of the ITI Treatment Guide. The ERA table isolated several medical, anatomical, and clinical factors that could have a significant influence on the potential for esthetic outcomes. When used during patient assessment, high-risk factors (both surgical and restorative) greatly influence the overall SAC Classification. An updated ERA table will be introduced in Chapter 3.2.

Successful application of the SAC Classification is based upon clinicians' knowledge, skill and experience and their ability to interpret objectively the clinical information that patients present. It does not fall within the scope of this Treatment Guide to re-publish the SAC Classification System, so we encourage the reader to explore this topic further in the full text.

For more in-depth information on the SAC classification, please check out the ITI Online Academy's learning module "The SAC Classification" by Dr. Anthony S. Dawson (charges apply). See what else the Online Academy has to offer at **academy.iti.org**

3.2 Esthetic Risk Assessment

The Esthetic Risk Assessment (ERA) table was developed to assist clinicians in the diagnosis and planning of treatment in the esthetic zone and to identify clinical situations that could contribute to an esthetic compromise. The ERA is easy to use and includes a comprehensive set of key clinical factors that contribute to treatment risk. This is why the ITI has adopted the ERA and integrated it into the SAC Classification textbook as one of the tools used in determining treatment difficulty. During the consultation phase of treatment, the ERA acts as a checklist and visual analog scale for the clinician and patient in determining the risk of achieving an esthetic outcome with treatment.

Since 2006, several advancements have been made in implant dentistry ranging from improvements in implant and abutment design, surgical and restorative materials to the introduction of digital diagnostic tools such as cone-beam computed tomography (CBCT) and digital planning software, which have necessitated an update to the existing ERA table. A careful effort was made not to rewrite the ERA, but to update it to a more current form based upon knowledge gained since 2006. Table 2 introduces the newly updated ERA table for the clinical assessment of the esthetic risk.

Table 2   Esthetic Risk Assessment (ERA)

Esthetic risk factors	Level of risk		
	Low	**Medium**	**High**
Medical status	Healthy, uneventful healing		Compromised healing
Smoking habit	Non-smoker	Light smoker (≤ 10 cigs/day)	Heavy smoker (> 10 cigs/day)
Gingival display at full smile	Low	Medium	High
Width of edentulous span	1 tooth (≥ 7 mm)[1] 1 tooth (≥ 6 mm)[2]	1 tooth (< 7 mm)[1] 1 tooth (< 6 mm)[2]	2 teeth or more
Shape of tooth crowns	Rectangular		Triangular
Restorative status of neighboring teeth	Virgin		Restored
Gingival phenotype	Low-scalloped, thick	Medium-scalloped, medium-thick	High-scalloped, thin
Infection at implant site	None	Chronic	Acute
Soft-tissue anatomy	Soft tissue intact		Soft-tissue defects
Bone level at adjacent teeth	≤ 5 mm to contact point	5.5 to 6.5 mm to contact point	≥ 7 mm to contact point
Facial bone-wall phenotype*	Thick-wall phenotype ≥ 1 mm thickness		Thin-wall phenotype < 1 mm thickness
Bone anatomy of alveolar crest	No bone deficiency	Horizontal bone deficiency	Vertical bone deficiency
Patient's esthetic expectations	Realistic expectations		Unrealistic expectations

* If three-dimensional imaging is available with the tooth in place
[1] Standard-diameter implant, regular connection
[2] Narrow-diameter implant, narrow connection

3.2.1 Medical Status

Dental-implant candidates undergo an assessment of their medical risk to determine if they are healthy enough for routine surgical procedures (Ata-Ali and coworkers 2014; Zadik and coworkers 2012; Michaeli and coworkers 2009; Moy and coworkers 2005; Buser and coworkers 2004; Morris and coworkers 2000). This assessment includes an evaluation of their past medical history, current medications, and allergies. The ERA assumes that a patient is healthy enough for dental implants, but applies a risk rating to the overall health of the patient based upon how it may influence the ability to achieve an esthetic outcome. For example, a patient who uses corticosteroids (oral inhaler) could get a compromised outcome when soft- or hard-tissue augmentation is performed, potentially compromising the esthetic result. Patients with compromised wound healing present a high esthetic risk.

3.2.2 Smoking Habit

The patient's smoking habits may have deleterious effects on grafting procedures, implant integration, and the long-term health of the peri-implant tissues (Buser and coworkers 2004). A recent systematic review of the literature reported that smokers had an increased risk of peri-implantitis (odds ratios from 3.6 to 4.6) and radiographic marginal bone loss (odds ratios from 2.2 to 10) compared to nonsmokers (Heitz-Mayfield and Huynh-Ba 2009).

The placement of implants in the esthetic zone is also often accompanied by hard- or soft-tissue augmentation procedures. Cigarette smoking may adversely affect wound healing, resulting in a higher risk in terms of grafting success. The heat as well as the toxic products of cigarette smoking such as nicotine, carbon monoxide and hydrogen cyanide have been implicated as risk factors for impaired healing and may thus affect the success of and result in complications related to surgical procedures (Levin and Schwartz-Arad 2005). In two studies on guided bone regeneration (GBR), smoking was associated with higher complication rates and poor treatment outcomes (Lindfors and coworkers 2010; Schwartz-Arad and coworkers 2005). Patients who smoke should be educated on or directed to cessation programs before implant therapy is initiated. A heavy smoker (> 10 cig/d) presents a high esthetic risk.

Clinical recommendation: Smoking is not a contraindication for implant placement. However, patients should be informed that the survival and success rates are lower in smokers. Heavy smokers should be informed that they are at greater risk of implant failure and loss of marginal bone. Patients who smoke should be informed that there is an increased risk of implant failure when sinus augmentation procedures are used (4th ITI Consensus Conference).

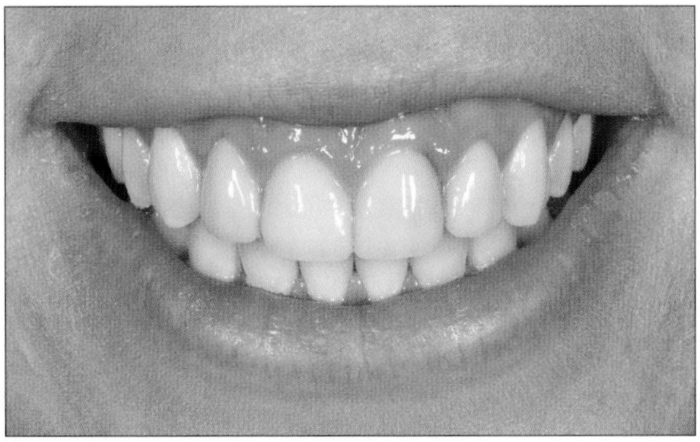

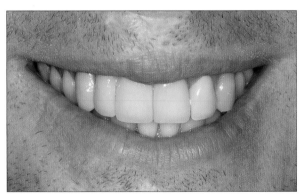

Fig 7   *High gingival display at full smile.*

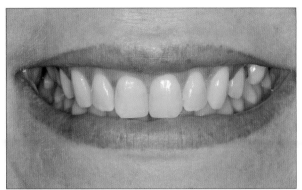

Fig 8   *Medium gingival display at full smile.*

Fig 9   *Low smile line with compromised outcome due to long contact areas on the prosthesis.*

3.2.3   Gingival Display at Full Smile

The smile is often considered the objective endpoint for rehabilitation in the esthetic zone. The basic components of smile analysis have been reported to consist of midline positioning, the presence or absence of the buccal corridor, the relationship of the maxillary incisal edges to the curvature of the lower lip, and clinical crown lengths displayed upon smiling (Kokich and coworkers 1999; Jensen and coworkers 1999; Hochman and coworkers 2012). The position of the lip line is associated with the amount of tooth substance and supporting tissues visible when the patient chews, speaks, or smiles. Tjan and coworkers (1984) defined three general categories of normalcy for smile type: low, average, and high smiles were defined based on the relative position of the vermillion border of the upper lip to the display of the clinical crown length and the associated gingiva. Patients characterized by a high gingival display at full smile will show the maxillary teeth in their entirety, as well as a significant portion of the supporting soft tissues (Fig 7). The esthetic risk for these patients is greatly increased, mostly due to the gingival tissue display and the need to maintain mucogingival symmetry with the adjacent teeth. Precise surgical and restorative techniques are necessary to develop healthy, symmetric, and well-contoured soft tissues, and any failures will be readily visible—particularly when restoring extended edentulous situations (Buser and coworkers 2004; Mitrani and coworkers 2005; Mankoo 2008).

The displayed gingival tissues and interdental papillae are often key determinants of treatment risk, as they are most difficult to replace when deficient (Vailati and Belser 2011). Patients who exhibit a medium gingival display typically display most of their anterior teeth and papillae and only very little of the supporting periodontal structures (Fig 8). Here the esthetic risk is increased and is more associated with factors affecting the appearance of the teeth and restorations. Particular attention should focus on the contours of the restoration; size, shape, color, texture, optical properties, and its proportions relative to the adjacent teeth. Restoration contours can be successfully managed by developing the incisal and gingival embrasures and addressing convexity in the teeth and surrounding structures (Spear and Kokich 2007).

It has been reported that the display of the interdental papillae during speaking and smiling represents the most important esthetic characteristic to be assessed, due to the frequency of visibility in patients with low smile lines (87%) (Hochman and coworkers 2012). The absence of the interdental papillae during smiling in patients with a low lip line can result in an unattractive smile, where the contact dimensions are usually increased (Fig 9). Special consideration should be given to the pre-treatment assessment of the position of the lip line and subsequent display of teeth, gingival tissues, and papillae and their potential impact on esthetic risk. If soft-tissue defects exist that cannot be addressed surgically, prosthetic planning for gingival-tissue replacement should be initiated before placing the dental implant(s). Vailati and Belser (2011) described the Pink Power Concept (PPC) as a new approach that fundamentally reevaluated the use of artificial gingiva as a structured implant-restorative strategy in the treatment of multi-unit gaps in the esthetic zone. This approach focuses on meticulous treatment planning, comprising optimal implant selection (design and size) and positions, planned before removing the teeth. Patient education is a key component of the PPC, as artificial gingiva carries a stigma of being unesthetic, which can greatly limit acceptance if not outlined before beginning treatment.

3.2.4 Width of the Edentulous Span

When evaluating edentulous spaces for restoration, careful attention should be given to the materials planned to replace the missing tooth structure and their space requirements for long-term durability. This will be referred to as prosthetic volume. For anterior single-tooth replacement in sites without tissue deficiencies, predictable treatment outcomes, including esthetics, can be achieved because tissue support is provided by the adjacent teeth (Belser and coworkers 2004; Buser and coworkers 2004; Belser and coworkers 2009; den Hartog and coworkers 2013; Furze and coworkers 2012). The esthetic risk is clearly lower if there is support for the papillae from the proximal crests of bone on the adjacent teeth and if the distance from this bone to the

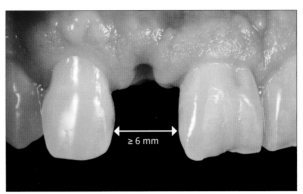

Fig 10   A single-tooth situation with adequate space for implant and restoration.

restoration's contact points above is short (Kan and coworkers 2003a; Kan and Rungcharassaeng 2003b; Degidi and coworkers 2008a; Lops and coworkers 2008). If interdental and inter-root space is adequate (≥ 7 mm for regular connection/diameter implants and ≥ 6 mm for narrow connection/diameter implants), sufficient support will be available for the peri-implant tissues and the prosthetic volume will be adequate for the abutment and restorative materials to create natural appearing contours (Fig 10).

The esthetic outcome can be compromised by unfavorable periodontal conditions or if inadequate prosthetic volume is available for implant placement and restoration. As the interdental and inter-root space decreases, the implant and restorative component options become limited and the prosthetic volume for ideal restoration emergence and contours suffer increasing the esthetic risk (Figs 11a-b).

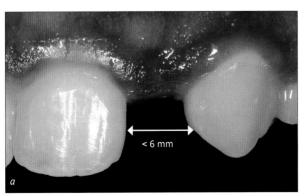 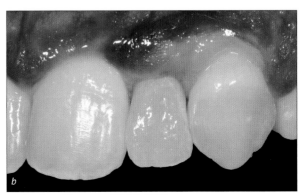

Figs 11a-b   A single-tooth situation with limited restorative space and resulting restoration with compromised contours.

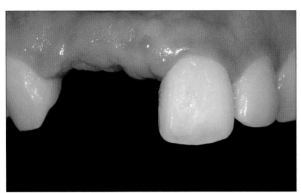

Fig 12   An extended edentulous situation highlighting a deficiency in soft- and hard-tissue support for implant restorations.

A minimum interimplant distance of 2 mm has been recommended to allow for preservation of the osseous crest and maintenance of the soft tissue when bone-level implants are used (Elian and coworkers 2007a; Elian and coworkers 2014; Koutouzis and coworkers 2015). In 2007, Priest presented the 3 × 3 × 3 PIE concept for adjacent implants (diameter 4 mm), recommending the following:

- Placement 3 mm apically from the planned restoration zeniths.
- Implant centers placed at least 3 mm palatally from the planned facial margin.
- Interimplant spacing of 3 mm, placing the straight-line emergence of the implant through the palatal incisal edge of the planned restorations.

Reports vary on the ideal distance between the implant body and the adjacent tooth root when it comes to preserving the interproximal tissue support (between 1.5 and > 3 mm), but it is clear that as the distance decreases, the risk of tissue loss increases (Buser and coworkers 2004, Lops and coworkers 2008). Efforts should be made to maximize this distance while not negatively influencing restorative material options (i.e., ceramic vs. titanium abutments).

When the edentulous space increases to include multiple missing teeth, the esthetic risk also increases due to the unpredictable nature of the interimplant soft- and hard-tissue support and the increased difficulty to maintain symmetric mucosal contours (Mitrani and coworkers 2005; Mankoo 2008) (Fig 12). The placement of adjacent implants must therefore not only be restoration-driven, but also biologically driven in an effort to promote the best sulcular anatomy through preservation of the soft and hard tissues after implant placement.

If extended edentulous spans are restored with adjacent implants, the morphology of the implants may cause the coronal aspect of the osseous crest between them to decrease, limiting the support for the soft tissues (Buser and coworkers 2004; Tarnow and coworkers 2003). For this reason, the restoration-based placement of dental implants to allow for maximum interimplant tissue support is paramount. Even small errors can be detrimental and lead to tissue deficits and limited space for establishing ideal emergence profiles of the restorations (Priest 2007).

Surgical variation in any of these parameters could significantly impair esthetic outcomes. Implant treatment planning for these patients should consider the increased risk posed by the adjacent implants and the need for surgical precision. As with all situations in the esthetic zone, appropriate implant selection is imperative, as the use of oversized implants can result in increased bone attrition and consequent facial and proximal tissue loss (Buser and coworkers 2004). When adequate soft and hard tissue exists, the selection of implants that will maximize circumferential bone support and allow for durable and esthetic abutments providing ideal prosthetic volume is recommended. Undersized implants can contribute to esthetic compromise in these situations when improperly used, i.e., shallow placement resulting in ridge-lap restorations with limitations to ideal emergence profiles.

Esthetic risk can be influenced by the location of the adjacent missing teeth, as extended spaces lateral to the midline increases the difficulty of maintaining harmonious tissue contours and restoration symmetry. Missing central incisors provide the best opportunity for an esthetic result due to potential "redundant" tissue located in the nasopalatine area and the symmetry of gingival architecture required after healing. When replacing a set of adjacent teeth that includes lateral incisors, the challenge is increased by the need to provide anatomically correct gingival zenith positions. Further, the emergence of appropriately contoured adjacent restorations through the peri-implant mucosa is critical if papillary support is to be gained, increasing the reliance on appropriate implant selection (size and shape). Consideration should be given to the prevention of the placement of adjacent implants in these spans where possible.

To achieve consistent outcomes, when a lateral incisor is involved adjacent to a missing central incisor or canine, cantilevering into the lateral site should be considered. This will allow the surgeon to place the implant in a position that maximizes interproximal tissue support while creating an ovate pontic at the lateral site. Patients with adjacent missing teeth including a lateral incisor present a maximum esthetic risk when adjacent implants are placed (Figs 13a-c).

When combined with additional risk factors such as high lip line or a thin gingival phenotype, the placement of adjacent implants in extended edentulous areas in the anterior maxilla often represents a maximum esthetic risk. Site development for patients in this category is often mandatory before or during implant placement. The results of such procedures vary, with horizontal augmentation gains often superior to gains achieved in the vertical dimension.

3.2.5 Shape of Tooth Crowns

One key to clinical outcomes in esthetic dentistry is the symmetry of the restorations, their shape, contours, and textures (Gallucci and coworkers 2007). If an implant restoration is mismatched with the adjacent tooth, this will greatly influence the appearance and final esthetic outcome. This situation is exacerbated when the implant restoration is located at the midline (Fig 14). The shape, contours, and texture of the restoration are key components in the white esthetic score (WES) index and can influence the patient's perception of the ideal (Belser and coworkers 2009; Jones and Martin 2014).

With the esthetic outcome strongly influenced by the symmetry of the final mucosal contours, the risk can often be reduced by the presence of square teeth (and, often, a thick gingival phenotype) (Stellini and coworkers 2013). Although implant-supported restorations in this environment are rarely associated with long and complete papillae, it should be noted that it is often in harmony with the patient's natural state (Figs 15a-b). Rectangular and triangular tooth shapes are associated with a higher risk level, most likely associated with the emergence anatomy and tissue support (Takei 1980; Gobbato and coworkers 2013). Triangular tooth shapes often have a corresponding soft-tissue architecture of the thin, high-scalloped type when associated with teeth in good periodontal health (Stellini and coworkers 2013; Peixoto and coworkers 2015) (Fig 16). A high esthetic risk is evident when a triangular tooth shape is associated with localized periodontal defects and the loss of interproximal papillae. These patients will often require a dental implant restoration that is rectangular-shaped

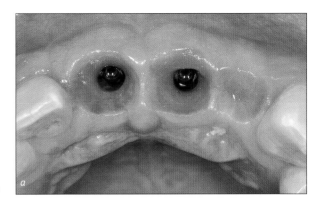

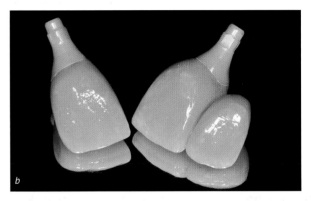

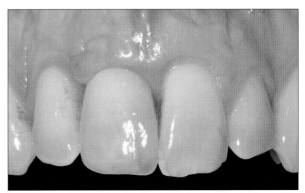

Figs 13a-c   An extended edentulous situation highlighting a single implant with a cantilevered restoration.

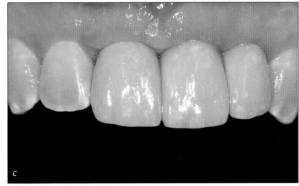

Fig 14   Implant restoration 11 with contours mismatched to those of the adjacent tooth.

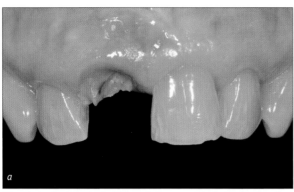 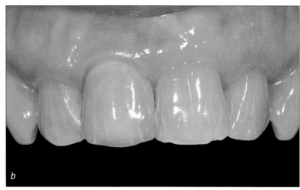

Figs 15a-b   Rectangular tooth morphology associated with short papillae and broad contact areas.

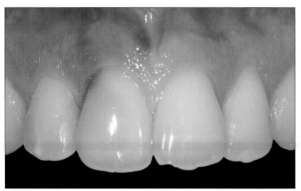

Fig 16   Triangular tooth shape associated with high-scalloped tissue architecture.

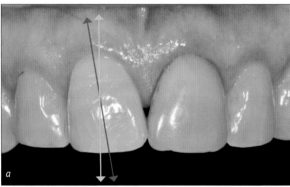 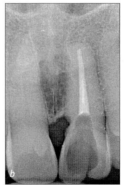

Figs 17a-b   A triangular tooth shape with an increased axis of inclination limiting the potential to maintain interproximal tissue contours upon removal of tooth 21.

with broad contact areas, potentially compromising the final appearance. When confronted with this situation, modifying the contours of the adjacent tooth to match those of the implant restoration might be an option to maintain symmetry and avoid black triangles. In a single-tooth implant study, Gobatto and coworkers (2015) reported that in an effort to achieve an esthetic outcome, they had to restore the adjacent tooth 65% of the time if the tooth form was triangular.

In situations where the adjacent triangular shaped tooth has a body angulation that moves the contact point coronal, consideration should be given to orthodontic correction in an effort to prevent a large papillary defect from occurring, as tooth-contour modification options may be limited (Figs 17a-b).

3.2.6 Restorative Status of Adjacent Teeth

The restorative status of teeth surrounding the edentulous space and planned surgical area can have an influence on esthetic outcomes and should be addressed in the treatment plan. If the teeth are virgin (non-restored), the esthetic risk can vary greatly, as their characteristics (thickness, translucency, optical properties) will play a role in the ability of the laboratory technician to create a restoration that accurately mimics the surrounding teeth. In situations where the adjacent teeth are thin in an orofacial dimension and are accompanied by increased translucency, accurate optical matching will be challenging (Figs 18a-b). When combined with other esthetic risk factors, e.g., a high smile line, the overall esthetic risk will be elevated.

If the adjacent teeth have restorations (crowns or veneers) that extend into the gingival sulcus and surgery is planned in the area, an elevated esthetic risk exists (Richter and Ueno 1973; Lindhe and coworkers 1987; Felton and coworkers 1991; Sanavi and coworkers 1998). Subgingival margins on adjacent teeth are often associated with recession subsequent to the placement of an implant, and esthetic complications can be associated with exposed restorative margins or an altered gingival architecture. This risk factor can be elevated if a periodontally involved tooth is located at the site planned for the implant, as recession can be noted after removal of the tooth, even in the absence of tissue reflection (Fig 19). For these patients, meticulous treatment planning is vital and may include the replacement of the adjacent restoration as part of the treatment, or modification of the surgical approach if indicated.

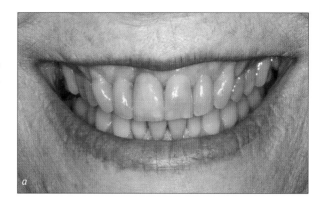

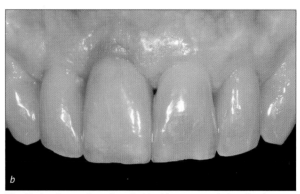

Figs 18a-b   Restoration of tooth 11 with a veneered zirconia abutment with a reduced orofacial thickness.

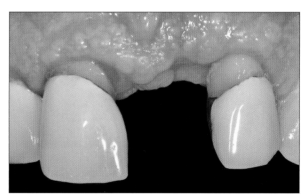

Fig 19   Exposure of crown margins of teeth 11 and 22 subsequent to extraction of tooth 21.

3.2.7   Gingival Phenotype

Phenotypes are the description of physical characteristics of an individual and are considered an expression of their genotype. The characteristics of the gingival phenotype (thick or thin) at an implant site can influence the treatment approach (surgical and restorative) as well as the ability to achieve an acceptable esthetic outcome. Several clinical methods of measurement have been reported to determine the gingival phenotype, ranging from photography, visual, direct measurement (after tooth extraction), and radiographic evaluation (CBCT) to sounding (manual or ultrasound) and probe visibility (Chappuis and coworkers 2015; Frost and coworkers 2015; Stellini and coworkers 2013; Müller and coworkers 2000; Kan and coworkers 2010; Egar and coworkers 1996).

Kan and coworkers (2010), reported that probe visibility ($p = 0.0117$) and direct measurement after extraction ($p = 0.0001$) were statistically significant in determining thick versus thin phenotypes when compared to visual assessment, whereas Frost and coworkers (2015) attempted and failed to determine a threshold measurement using probe visibility to determine thick vs. thin phenotypes and correlating them with facial-plate thickness. But they were able to conclude that thinner measurements of gingival thickness showed a tendency towards a thinner facial plate.

There are numerous reports of the shape of the tooth being directly correlated to the gingival phenotype, square tooth morphology being associated with thick, triangular more often associated with thin (Peixoto and coworkers 2015; Stellini and coworkers 2013; Müller and coworkers 2000; Olsson and Lindhe 1991). A more definitive measurement of the gingival phenotype and facial plate thickness can be obtained by CBCT combined with lip retraction, which can provide a clear visualization of the soft and hard tissues surrounding the tooth in question (Januário and coworkers 2008) (Figs 20a-b).

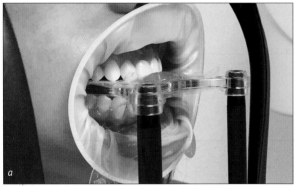
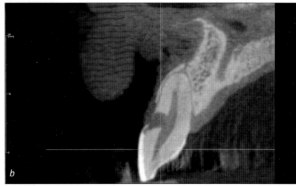

Figs 20a-b   Lip retractors used during CBCT to elevate the lip away from the facial tissue, allow clear visualization of the soft- and hard-tissue thickness.

Thick gingival phenotype. A thick gingival phenotype presents a low esthetic risk when replacing single missing teeth in the anterior area. The gingival tissue in these patients is often characterized by a predominance of thick, broad-banded keratinized tissue that is typically resistant to recession after surgical procedures (Chen and Buser 2014; Chen and coworkers 2009b; Kan and coworkers 2003a; Kois 2001) (Fig 21).

The thickness of the gingival tissue effectively masks the color of the implant(s) and any subgingival metallic components, reducing the risk of mucogingival discoloration. The phenotype clearly favors the long-term stability of the esthetic peri-implant soft tissues (Chen and Buser 2014). For patients with an extended edentulous space in the esthetic zone, a thick gingival phenotype can be both favorable and detrimental. Thick gingiva remains predictable in terms of position and appearance and resistant to recession. However, the character of the tissue reduces the likelihood of papillae developing when multi-tooth edentulous areas are present (Fig 22)

Medium gingival phenotype. To date, the available body of literature has not defined a medium gingival phenotype. It is the authors' experience that there is a significant patient population that display some of the characteristics of a thick phenotype—most often the presence of thick attached tissues—and those of a thin phenotype: long, thin or blunted dental papillae. And these characteristics are often found in patients with square-triangular tooth shapes. In these cases, surgical outcomes have more variability resulting in more challenging restorative procedures with somewhat less esthetic predictability over the long term, so the esthetic risk is increased.

Thin gingival phenotype. A thin gingival phenotype is characterized by a high-scalloped gingival architecture that is often associated with attractive single-tooth implant outcomes. The successful maintenance of the soft-tissue architecture depends on the support of facial bone and the periodontal support from the adjacent teeth (Cardaropoli and coworkers 2004; Kan and coworkers 2003a; Kois 2001; Weisgold 1977). The health and proximity of adjacent structures as they traverse the connective tissues and epithelium is important to establishing and maintaining papillae. The propensity for these tissues to respond to stimuli with recession cannot be ignored as a significant risk to a satisfactory esthetic outcome (Fig 23).

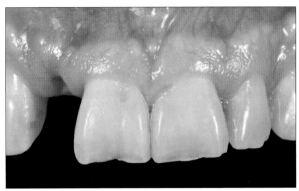

Fig 21   Example of a thick gingival phenotype.

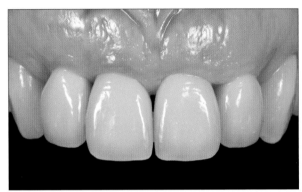

Fig 22   Twelve-year follow-up of implants 12 to 22 in a thick gingival phenotype patient.

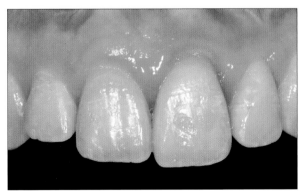

Fig 23   Recession of the gingival margin facial to tooth 21, secondary to facial resorption of bone following internal resorption.

The thin and friable nature of the soft tissues is conducive to the formation and maintenance of natural and predictable interproximal papillae, but an increased esthetic risk is associated with the possibility of mucosal recession in situations where immediate implants are used (Chen and Buser 2014, Chen and coworkers 2009b). In a study of type I implant placement using a flapless surgical approach and immediate provisional restoration, thin-phenotype sites had significantly more recession than thick-phenotype sites after 1 year (0.75 ± 0.59 mm vs. 0.25 ± 0.33 mm, respectively) (Brown and Payne 2011). In a retrospective study of type I implant placement using a conventional surgical approach and loading protocol, a higher frequency of recession of the mid-facial mucosa of 1 mm or more was observed for thin-phenotype sites (11 of 24 sites) compared to thick-phenotype sites (6 of 18) (Evans and Chen 2008). Of the sites that developed recession, 6 of the 11 thin-phenotype sites showed severe recession of more than 2 mm.

In contrast to these observations, Kan and coworkers (2009b) reported no differences between thick- and thin-phenotype sites when CT grafts were incorporated in the surgical protocol of flapless implant placement and immediate restoration. Predictable maintenance of the mucosal margin (> 3 years) has been reported in situations where early implant placement (type II) was combined with contour augmentation by guided bone regeneration at the time of placement (Buser and coworkers 2011). Long-term predictability requires careful attention to detail with particular regard to implant position and adequate supporting bone, restoration emergence profile, and technical adaptation and contour (Chu and Tarnow 2013).

Patients with an extended edentulous situation with a thin gingival phenotype often require surgical procedures to alter the characteristics of the tissue before or during implant treatment. The danger of recession and tissue discoloration (from the underlying implant and prosthetic components) is further increased in patients with adjacent missing teeth as implant positioning and restoration contours become more critical. Restorative and surgical planning for these patients requires implants to be placed further palatally (remaining in the orofacial comfort zone), allowing for maximum hard-tissue and soft-tissue coverage of the implant surface (Buser and coworkers 2004).

3.2.8 Infection at the Implant Site

Clinically examining the area at and near the planned implant site for infection is an important part of the preoperative evaluation of the esthetic risk. Local infection associated with periodontal disease, endodontic lesions, posttraumatic lesions (root fractures, root resorption, ankylosis), or foreign bodies (amalgam residue, infected root remnants), are capable of directly reducing the quantity and quality of the hard and soft tissues at potential implant sites or adjacent to them (Martin and coworkers 2006). The infection should be resolved, as it might be associated with an additional loss of esthetically important tissues, particularly the crestal bone levels on the adjacent teeth or soft-tissue shrinkage resulting in gingival recession. During the planning stage, the characteristics of the infection (acute or chronic) may affect its impact on the hard and soft tissues and the resulting esthetic risk. In the context of a local infection, the highest esthetic risk is associated with acute infections with suppuration and local swelling. Chronic infections, especially chronic periapical lesions of teeth to be replaced with implants, bear a medium risk for complications with esthetic significance if not resolved before implant placement (Lindeboom and coworkers 2006; Waasdorp and coworkers 2010; Montoya-Salazar and coworkers 2014; Villa and Rangert 2007) (Figs 24a-b). Meticulous cleaning, socket curettage/debridement and a 0.12% chlorhexidine rinse has been reported as a critical aspect of successfully placing implants at infected sites (Chrcanovic and coworkers 2015).

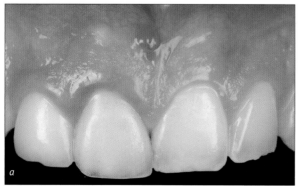 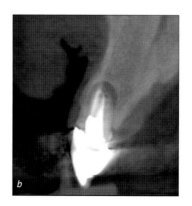

Figs 24a-b Peri-apical pathology associated with tooth 11.

Identifying patients with increased periodontal susceptibility or an increased risk for advancing or refractory periodontal disease is also critical. The literature shows increasing evidence that these patients are more prone to biological complications (peri-implantitis or implant failure), which are exacerbated when combined with smoking (Heitz-Mayfield and Mombelli 2014a; Heitz-Mayfield and coworkers 2014b; Heitz-Mayfield and Huynh-Ba 2009). Thus, periodontal disease must be resolved before implant therapy is initiated and should be considered to influence the esthetic risk.

> **Clinical recommendation:** A history of treated periodontitis is not a contraindication for implant placement. However, patients with a history of treated periodontitis should be informed of an increased risk of implant failure and peri-implantitis. Patients with a history of periodontitis should receive individualized periodontal maintenance and regular monitoring of peri-implant tissue conditions (4th ITI Consensus Conference).

3.2.9 Soft-tissue Anatomy

Soft-tissue deficiencies around teeth or in edentulous spans can pose an increased esthetic risk. The diagnosis of the soft- or hard-tissue defect needs to be determined prior to establishing risk. Evaluation of the soft tissues should commence with a smile analysis, to include the position and symmetry of the gingival margins, papillae, and contours of the facial keratinized mucosa. If the gingival margins are symmetrical and the defect resides in the underlying support for the soft tissue, then the defect would be considered favorable, as it would be managed with hard tissue. In these situations, if the adjacent

structures are healthy, if extractions (if required) are performed with a minimum of trauma to the bone and surrounding soft tissues, and if the defect is restricted to the horizontal dimension, site enhancement is predictable, and an esthetic outcome can be expected (Hämmerle and Jung 2003; Hermann and Buser 1996).

A new and interesting soft-tissue aspect has been reported by Chappuis and coworkers (2015) in a recent CBCT study in post-extraction single-tooth sites. The authors observed spontaneous sevenfold increase soft-tissue thickening in sites with a thin-wall phenotype within an eight-week healing period, resulting in a thick facial mucosa. Such a thick mucosal flap provides an advantage for the concept of early implant placement (type II), potentially reducing the need for additional soft-tissue grafting using a connective-tissue graft.

If soft-tissue defects are present prior to implant placement, in particular a lack of sufficient keratinized mucosa, an increased esthetic risk should be recognized (Fig 25). Several techniques to improve the soft tissue (connective-tissue grafts, CTG; vascularized pedicle grafts, VPG; free gingival grafts, FGG; orthodontic extrusion) have been described in the literature that vary in required treatment time and esthetic outcomes (Akcalı and coworkers 2015; Kaitsas and coworkers 2015). Of important note, these grafting procedures are dependent upon good underlying bone support and should not be considered a replacement of bone augmentation.

The timing of the soft-tissue graft will have great influence on the esthetic risk and long-term esthetic outcome. If soft-tissue defects exist after implant placement, attempts to improve outcomes may lead to short-term resolution but present a risk of recession following the healing of the graft and maturation of the tissue (Levine and coworkers 2014).

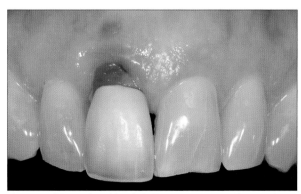

Fig 25   Facial recession of the gingival margin at a planned implant site 11.

3.2.10 Bone Level at the Adjacent Teeth

The replacement of single missing teeth requires careful evaluation of the soft and hard tissues at the implant site as well as the periodontal health of the adjacent teeth. Maintenance of the interproximal tissue (papillae) adjacent to the implant depends on the level of the bone crests on the adjacent teeth and their relationship to the contours of the restoration to the contact point (Choquet and coworkers 2001; Kan and coworkers 2003a; Degidi and coworkers 2008b; Schropp and Isidor 2015) (Figs 26a-b). Where local infections have resulted in vertical bone loss around adjacent teeth, the risk of a compromised esthetic outcome is greatly increased. The probability of a space (black triangle) arising between a properly contoured restoration and the adjacent tooth increases with more observed crestal bone loss on the adjacent roots. Furthermore, the regeneration of crestal bone along a previously infected root surface is not predictable, and is unlikely with current available treatment options.

The design of the dental implant and its distance from the adjacent tooth can influence the maintenance of the bone crest on the tooth surface. It has been stated that implants should be no closer than 1.4 mm to the adjacent tooth root in order to maintain crestal bone height (Tarnow and coworkers 2000). In contrast, Vela and coworkers (2012) reported that platform switched implants can be placed closer (1 mm) to the adjacent tooth while maintaining the proximal bone crest. This finding should be interpreted with caution, as the use of oversize implants in single-tooth sites should be avoided, and implant selection should focus on maximizing bone volume if restorative abutments and materials permit.

3.2.11 Facial Bone-wall Phenotype

Patients with a tooth requiring extraction and replacement with a dental implant are often considered for immediate implant placement. Several clinical factors must be considered before pursuing the immediate option: presence and type of localized infection, health of the adjacent teeth, ability to achieve primary stability, soft- and hard-tissue phenotypes. Esthetic compromise in the form of mid-facial recession can be a result if immediate implants are placed when the facial bone is thin (≤ 1 mm) or missing (Levine and coworkers 2014; Chappuis and coworkers 2013b; Chen and Buser 2014). Therefore, preoperative planning for immediate implants should include a local CBCT that highlights the presence and thickness of the facial bone (Vera and coworkers 2012) (Figs 27a-b). Lip retractors will help visualize the facial plate and determine the phenotype (Januário and coworkers 2008).

Dimensional alterations of the facial bone wall following tooth extraction in the esthetic zone can have a profound effect on the treatment outcomes. In a 3D analysis with CBCT, Chappuis and coworkers (2013b) identified a facial bone wall thickness of ≤ 1 mm as a critical factor associated with bone resorption. In addition, they reported that thin-wall phenotypes (≤ 1 mm) displayed pronounced vertical bone resorption (median bone loss: 7.5 mm) when compared to thick-wall phenotypes (median bone loss: 1.1 mm) (Figs 28a-b). Januário and coworkers (2011) evaluated the thickness of the facial bone wall in a CBCT study of the anterior maxilla of 250 patients, reporting that most locations in all tooth sites were ≤ 1 mm thick and that close to 50% of the sites were ≤ 0.5 mm thick. A CBCT study in 125 patients by Braut and coworkers (2011) showed that in central incisor sites, less than 5% of the sites had a thick-wall phenotpye (> 1 mm), whereas the prevalence of thick-wall phenotypes was much higher for first premolars, at 27.5%.

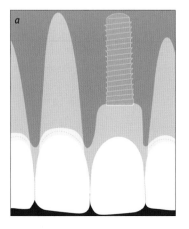
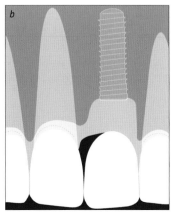

Figs 26a-b Ideal bone support on adjacent teeth (a) and bone loss on the adjacent tooth (b), which may lead to decreased support for the papilla.

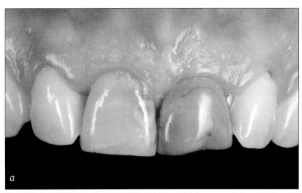
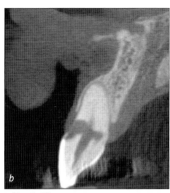

Figs 27a-b   CBCT evaluation of facial bone thickness and degree of resorption of tooth 11.

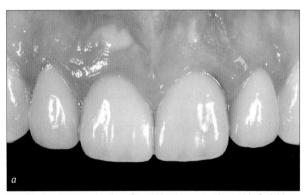
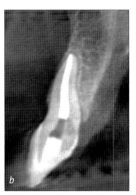

Figs 28a-b   CBCT evaluation of tooth 21 demonstrating a thin facial bone phenotype.

While successful esthetic results have been reported with implants placed after the extraction of anterior teeth, an increased esthetic risk exists in situations where the facial bone is 1 mm or less in thickness and an immediate implant is considered (Chen and Buser 2014). In these instances, early implant placement (types II and III) should be pursued with formal or simultaneous grafting once initial soft-tissue healing of the socket has completed, as this approach has shown to be more predictable in maintaining mucosal contours (Chen and Buser 2014; Chen and coworkers 2009a).

3.2.12 Anatomy of the Alveolar Crest

Deficiencies in horizontal and vertical bone dimensions will increase the esthetic risk, as augmentation procedures can vary in their ability to fully restore the ridge contours. Unfavorable local conditions of the alveolar ridge due to atrophy, periodontal disease, or traumatic sequelae may provide insufficient bone volume or unfavorable vertical, horizontal, or sagittal intermaxillary relationships, which may render implant placement impossible or unsuitable from a functional and esthetic viewpoint (Chiapasco and coworkers 2009) (Figs 29a-b).

Horizontal ridge augmentation has proven successful using of a variety of regenerative procedures, with no specific approach being superior in terms of technique and materials (Kuchler and von Arx 2014). The primary aim of horizontal ridge augmentation in the anterior maxilla is to facilitate a better implant position in order to improve the functional and esthetic outcome.

The position and the shape of the augmented bone will influence the soft-tissue profile, which should follow the contour of the neighboring teeth (Chen and coworkers 2014). Little information is given in the literature regarding the stability of the bone and esthetic outcomes in the anterior maxilla, as several confounding variables are associated with treatment in this region (Buser and coworkers 2009; Chiapasco and coworkers 2009; Kuchler and von Arx 2014). If horizontal augmentation is successful, survival and success rates of implants placed in the augmented bone will not be different from those placed in native bone with adequate width (Kuchler and von Arx 2014). A recent ten-year study by Chappuis and coworkers (2017) reported a 98.1% success rate after ten years following implant placement into augmented bone. Bone augmentation was performed with an autologous block graft, a superficial layer of bovine DBBM particles and non-crosslinked collagen membranes. Patients that present with these defects are considered to present a moderate esthetic risk.

A loss of vertical bone in the edentulous space magnifies the esthetic risk, as augmentation procedures able to address this condition are much more difficult in terms of technique and predictability. Vertical defects are commonly accompanied by a horizontal component. In these situations, the preoperative diagnosis of the degree and

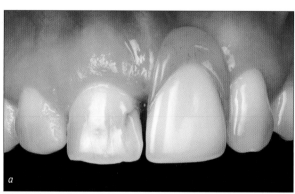
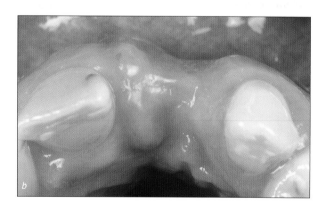

Figs 29a-b Horizontal defect at site 21 after tooth loss due to trauma.

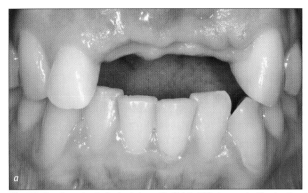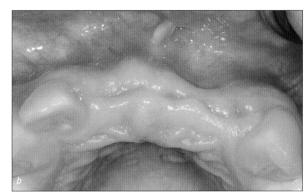

Figs 30a-b   An extended edentulous site (11 to 22) demonstrating horizontal and vertical bone deficiencies.

location of the atrophy is critical to select the most appropriate treatment approach. These types of defects are often found in extended edentulous spaces where the support of bone crests adjacent to teeth has been lost, resulting in resorption of the ridge crest and supporting soft tissues (Figs 30a-b). A diagnostic wax-up highlighting the tissue deficiencies based upon an ideal tooth form will aid the clinical team in this difficult decision (Fig 31).

Patients who exhibit vertical hard-tissue loss are associated with the highest esthetic risk. One treatment option is vertical ridge augmentation, which is best documented by the use of autologous particulate grafts, combined with a barrier membrane and xenographic bone fillers (Simion and coworkers 2007; Urban and coworkers 2014; Urban and coworkers 2015; Rochietta and coworkers 2016). However, higher complication rates have to be anticipated with these techniques (Simion and coworkers 2004). Another treatment alternative is horizontal ridge augmentation using the GBR technique and compensation of the vertical defect component by prosthetic means, using pink ceramics. An important prerequisite for this approach relies on the pink margin of the restoration being hidden below the lip line at full smile. Utilizing this artificial tissue allows for establishment of more harmonious gingival contours, as highlighted by the Pink Power Concept (PPC) (Vailati and Belser 2011). Of important note, vertically deficient sites next to periodontally involved teeth cannot be enhanced without addressing the periodontal disease itself. If periodontally compromised teeth are involved in future implant sites, tooth extrusion can be another treatment alternative (Salama and coworkers 1996).

Only few situations will force vertical ridge augmentation to be seriously considered. One of them is if the position of the lip line at full smile is too high for the PPC approach. Selecting younger, healthy patients and

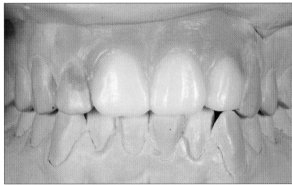

Fig 31   Diagnostic wax-up capturing the soft- and hard-tissue defects related to the planned restorations.

having highly experienced clinicians perform these very complex surgical procedures will help achieve acceptable treatment outcomes.

The Proceedings of the 5th ITI Consensus Conference highlight pertinent Consensus Statements:

- Horizontal bone augmentation in the anterior maxilla is a reliable treatment option to enable the proper placement of implants.
- Mean horizontal bone gain in the staged approach (measured at the time of implant placement) ranged from 2.2 to 5 mm. The included studies did not provide information about the long-term stability of horizontal ridge augmentation.
- There is not enough data available to indicate superiority of one method or material over another.
- Survival and success rates of implants placed in horizontally augmented bone were not different from those reported for implants placed in native bone with adequate width.

3.2.13 Patients' Esthetic Expectations

Upon completion of the ERA table, the visual impact of low, medium, and high esthetic risk will educate the clinician and patient on the overall treatment risk for achieving an ideal implant supported restoration. The esthetic risk factor that can determine whether the treatment should proceed is the patients' expectations. With patients who have high or unrealistic expectations combined with a high esthetic risk, treatment should be avoided, or the patient should be advised of the potential shortcomings in treatment with an attempt to move their expectations to more realistic. It is not uncommon to have patients presenting a high esthetic risk that understand the limitations to treatment and are willing to accept a compromised esthetic outcome (i.e., longer contacts, closed embrasures, pink ceramics) (Figs 32a-b).

With regards to implant success, patients presenting with a high esthetic risk should be informed of the challenges associated with the treatment. Alternative restorative methods should be duly considered before planning implant for dental implant therapy. Patients who qualify for surgical implant procedures from a medical point of view and whose esthetic expectations are high should always undergo a detailed examination not only of the edentulous space, but also of the supporting hard and soft tissues. Adjacent teeth, periodontal support, and existing hard and soft tissues are all critical factors when planning for a predictable esthetic result. Together, these factors constitute an assessment of esthetic risk.

When advising patients with high esthetic expectations, informing them of limitations in outcomes before the treatment is considered a risk in itself. But failure to inform patients of treatment limitations before treatment can lead to compromised esthetic outcomes being interpreted by the patient as a complication and will therefore be unacceptable in many cases. Using the ERA table during consultation can be a valuable tool achieving consistent esthetic implant outcomes in the dental practice, but more importantly, spare dentists from having to deal with unexpected esthetic complications and unhappy patients.

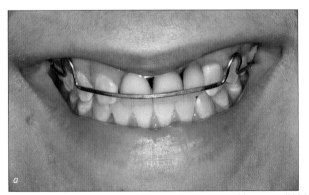
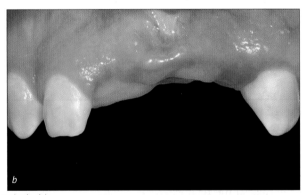

Figs 32a-b   Patient missing teeth 11 to 22 that presents with an overall high esthetic risk.

For more in-depth information on the assessment of esthetic risks, please check out the ITI Online Academy's learning module "Esthetic Risk Assessment" by Dr. William Martin (charges apply). See what else the Online Academy has to offer at **academy.iti.org**

For more in-depth information on risk factors in esthetics, please check out the ITI Online Academy's congress lecture "Esthetics: An Overview of Risk Factors" by Dr. William Martin (charges apply). See what else the Online Academy has to offer at **academy.iti.org**

3.3 Treatment Planning

The restoration of single and extended edentulous sites in the esthetic zone is a demanding process that requires the treatment team to focus their attention on details while having a thorough understanding of treatment risk and potential outcomes. Every consultation should start with the end-point in mind, as the final restoration will drive the planning and treatment process similar to that of a blueprint with a house. The dimensions of the final restoration will highlight the necessary interdental and interocclusal space requirements as well as the contours of the soft and hard tissues. When adequate restorative space and tissue support is determined, the restoration will drive the 3D positioning of the implant placement in the orofacial (body and angulation), vertical, and mesiodistal positions (Buser and coworkers 2004). (Implant positioning is covered in more detail in Chapter 4.2.6.)

The selection of the implant design will influence these positions to maximize prosthetic volume for an acceptable esthetic restoration. The key reference points in proper 3D placement are the shoulder and body of the implant and their relationship to the restoration and anatomy, allowing for adequate space for restorative materials so the technician can create ideal emergence profiles and restoration contours (Figs 33a-b).

Once the implant is placed, the volume of peri-implant tissue between the implant shoulder and the mucosal margin is referred to as the transition zone (Martin and coworkers 2006) (Fig 34). In most situations, the anatomy of the transition zone around anterior implants poses a challenge when seeking access to the shoulder of the ideally placed implant. It is not uncommon to find an implant 3 mm submucosally at the midfacial aspect and ≥ 5 mm submucosally at the interproximal aspect.

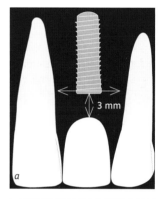

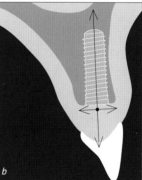

Figs 33a-b 3D positioning of a bone-level implant to allow for adequate prosthetic volume.

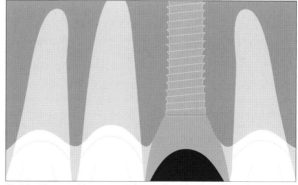

Fig 34 The transition zone. Volume of peri-implant tissue from the implant shoulder to the mucosal margin.

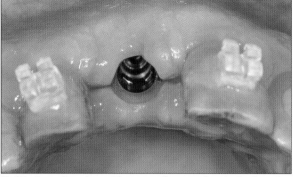

Fig 35 An unshaped transition zone after removing the healing abutment.

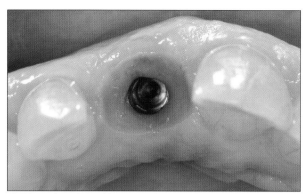

Fig 36 A shaped transition zone after removing the provisional restoration.

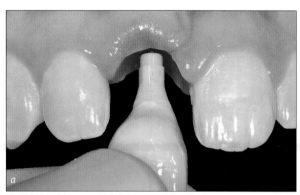

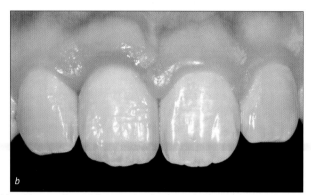

Figs 37a-b A screw-retained, one-piece zirconia abutment veneered with feldspathic ceramics at delivery and at the three-year follow-up.

The transition zone often heals after implant placement under the influence of healing abutments that do not represent the ideal emergence contours of a restoration (Fig 35). Taking an impression of the unshaped transition zone can then lead to difficulty in determining accurate emergence profiles, abutment contours, margin position, and contact points for the definitive restoration. The transition zone can be shaped with a custom healing abutment or a provisional restoration that establishes the ideal contours from the implant shoulder to the contact points of the adjacent teeth. In the Proceedings of the 5th ITI Consensus Conference, a clinical recommendation was made to use implant-supported provisional restorations to shape the transition zone prior to fabrication of the final restoration in all esthetically relevant areas (Morton and coworkers 2014) (Fig 36).

When cemented restorations are desired, it is critical to create an abutment that raises the cement line to a more accessible position for removal at the time of delivery. The deeper the position of the cement line (> 1 mm), the greater the hazard of cement residual remaining after cleaning, which can lead to mucositis and eventually peri-implantitis if not addressed (Linkevičius and coworkers 2011; Linkevičius and coworkers 2013; Wadhwani and coworkers 2012b; Wilson 2009).

Screw-retained restorations eliminate cement while offering retrievability. The method of retention has no bearing on the esthetic outcomes, as durable, esthetic materials that allow for screw retention have come to the forefront in modern implant dentistry (Sailer and coworkers 2009a) (Figs 37a-b).

For more in-depth information on structured case assessment and treatment planning, please check out the ITI Online Academy's learning module "Structured Assessment and Treatment Planning" by Dr. Hans-Peter Weber (charges apply). See what else the Online Academy has to offer at **academy.iti.org**

3.3.1 Anatomical Considerations

The anterior region of the mouth poses esthetic challenge as a difficult pre-existing anatomy can be coupled with high patient expectations. This region is often prone to tissue deficiencies caused by various conditions, which can be anatomic or pathologic in nature (Buser and coworkers 2004) (Table 3). These tissue deficiencies will often require bone augmentation such as guided bone regeneration to rebuild deficient sites before implant placement or contour augmentation procedures when performed simultaneous with implant placement (Buser and coworkers 2013b). Understanding the ridge anatomy, which includes the soft tissue and bone in all dimensions, and the role they play for the long-term prognosis of the implant is a critical factor in determining the optimum treatment approach.

Once a tooth has been extracted, the alveolar ridge undergoes a remodeling process that can result in a decrease in ridge width (3.87 mm) and crestal height (1.53 mm) (Van der Weijden and coworkers 2009). The extent of bone resorption also depends on the thickness of the facial bone wall, as thin-wall phenotypes (≤ 1 mm) were reported to lose 62.3% or 7.5 mm (median) of mid-facial vertical bone height, while thick bone phenotypes lost only 1.1 mm (Chappuis and coworkers 2013b). The resorption, however, mainly took place in the mid-facial area, whereas approximal areas showed only minimal changes within 8 weeks of healing. This post-extraction remodeling process not only changes the underlying bone, but also the supporting soft-tissue architecture. Chappuis and coworkers (2015) reported on soft-tissue alterations in post-extraction sites in the esthetic zone. They reported a sevenfold increase in soft-tissue thickness for thin-wall phenotypes (≤ 1 mm) at 8 weeks, whereas the soft-tissue thickness remained unchanged with thick-wall phenotypes (> 1 mm). A key conclusion was that the observed spontaneous soft-tissue thickening in the thin-wall phenotypes resulted in vertical soft-tissue loss of only 1.6 mm, which concealed the vertical bone resorption of 7.5 mm. The result is that the thickening of the soft tissue is able to mask the underlying bone defect, but may offer advantages for the clinician in providing a thick flap with better vascularity and less need for connective-tissue grafting in standard sites (Chappuis and coworkers 2015).

In single-tooth situations, some of the support for the tissues is gained from the adjacent teeth, but the proposed implant site first needs to be assessed in the orofacial dimension, determining if there is sufficient crest width and if facial-bone atrophy is present or absent. This dimension can be evaluated by bone sounding or

Table 3   Clinical conditions associated with tissue deficiencies in the anterior maxilla (Buser and coworkers 2004)

Conditions	Remarks
Anatomic:	
Narrow alveolar crest and/or facial undercut of alveolar process	Congenitally missing teeth
Pathologic:	
Dental trauma	Tooth avulsion with fracture of the facial bone plate
Posttraumatic conditions	Root ankyloses with infraocclusion, root resorption, root fractures
Acute or chronic infections	Periodontal disease, periapical lesions, endo/perio lesions
Disuse bone atrophy	Long-standing tooth loss

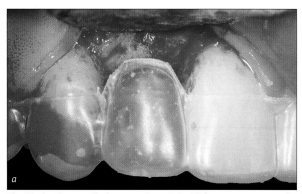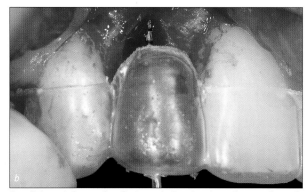

Figs 38a-b Bone scalloping procedure at site 12 for a narrow-connection implant (3.3 mm). 3 mm of scalloping apical to the planned mucosal margin are indicated by the vacuform template.

CBCT imaging. The mesiodistal dimension is determined by evaluating of the diagnostic wax-up or the adjacent and contralateral teeth. A deficiency in this dimension should be addressed by orthodontics, enameloplasty, or modification by restoration throughout the course of the treatment (Kan and coworkers 2009b). The most critical assessment remains the coronoapical dimension. Deficiencies here can result from several factors: periodontal disease of the adjacent tooth/teeth, atrophy, trauma, infection or congenital abnormality (Buser and coworkers 2004). Managing a deficit in this dimension is difficult and will require careful attention to procedures that recapture the vertical height and present a high anatomical risk.

Clinical scenarios exist (congenitally missing teeth) where there is a vertical excess of hard tissue. To address this, bone-scalloping procedures will need to be incorporated into the surgical treatment to prevent shallow placement of the dental implant (Figs 38a-b). A surgical template that highlights the proposed mucosal margin of the restoration will dictate the degree of scalloping needed to position the implant in the correct submucosal position, allowing for an ideal emergence profile of the restoration. Lastly, the determination of the location of the nasopalatine canal, floor of the nose, and adjacent tooth roots are necessary in the selection of the dental implant. This assessment can be performed through the use of plane-film radiography (periapical) or sectional imaging when needed (CBCT).

For more in-depth information on anatomical considerations in implant dentistry, please check out the ITI Online Academy's learning module "Anatomy with Relevance to Implant Surgery" by Dr. Vivianne Chappuis (charges apply). See what else the Online Academy has to offer at **academy.iti.org**

3.3.2 Indications for CBCT in the Esthetic Zone

The successful placement and restoration of dental implants in the esthetic zone depends on accurate preoperative planning, followed by surgical and restorative procedures embracing validated treatment protocols. The use of specific imaging techniques to assist in the planning process is based on the patient's clinical presentation and the clinician's professional judgment in order to formulate a diagnosis (Harris and coworkers 2002; Harris and coworkers 2012). Bornstein and coworkers (2014a) reported that imaging modalities for presurgical implant planning should be adequate to provide three types of information:

- ***Morphologic characteristics of the residual alveolar ridge.*** The morphology of the residual alveolar ridge (RAR) includes considerations of bone volume and density. Vertical bone height, horizontal width, and edentulous saddle length determine the amount of bone volume available for implant placement.
- ***Orientation of the residual alveolar ridge.*** The orientation and residual topography of the alveolar-basal bone complex should be assessed to determine deviations of the RAR that compromise alignment of the implant body with respect to the restorative plan.
- ***Local anatomic or pathologic boundaries within the RAR limiting implant placement.*** Numerous internal anatomic features of the jaws (e.g., nasopalatine fossa and canal, nasal fossa, mental foramen, submandibular gland fossa, inferior alveolar or mandibular canal) compromise and limit implant placement or risk involvement of adjacent structures. Anatomic anomalies and local pathologies (e.g., retained root tips, sinus disease, or adjacent inflammatory processes) may also prevent or restrict implant placement.

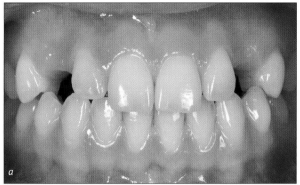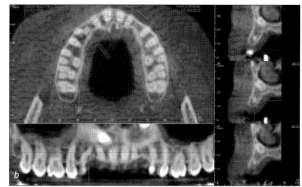

Figs 39a-b   Cross-sectional imaging provides detailed information on the position of root 14 and impacted tooth 13 in respect to the edentulous space 13.

For over thirty years, the information required to satisfy these goals has been obtained from clinical examination and, most commonly, two-dimensional (2D) imaging such as panoramic, peri-apical, lateral cephalometric radiography, which has resulted in predictable treatment and high success rates in clinical practice (Bornstein and coworkers 2014a). The introduction and widespread use of cross-sectional CBCT imaging in implant dentistry over the last fifteen years has enabled clinicians to diagnose and evaluate the jaws in three dimensions, providing more precise and better information of the type that often cannot be provided by clinical examinations, study casts, and conventional imaging alone (Figs 39a-b).

There are today no clearly defined indications or contra-indications for 3D imaging (CBCT) for implant planning in the esthetic zone. Most published national and international guidelines do not offer evidenced-based action statements developed from a rigorous systematic review. The majority of the information is derived from clinical trials, either cohort or case-controlled studies, and are often presented as consensus-based recommendations derived by a limited methodological approach with only partial retrieval or analysis of the literature or contain even generalized or case-unspecific statements (Bornstein and coworkers 2014a). One particular note comes from Harris and coworkers (2012), in a summary of the EAO Consensus Conference, where they stated that cross-sectional imaging is not indicated for situations "if the clinical assessment of implant sites indicates that there is sufficient bone width and the conventional radiographic examination reveals the relevant anatomical boundaries and adequate bone height and space." This statement highlights the need for the clinician to perform a comprehensive clinical examination before selecting the imaging method for a given clinical scenario.

The 5th ITI Consensus Conference published treatment guidelines with respect to CBCT imaging in dental implant therapy (Bornstein and coworkers 2014b):

- The clinician performing or interpreting CBCT scans for implant dentistry should take into consideration current radiologic guidelines.
- The decision to perform CBCT imaging for treatment planning in implant dentistry should be based on individual patient needs following thorough clinical examination.
- When cross-sectional imaging is indicated, CBCT is preferable over CT.
- CBCT imaging is indicated when information supplemental to the clinical examination and conventional radiographic imaging is considered necessary. CBCT may be an appropriate primary imaging modality in specific circumstances (i.e., when multiple treatment needs are anticipated or when jawbone or sinus pathology is suspected).
- The use of a radiographic template in CBCT imaging is advisable to maximize surgical and prosthetic information.
- The field of view (FOV) of the CBCT examination should be restricted to the region of interest (ROI) whenever possible.
- Patient- and equipment-specific dose reduction measures should be used at all times.
- To improve image data transfer, clinicians should request radiographic devices and third-party dental implant software applications that offer fully compliant DICOM data export.

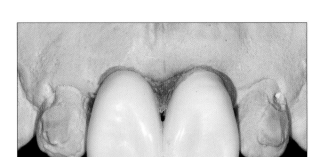
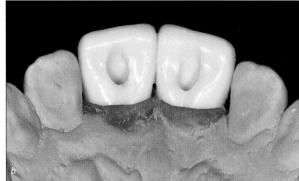
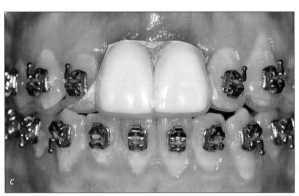
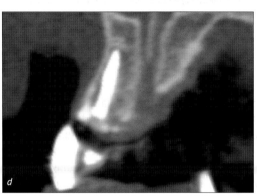

Figs 40a-d Radiopaque teeth (Ivoclar Vivadent, Amherst, NY, USA) are trimmed to ideal contours with access holes placed through the center of the tooth, then picked up in a thin vacuform that can be worn during the CBCT. During planning, the slice that highlights the hole in the tooth will assure the proper cross-section for planning.

When planning for dental implants and using CBCT imaging, the placement of a radiopaque tooth in the planned implant site through the use of a radiographic template or a post-scan digital wax-up highlighting the ideal contours creates an important reference point for crown-down planning and site evaluation (Figs 40a-d).

For more in-depth information on the use of CBCT in implant dentistry, please check out the ITI Online Academy's congress lecture "Indications and Recommendations for CBCT in Implant Dentistry" by Dr. Michael M. Bornstein (charges apply). See what else the Online Academy has to offer at **academy.iti.org**

3.3.3 Digital or Conventional Planning

During the past several years, digital technologies have become commonplace in all aspects of implant dentistry, including radiographic imaging, digital planning, template fabrication, implant placement, impression-taking, and abutment/restoration fabrication. The incorporation of critical patient data into the digital realm allows for precise planning that is portable between the members of the treatment team. This digital information can create synergies between the surgeon, restorative dentist and technician so all members can visualize and manipulate the planned treatment from different locations. This process can improve the preoperative diagnosis of the planned implant sites (general anatomy) and allow for virtual prior to live surgery.

In addition, digital technology can improve the accuracy of the surgical templates and quality of the final restorations through enhanced control over the design of the provisional and final reconstructions, with the possibility to manufacture with industrially controlled fabrication processes (Tahmaseb and coworkers 2014; Hämmerle and coworkers 2015).

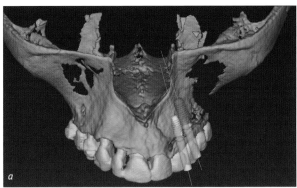
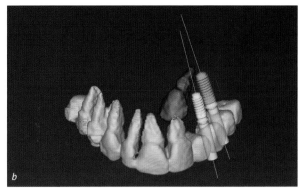

Figs 41a-b Digital planning for treatment options to replace the missing teeth 12 to 14 with implants while avoiding an impacted canine.

The conventional approach to implant planning begins with a thorough clinical examination, diagnostic casts, digital photography, and radiographic evaluation (plane film and CBCT). Treatment planning for the implant is determined by a diagnostic wax-up highlighting the hard- and soft-tissue deficiencies and their relationship to the planned restorations. This wax-up is an analog representation of the proposed treatment and will drive the planning, leading to the surgical procedures needed to position the implant in an ideal 3D position. Templates are fabricated on gypsum casts based upon surface contours and an interpretation of the critical anatomy as isolated on the radiographs. A limitation to this process is appreciated when anatomical situations are present that cannot be accounted for in detail, as all decisions on implant positioning are arbitrarily determined by the drilling into the cast.

The introduction of digital planning has created a software environment where the patient's imaging (CBCT) data can be merged with clinical data (surface scans) for a 3D evaluation of the implant site and localized anatomy. This information allows for thorough pre-operative planning of the implant(s) to be placed by type, size, position, and inclination with respect to the planned restoration (Vercruyssen and coworkers 2015). Deficits in soft and hard tissues, limiting anatomical situations, and localized pathology can be clearly visualized and be planned prior to the surgery (Figs 41a-b). Upon completion of the digital planning, the treatment can be streamlined through the fabrication of stereolithographic templates that assist in the precise placement of the implants.

A major advantage of digital planning over conventional planning is better patient communication. The ability to review the planned procedure ahead of the treatment is a powerful tool for showing patients options for their treatment and the required procedures to achieve an ideal esthetic result.

For more in-depth information on digital planning, please check out the ITI Online Academy's congress lecture "How is the Digital Workflow Integrated into Patient Treatment" by Dr. German Gallucci (charges apply). See what else the Online Academy has to offer at **academy.iti.org**

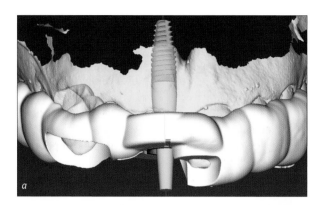

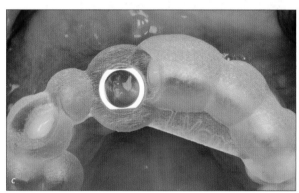

Figs 42a-c   Virtual planning and template design for implant 11 and printed stereolithographic template.

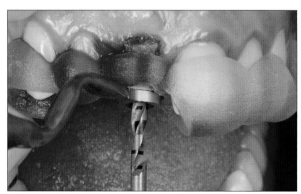

Fig 43   Fully guided flapless placement of implant 11.

3.3.4   Surgical Templates for Implant Placement

The placement of dental implants in the esthetic zone requires precise positioning in 3D based upon a restorative plan, as deviations in any of the dimensions can result in negative esthetic outcomes (Buser and coworkers 2004). Surgical templates to guide the placement of the implant can help minimize damage to the surrounding tissues, teeth, and prosthetic volume of the definitive restoration.

The introduction of CBCT as a 3D imaging tool in implant dentistry has led to its incorporation into planning software, making it possible to virtually plan optimal implant positions relative to vital anatomic structures and the planned restoration (Tahmaseb and coworkers 2014). The digital plan can then be used to fabricate a surgical template, transferring the proposed implant position from the computer to the patient, with the template directing the implant osteotomy and final positioning without damage to the surrounding anatomic structures (Widmann and coworkers 2010).

Surgical templates can be classified into two groups based upon their method of use, static or dynamic (Jung and coworkers 2009). Static systems are those that communicate predetermined sites using surgical templates or implant guides in the operating field. Static guides can be fabricated using gypsum casts and plane film radiography or by virtual planning using CBCT imaging and a stereolithographic process (Higginbottom and coworkers 1996; Ersoy and coworkers 2008; Di Giacomo and coworkers 2005) (Figs 42a–c). Dynamic systems communicate the planned implant positions to the operative field using visual imaging tools on a computer monitor instead of rigid intraoral guides. The dynamic systems include surgical navigation and computer-aided navigation technologies and allow the surgeon to modify the surgical procedure and implant positions in real time using the anatomical information available from the preoperative plan and a CT or CBCT scan (Tahmaseb and coworkers 2014).

In a systematic review by Jung and coworkers (2009), the static systems tended to be more accurate than the dynamic approaches. However, this outcome should be interpreted with some caution, as most of the publications on navigation were clinical studies, whereas the majority of studies on static protocols were preclinical (models, cadaver, etc.), where more accurate measurements are possible. The greater accuracy of these latter studies can be explained by better access, greater visual control of the axis of the osteotomy, absence of movement in a cadaver, and the absence of saliva or blood in the preclinical models (Tahmaseb and coworkers 2014). In general, given the variation in available data, no one approach can be deemed superior to the other. Nevertheless, the accuracy of guided approaches should be considered superior to that of freehand placement when a fully guided approach is used.

The use of surgical templates obtained with virtual planning is indicated in situations with anatomical limitations and where a flapless approach is desired (Fig 43). This will ensure that maximum diligence is applied to the preparation of the osteotomy, and the implant is placed a comfort zone that allows for ideal bone support and avoids long-term esthetic compromise.

The Proceedings of the 5th ITI Consensus Conference defined treatment guidelines for using templates for the placement of implants:

- Guided surgery should be viewed as an adjunct to, not a replacement for, appropriate diagnosis and treatment planning.
- Guided surgery should always be prosthetically driven. This includes either a radiographic template generated from a wax-up, or appropriate software applications to create a digital wax-up.
- Information to be gathered from the combination of high-quality CBCT images and digital planning should include locations of vital structures, desired implant positions and dimensions, the need for augmentation therapy, and the planned prostheses.

- Due to the reported mean deviations, an additional 2 mm should be taken into consideration when planning implant position with relation to vital structures and adjacent implants in all directions. In borderline cases, an intraoperative periapical radiograph should be taken as a safety measure.
- Guided surgery may be utilized with a flapless or raised flap approach.
- Only mucosally and/or tooth- or implant-supported surgical templates should be used.
- For improved accuracy, implants should be inserted in a fully guided manner (vs. guided implant-bed preparation alone) whenever possible.
- Guided surgery may be used with different loading protocols, in partially and fully edentulous indications.
- Indications for guided surgery include: to aid in treatment planning, when encountering complex anatomy, to perform minimally invasive surgery, and to improve patient understanding of therapeutic needs and treatment options.

For more in-depth information on guided surgery, please check out the ITI Online Academy's congress lecture "The Precision of Guided Surgery" by Dr. Ali Tahmaseb (charges apply). See what else the Online Academy has to offer at **academy.iti.org**

4 Selecting Biomaterials for Implant Procedures

V. Chappuis, S. S. Jensen, D. D. Bosshardt, D. Buser

4.1   Ceramic vs. Titanium Implant Materials

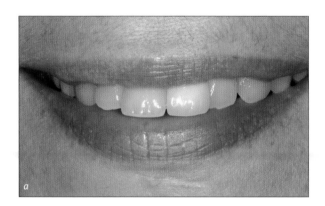

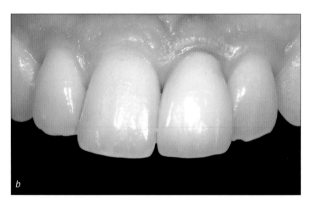

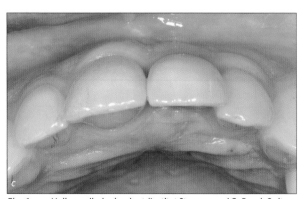

Figs 1a-c   Hollow-cylinder implant (Institut Straumann AG, Basel, Switzerland) at site 21 with a 21-year follow-up in a 50-year-old female patient. The implant revealed healthy peri-implant conditions with no signs of biological or technical complications. A slightly grayish shade is visible at the crown margin.

4.1.1   Commercially Pure Titanium Implants

The introduction of osseointegrated titanium (Ti) implants (Brånemark and coworkers 1969; Schroeder and coworkers 1976) initiated a major paradigm shift in reconstructive dental medicine. During the development phase of this new treatment approach in the 1970s and 1980s, two implant surfaces dominated the market—a machined, rather smooth surface and a coated, titanium plasma-sprayed (TPS) surface, which was rather rough and microporous. For both implant surfaces, satisfactory survival and success rates were reported after up to twenty years of follow-up (Adell and coworkers 1981; Buser and coworkers 1997; Lekholm and coworkers 1999; Jemt and Johansson 2006; Jacobs and coworkers 2010; Chappuis and coworkers 2013). Depending on the duration of the follow-up period, the survival rates ranged from 90% to 95% in most studies (Figs 1a-h).

In the last two decades, the surface topography of implants, mainly consisting of commercially pure titanium (cpTi), has been thoroughly investigated and markedly improved (Buser and coworkers 1998; Gotfredsen and coworkers 2000). Today, cpTi implants with a micro-rough surface produced with various techniques such as sandblasting and/or acid-etching dominate the market and are considered the "gold standard" for dental implants due to their corrosion resistance and biocompatibility. They are produced using various techniques, such as sandblasting, acid-etching, or a combination (Wennerberg and coworkers 2009).

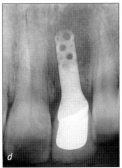 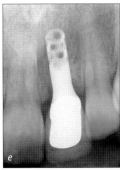 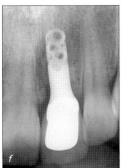 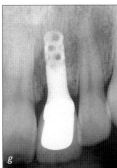 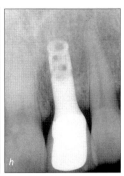

Figs 1d-h   The implant with a rough TPS surface yielded stable peri-implant bone levels at one (d), three (e), five (f), eight (g), and twenty (h) years. Only minor bone loss (0.02 mm) was observed between the one-year and the twenty-year examination.

Significantly enhanced bone/implant contact (BIC) was found when the initial sandblasted and acid-etched cpTi surface (SLA) was made hydrophilic by chemical modification (SLActive) (Buser and coworkers 2004; Ferguson and coworkers 2006). These studies revealed increased BIC and a higher removal torque during initial healing and allowed for shorter healing times (Bornstein and coworkers 2009a) (Figs 2a-h).

Dental implants made of cpTi placed under favorable conditions in healthy partially edentulous patients have shown success rates of 97% after ten years and 90% after twenty years (Buser and coworkers 2012; Chappuis and coworkers 2013).

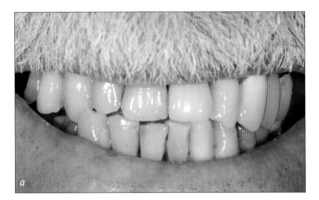

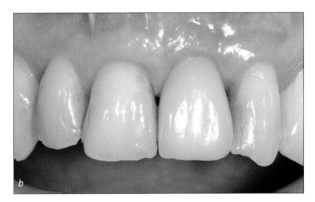

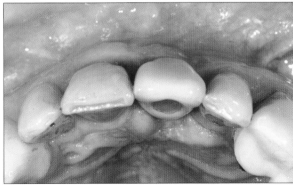

Figs 2a-c   An SLA implant (Institut Straumann AG) in a male patient at site 21 with eleven-year follow up. The implant revealed healthy peri-implant conditions with no signs of biological and technical complications. A slight grayish shade is visible at the crown margin.

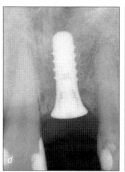
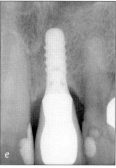
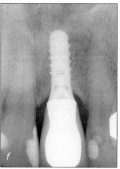
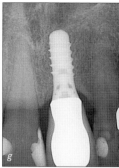
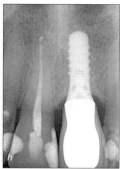

Figs 2d-h   The implant surface exhibiting a SLA surface yielded stable peri-implant bone levels at one (d), three (e), five (f), eight (g), and twenty (h) years. Only minor bone loss (0.02 mm) was observed between the one-year and the twenty-year examination.

Yet in spite of these excellent outcomes, technical, biological, and esthetic complications do occur. In a recent systematic review with a mean follow-up time of five years of implant-supported single crowns, technical complications occurred in 16.4%, biologic complications in 7.1%, and esthetic complications in 7.1% of cases after five years (Jung and coworkers 2012). One of the complications observed was fatigue fracture of narrow-diameter implants, usually after several years of implant function (Zinsli and coworkers 2004). Thus, research focused on overcoming these drawbacks by improving the mechanical properties of the implant materials (Figs 3a-f).

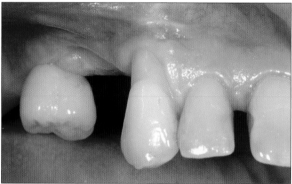

Fig 3a   A 63-year-old male patient with multiple implant fractures at sites 14, 15, and 16 only five months after implant placement.

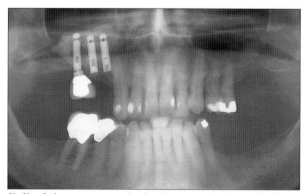

Fig 3b   Orthopantomogram. Previously augmented sinus graft with two fractured implants.

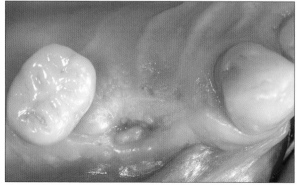

Fig 3c   The intraoral view. Loosened crown on the first molar and a fistula at the second premolar site.

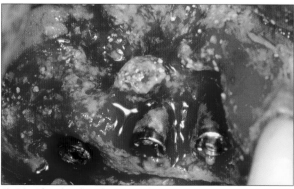

Fig 3d   After elevation of a mucoperiosteal flap. Three fractured implants and an infection of the grafted area.

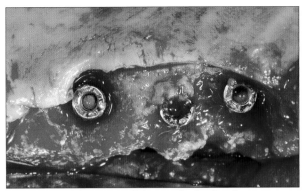

Fig 3e   Occlusal view. Fractured abutment-implant interface.

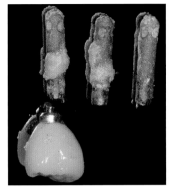

Fig 3f   The implants were ultimately removed.

4.1.2   Titanium-alloy Implants

New titanium alloys were developed to improve the mechanical properties of implants—not only to minimize the risk for implant fracture but also to expand the indications for narrow-diameter implants (NDI) at sites with limited bone volume (Engfors and coworkers 2004; Müller and coworkers 2015; Sohrabi and coworkers 2012; Ioannidis and coworkers 2015) (Table 1).

Table 1   New implant materials with optimized mechanical properties compared to commercially pure titanium Grade 4 (cpTi Grade 4).

	Commercially pure titanium Grade 4 (cold-worked)	Ti-6 Al-4 V	Straumann Roxolid	Zirconia[1] (3Y-TZP)
Composition (wt. %)	N ≤ 0.05 C ≤ 0.08 H ≤ 0.015 Fe ≤ 0.5 O ≤ 0.4 Ti = balance	N ≤ 0.05 C ≤ 0.08 H ≤ 0.012 Fe ≤ 0.25 O ≤ 0.13 Al 5.5 to 6.5 V 3.5 to 4.5 Ti = balance	13% Zr Ti = balance Impurities below the level of titanium Grade 4	ZrO_2 + HfO_2 + Y_2O_3 ≥ 99.0 Y_2O_3 ≥ 4.5 to ≤ 5.4 HfO_2 ≤ 5.0 Al_2O_3 ≤ 0.3 Other oxides < 0.5
Elasticity (GPa)	102	114	98	200 – 220
Strength (MPa)	860[2] (≥ 550[3])	1,000[2] (≥ 860[3])	990[2]	1,500[4] (≥ 800[5])

[1] Data applies to implant material only.
[2] Typical values for tensile strength.
[3] Minimum value for tensile strength as per ASTM standard for surgical implants.
[4] Typical values for 4-point bending strength.
[5] Minimum values as per ISO 13356.

To enhance its strength, Ti can be alloyed with other elements, such as aluminum (Al), vanadium (V), or zirconium (Zr). Although the same surface modifications—sandblasting and acid-etching—can be applied to cpTi (SLActive) and some titanium alloy implants, it is possible that these new implant materials may end up with different surface characteristics (e.g., roughness, hydrophilicity and wettability). The physico-chemical surface characteristics of titanium alloy implants might thus elicit different tissue responses (Saulacic and coworkers 2012). The two following titanium alloys have been mainly used in the dental and medical field.

- **Titanium alloys** containing titanium-6-aluminum-4 vanadium (Ti-6Al-4V) were mainly used in orthopedics due to its superior mechanical and physical properties compared to cpTi (Williams 2001). Even though Ti-6Al-4V has an excellent biocompatibility (Velasco-Ortega 2010), its corrosion resistance and biocompatibility remains inferior to cpTi (Ikarashi and coworkers 2005). Conflicting results have been reported for dental applications. Whereas high survival and success rates of 98% were shown after five years in implants with a diameter of 3.75 mm and different lengths in a variety of indications (De Leonardis and coworkers 1999), experimental studies revealed significantly reduced removal torque values and/or a less favorable bone response (Han and coworkers 1998; Johansson and coworkers 1998; Stenport and coworkers 2008; Saulacic 2012). Aluminum ion leakage was suggested as one possible explanation for these results (Johansson and coworkers 1998).
- **A titanium-zirconium alloy (TiZr)** was recently developed that consists of Ti alloyed with 13%–15% Zr and showed better tensile and fatigue strength than commercially pure titanium (Kobayashi and coworkers 1995; Ho and coworkers 2008). In preclinical investigations, TiZr implants performed similarly to cpTi implants with respect to osseointegration (Thoma and coworkers 2011; Gottlow and coworkers 2012; Jimbo and coworkers 2015). The clinical performance of narrow-diameter TiZr implants was investigated in several clinical trials with short-term observation periods up to three years in partially edentulous patients (Al-Nawas 2012; Chiapasco and coworkers 2012; Benic and coworkers 2013; Ioannidis 2015). The clinical question remains, however, whether narrow-diameter implants made of TiZr represent a valid alternative to the cpTi regular-diameter implants, which are considered the gold standard for single-tooth replacements in the anterior and premolar regions. More long-term investigations are needed on the survival and success rates of narrow-diameter implants, analyzing the risk for biomechanical and other potential complications (Ioannidis and coworkers 2015).

4.1.3 Ceramic Implants

New paradigms on the nature of biomaterials have emerged in recent years (Williams 2008). Strategies for their design focus not only on improved strength and toughness but also on tailoring their surfaces to systematically targeting a specific cell response (Franz and coworkers 2011).

More recently, yttria-stabilized zirconia was brought to the market as a new dental implant material. Similar to Ti implants, one- and two-piece zirconia implants have been developed (Kohal and coworkers 2004; Gahlert and coworkers 2007; Oliva and coworkers 2010; Depprich and coworkers 2008; Cionca and coworkers 2015; Payer and coworkers 2015).

Ceramic implants made of zirconia (ZrO_2) appear to be a highly interesting biomaterial for medical applications (Hisbergues and coworkers 2009). Zirconia implants have been proposed as a new potential alternative to Ti (Andreiotelli and coworkers 2009). However, ZrO_2 implants have so far demonstrated less favorable clinical survival and success rates than Ti implants (Andreiotelli and coworkers 2009; Siddiqi and coworkers 2015; Depprich and coworkers 2014; Cionca and coworkers 2015). A potential weakness of zirconia is its low temperature degradation, often referred to as "aging" (Chevalier and coworkers 2006; Lughi and Sergo 2010).

Adding aluminum oxide (Al_2O_3, alumina) diminishes the conversion rate from the tetragonal to the monoclinic phase and therefore improves the mechanical properties of ZrO_2 (Chevalier and coworkers 2006). Aluminum has also been added to Ti, with histologic specimens revealing more multinucleated giant cells (MNGCs) and less bone formation on these implant surfaces, which raises

concerns about biocompatibility (Saulacic and coworkers 2014; Albrektsson and coworkers 2014). Well-conducted long-term studies are urgently needed to permit a meaningful assessment of the survival or success rates of ceramic implants and a statement concerning their application as an alternative to Ti (Depprich and coworkers 2014) (Figs 4a-e; Table 1).

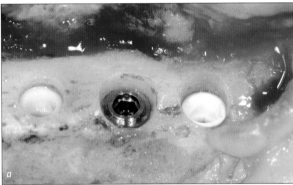
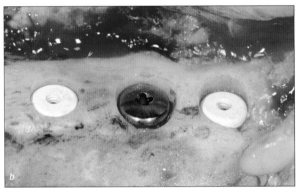

Figs 4a-b   An experimental study in the anterior maxilla of minipigs (Chappuis and coworkers 2016b). Two ceramic implants—yttria-stabilized zirconia (TZP, left implant) containing 5% yttria and alumina-toughened zirconia (ATZ, right implant) containing 4% yttria and 20% alumina—were placed and compared to a commercially pure titanium implant with a hydrophobic surface (cpTi, center) (a). Cover screws were inserted; primary would closure allowed undisturbed healing (b).

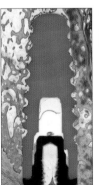
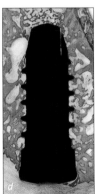
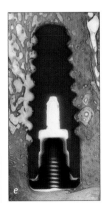

Figs 4c-e   After a four-week healing period, the ceramic implants—TZP (c) and ATZ (e)—revealed comparable results regarding osseointegration compared to commercially pure titanium Grade 4 (d).

For more in-depth information on the evolution of dental implants, please check out the ITI Online Academy's congress lecture "The Evolution of Dental Implants and the ITI" by Dr. David L. Cochran (charges apply). See what else the Online Academy has to offer at **academy.iti.org**

For more in-depth information on the integration of dental implants, please check out the ITI Online Academy's learning module "Tissue Integration of Dental Implants" by Dr. David L. Cochran (charges apply). See what else the Online Academy has to offer at **academy.iti.org**

4.2 Bone Grafts and Bone Substitute Materials

Autologous bone grafts remain the ideal material for regenerating bone defects, but their availability is limited, and harvesting can be associated with complications. Recent advances in biotechnology provided a great variety of bone grafting materials and the possibility to simplify the treatment (Hallman and Thor 2008).

The ideal bone substitute material is biocompatible, bioresorbable, osteoconductive, osteoinductive, structurally similar to bone, easy to use, and cost-effective (Kolk and coworkers 2012). Even though the ideal bone substitute with all these inherent characteristics has not yet been discovered, a key property is to facilitate new bone formation and subsequently undergo gradual substitution by newly formed bone (Hjørting-Hansen 2002). Of crucial importance for the clinical success of bone substitutes is their interaction with the adjacent tissue and cells due to a macroporous interconnecting pore size of > 300 µm diameter favoring cell infiltration, bone growth, and vascularization (Karageorgiou and coworkers 2005). Differences in material composition and surface characteristics will lead to distinct properties in terms of osteogenic, osteoinductive, and osteoconductive features, biodegradability, and handling (Table 2).

Table 2 Grafting materials of different origin and their osteogenic and osteoconductive potential and biodegradability

	Osteogenic/osteo-inductive potential	Osteoconductive potential	Biodegradability
Autografts (bone from the same individual)	+++	++	++/+
Allografts (bone from the same species but from a different individual) • Fresh frozen bone allograft • Freeze-dried bone allograft • Demineralized freeze-dried bone allograft • Deproteinized bone allograft	–	++	++
Xenografts (material of a biologic origin but from another species) • Bone mineral from animal bone • From calcifying corals • From calcifying algae	–	++	++
Alloplasts (material of synthetic origin) • Calcium phosphate • Polymers • Bioactive glasses	–	++	++/+

+++: high potential/biodegradability; ++: moderate potential/biodegradability; +: low potential/biodegradability

To achieve successful bone regeneration, bone grafts and bone substitute materials are used, for different purposes: (1) to enhance and support bone healing in order to bridge small and large defects; (2) to support and stabilize barrier membranes in guided bone regeneration (GBR) to reduce the risk of membrane collapse; and (3) to prevent the risk of bone resorption.

Most important, bone grafts and bone substitutes must be safe and biocompatible and should not transfer pathogens to the host. They can be incorporated as particulate grafts or as blocks, depending on the clinical situation. To further categorize the biologic characteristics, bone graft materials can be classified into four groups: autografts (same individual), allografts (same species), xenografts (other species), and alloplasts (synthetically produced) (Figs 5a-d; Table 2).

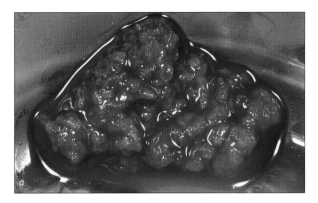

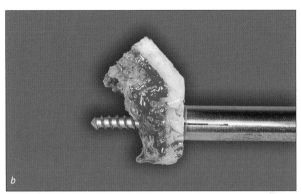

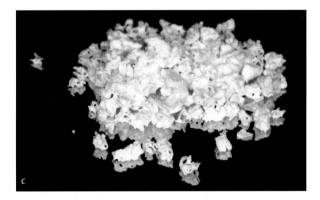

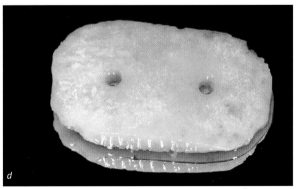

Figs 5a-d   Bone graft and bone substitute materials: Autologous bone chips (a), corticocancellous autologous bone block (b), deproteinized bovine bone mineral (DBBM) (c), allograft bone block (d).

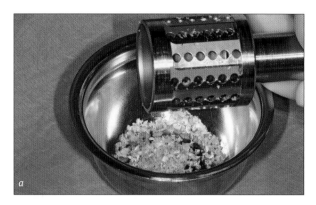

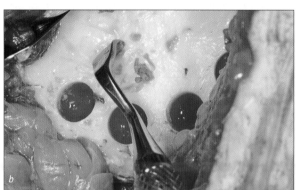

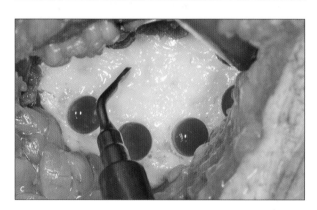

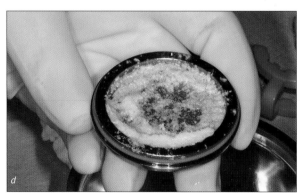

Figs 6a-d   Bone-harvesting techniques: bone mill (a), bone scraper (b), piezosurgery (c), and bone trap (d).

4.2.1   Autologous Bone Grafts

Autologous bone grafts remain the gold standard and therefore the first choice for most clinicians, as they are the only osteogenic and osteoinductive grafting material. Autografts are composed of an inorganic scaffold mainly composed of carbonated hydroxyapatite (LeGeros 2008) and an organic component comprising cells and extracellular matrix proteins. The cells include osteoprogenitor cells, osteocytes, osteoblasts, osteoclasts, bone-lining cells and endothelial cells.

Cortical or corticocancellous grafts consist mainly of osteocytes, which constitute over 90% of all bone cells in the adult skeleton (Lanyon 1993). Recent research suggests that it is the osteocytes that control and regulate bone formation, not the osteoblasts present on the bone surface (Bonewald 2011). Osteocytes seem to play a fundamental role in bone remodeling by secreting signaling factors implicated by the mechanisms of chemotaxis, differentiation, and apoptosis that appear to communicate with the bone surface by controlling the cellular activity of osteoblasts, osteoclasts, and bone-lining cells (Bonewald 2011).

The extracellular matrix proteins include mainly type I collagen, but importantly also the non-collagenous proteins osteopontin, bone sialoprotein, osteocalcin, fibronectin, and the group of bone-morphogenetic proteins, which induce new bone formation leading to graft incorporation into host bone (Urist 1965; Urist and coworkers 1967; Burchardt 1983; Goldberg and Stevenson 1993; Colnot 2009; Tsuji and coworkers 2006; Gorski 2011; Chappuis and coworkers 2012). These non-collagenous proteins are released gradually during remodeling of the grafted bone. The characteristics of autologous bone grafts depend on the general condition of the patient, the embryonic origin of the graft, the harvesting technique, and the handling and processing of the graft. In addition, autologous bone can be used either as particulated bone chips or as a bone block for larger defects. The major limitations of autologous bone are availability and increased morbidity, especially if a larger amount of grafting material is needed.

Particulated autologous bone. Today, autologous bone chips are routinely harvested locally from the surrounding surgical site by a bone scraper or bone chisel. This local technique of harvesting bone from the surgical site itself reduces morbidity, saves time and lowers the cost.

Bone chips harvested by a bone scraper or a bone mill have shown significantly higher number of live cells compared to particles collected with piezosurgery or bone filters connected to the suction device (Springer and coworkers 2004; Miron and coworkers 2011) (Fig 6). In addition, significantly higher expression of growth factors such as bone morphogenetic protein-2 and vascular endothelial growth factor were found using bone scrapers or bone mills (Miron and coworkers 2013). It is speculated that vibration and constant irrigation during the harvesting procedure may be the reason for the compromised cell viability (Miron and coworkers 2011). Even though viable osteocyte and osteoblasts can be harvested by bone filters, the concentration of growth factors is significantly reduced (Chiriac and coworkers 2005; Miron and coworkers 2011). In addition, several studies have revealed a risk of bacterial contamination of the collected bone (Young and coworkers 2001; Manzano-Moreno and coworkers 2015).

If small autograft particles are utilized, they will present with a favorable volume to surface ratio with large exposed surface areas, which increases the expression of growth factors but also the rate of resorption compared to larger particles (Pallesen and coworkers 2002). These paracrine function of growth factors released from autologous bone chips into the surroundings have been called bone-conditioned medium (BCM) (Caballé-Serrano and coworkers 2014). A proteomic analysis revealed that BCM contains more than 150 different growth factors, which might contribute to the overall process of graft consolidation (Caballé-Serrano and coworkers 2014).

It is still unclear how these autologous bone chips alter their signaling parameters over time following implantation into the bone defect, but they can influence the local environment by releasing a variety of growth factors and cytokines to favor new bone formation at the defect site (Figs 6a-d).

Autologous bone blocks. The reconstruction of larger alveolar defects in esthetic sites arising from trauma, disease, or post-extraction ridge alterations remains a challenge in implant dentistry. An effective treatment protocol for the reconstruction of large horizontal bone defects is the use of autologous corticocancellous bone blocks from the ramus or the symphysis (Buser and coworkers 1996; von Arx and Buser 2006; Chiapasco and coworkers 2006; Nyström and coworkers 2009; Cordaro and coworkers 2011; Khoury and Hanser 2015). Bone blocks have been shown to be mechanically more stable, resulting in significantly better preservation of the augmented volume compared to particulated autografts (Rocchietta and coworkers 2016).

There are several drawbacks related to autologous bone-block grafting: (1) the additional morbidity associated with block harvesting; (2) the lack of long-term studies, and (3) the significant graft resorption (18% to 60%) of the originally augmented volume (Widmark and coworkers 1997; Ozaki and Buchman 1998; Antoun and coworkers 2001; Cordaro and coworkers 2002; Araújo and coworkers 2002; Donos and coworkers 2002; Maiorana and coworkers 2005; Sbordone and coworkers 2009; Cordaro and coworkers 2011; Dasmah and coworkers 2012).

In order to prevent the resorption phenomenon, graft protection by a non-crosslinked collagen membrane and inorganic bovine bone mineral (ABBM) has been proposed (Proussaefs and Lozada 2003; Maiorana and coworkers 2005; von Arx and Buser 2006; Cordaro and coworkers 2013). A recent ten-year study on implants inserted in ridges previously augmented with autologous block grafts and using the GBR technique showed favorable results with a success rate of 98.1% and a graft resorption rate of only 7% (Chappuis and coworkers 2017). The use and application of autologous bone blocks were described in detail in Volume 7 of the ITI Treatment Guide (Cordaro and Terheyden 2014) (Figs 7a-y).

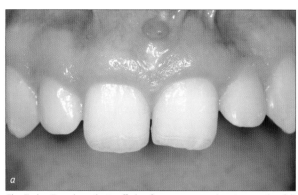
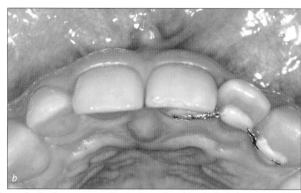

Figs 7a-b Female patient suffering from pronounced root resorption following orthodontic treatment. She had a rather thin gingival phenotype with a low-scalloped gingival margin. Tooth 22 showed progressive loosening despite being splinted to the neighboring dentition).

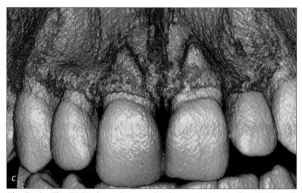
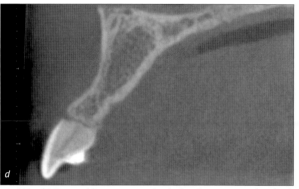

Figs 7c-d The CBCT showed a completely resorbed root of tooth 22 and a crest width of 2.2 mm with a pronounced apical undercut, preventing simultaneous implant placement.

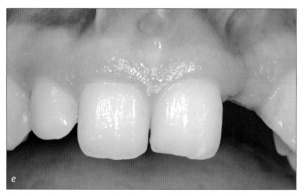
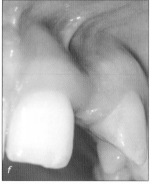

Figs 7e-f Six weeks after the flapless extraction of tooth 22, the soft tissues had healed completely, showing the pronounced flattening of the alveolar ridge especially in the apical area.

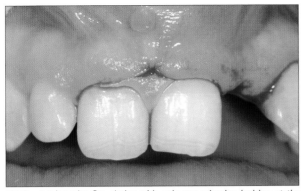

Fig 7g A triangular flap design with only one releasing incision at the distal line angle of the canine was chosen combined with a papilla-base incision at site 11–21 to gain sufficient access to the surgical field.

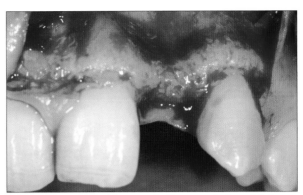

Fig 7h A mucoperiosteal flap was raised to expose the bone defect.

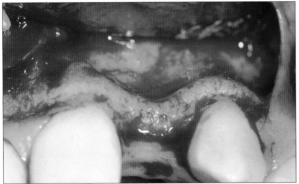

Fig 7i The insufficient crest width, with a significant apical bone deficiency, did not allow correct 3D restoration-driven implant placement.

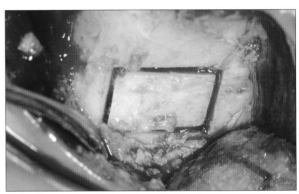

Fig 7j An autologous block was harvested from the chin.

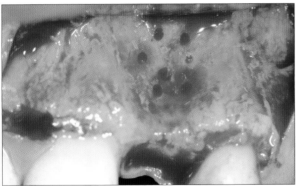

Fig 7k The cortical bone of the recipient site was perforated with a small round bur with a diameter of 1 mm.

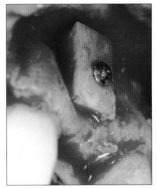

Fig 7l The bone block was secured using a traction-screw system (Medartis, Basel, Switzerland).

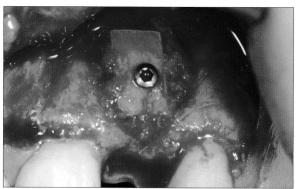

Fig 7m   The voids between the bone block and the recipient site were filled with autologous bone chips.

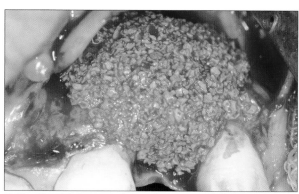

Fig 7n   To minimize resorption at the augmented site, the autologous block was protected by a layer of biomaterial with a low bone substitution rate (Bio-Oss; Geistlich Pharma, Wolhusen, Switzerland).

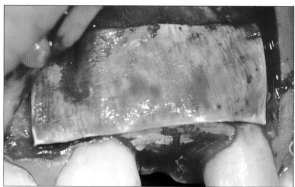

Fig 7o   A non-crosslinked collagen membrane was applied as a double layer to provide a long-term temporary barrier.

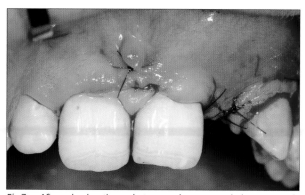

Fig 7p   After releasing the periosteum, primary wound closure was obtained to protect the grafted site.

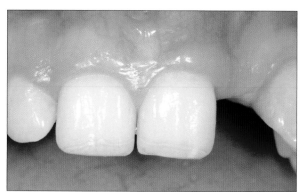

Fig 7q   After six months of uneventful healing producing sufficient bone and soft-tissue volume, reentry was planned.

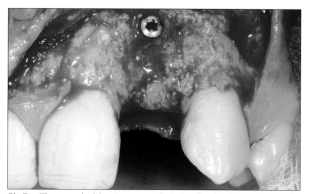

Fig 7r   The same incision type was selected as for the first surgery, and a mucoperiosteal flap was raised to expose the site. Minimal bone resorption had taken place in most crestal areas, whereas at the augmented site revealed minimal volume change.

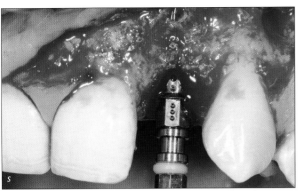

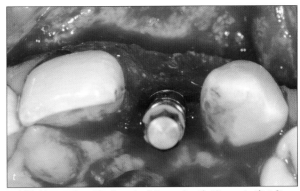

Figs 7s-t   An implant was inserted using a restoration-driven placement protocol (BL Narrow CrossFit, diameter 3.3 mm, length 10 mm; Institut Straumann AG). The implant shoulder was placed 3 mm below the suture (s) and 1 mm palatally of the incisal edge (t).

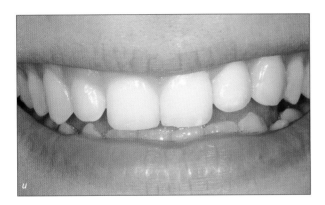

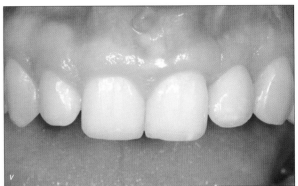

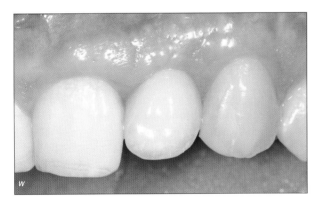

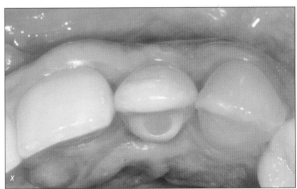

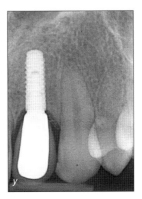

Figs 7u-y   Good esthetics at the three-year follow-up with a nice prosthetic restoration and a stable facial contour of sufficient height and thickness. The radiograph showed stable peri-implant bone levels.

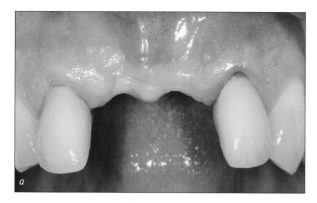

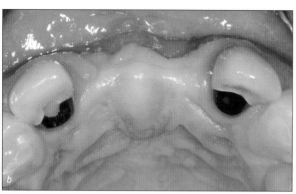

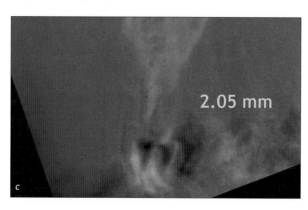

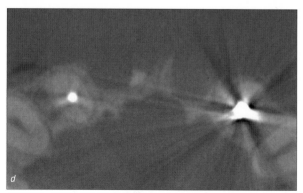

Figs 8a-d   Male patient suffered from a dental trauma with loss of the two central incisors. The patient had a rather thin gingival phenotype with a low-scalloped gingival margin. The CBCT revealed insufficient crest widths of only 2 mm, including a pronounced incisive foramen.

4.2.2   Allografts

Bone allografts overcome the limitations of harvesting autologous bone such as availability issues and morbidity, but they have other limitations, such as host dissimilarities and or high cost (Gruskin and coworkers 2012).

There is an ongoing debate about the association between the use of allogeneic material and the risk of disease transmission (Palmer and coworkers 1999; Traore and coworkers 2013). Elimination of this major concern of allogeneic material requires tissue processing, sterilization, and protein deactivation. Frozen allografts are therefore exposed to temperatures below −70°C to induce a stronger immune response than freeze-dried allografts (Ehrler and Vaccaro 2000; Shegarfi and Reikeras 2009). In freeze-dried bone allografts (FDBA), the bone is frozen, defatted, and dehydrated. Finally, in demineralized freeze-dried bone allograft (DFDBA), inorganic structural bone mineral is removed using hydrochloric acid to expose the osteoinductive molecules deposited in the bone matrix (Holtzclaw and coworkers 2008). However, DFDBA results in a loss of mechanical resistance due to the removal of the bone mineral and is therefore unsuitable where mechanical stability must be considered.

In summary, the more aggressively the allograft is processed, the less intense will be the immunological response. However, the osteoinductive and osteoconductive properties will decrease (Kolk and coworkers 2012).

Allografts are available in many different shapes: from corticocancellous or cortical grafts, as cancellous chips, or as demineralized bone matrix. Allografts can be either derived from cadaveric bone sources or harvested from live donors during arthroplasty. Even though allografts lack viable cell material, growth factors such as BMPs are present in the extracellular matrix (Reddi 2000). Urist made the key discovery that demineralized, lyophilized segments of rabbit bone, when implanted intramuscularly, induced new bone formation (Urist 1965). Therefore, demineralized allograft materials can be considered osteoinductive. However, the concentration of BMPs is lower than in autografts. It has been debated whether the concentration is of any clinical significance (Boyan and coworkers 2006; Chappuis and coworkers 2012).

Particulate allografts. The successful use of freeze-dried bone and demineralized freeze-dried bone for bone augmentation with simultaneous implant placement has been reported in several studies (Fugazzotto 1997; Park and coworkers 2008). In the United States, allografts are widely used; in Europe, regulations restrict the collection of human bone, which has limited the popularity of particulate allografts among clinicians.

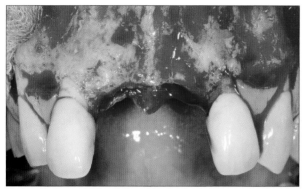

Fig 8e A trapezoidal flap design with releasing incisions at the distal line angle of the canines was chosen, combined with a papillary base incision to gain sufficient access to the surgical site.

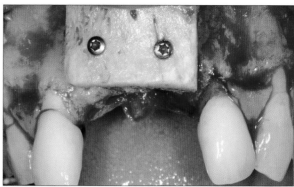

Fig 8f An allograft bone block was adapted to the surgical site after perforating the cortical bone with a small round bur and fixated with a traction-screw system (Medartis).

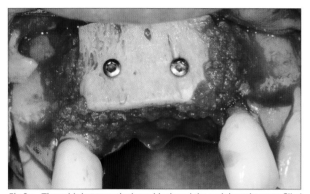

Fig 8g The voids between the bone block and the recipient site were filled with autologous bone chips.

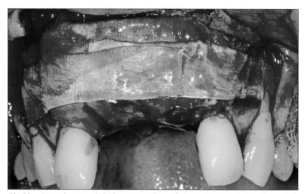

Fig 8h In order to minimize resorption of the augmented site, the autologous block was protected by a layer of biomaterial exhibiting a low bone substitution rate and subsequently with a double layer of non-crosslinked collagen membrane (Bio-Oss/Bio-Gide; Geistlich Pharma).

Allograft bone blocks. Mineralized block allografts in conjunction with the placement of a resorbable membrane, may be a viable treatment option for ridge augmentation in two-stage implant placement procedures (Keith and coworkers 2006; Nissan and coworkers 2011). However, recent data indicate a high incidence of late sequestrations with partial or total graft loss around implants placed in allogeneic block grafts (Chiapasco and coworkers 2015a; Chiapasco and coworkers 2015b).

A recent comparison of fresh-frozen allogeneic block grafts with autologous block grafts yielded that the block architecture influences significantly bone incorporation and remodeling. Cortical allograft blocks seem to show the least amounts of vital bone, while corticocancellous autologous blocks seem to undergo more resorption over time. Compared to autologous block grafts, only a small portion of the allograft blocks consists of vital bone six to eight months after grafting (Spin-Neto and coworkers 2015).

A systematic review concluded that clinical studies on allograft blocks included a relatively small number of interventions and implants without long-term follow-up periods. Therefore, allograft blocks do not provide sufficient evidence to establish treatment efficacy relative to graft incorporation, alveolar ridge augmentation and long-term dental implant survival (Waasdorp and Reynolds 2010) (Figs 8a-d).

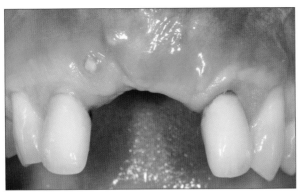

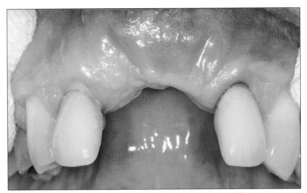

Fig 8i   At four months, a very small dehiscence was observed with a partial loss of the allograft block particles.

Fig 8j   At six months, the site had healed and showed sufficient bone and soft-tissue volume.

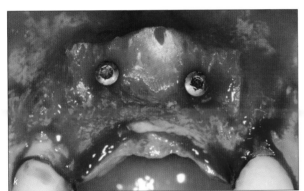

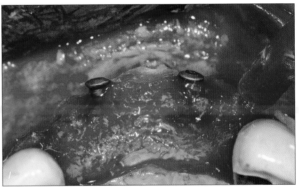

Figs 8k-l   The same incision design was selected as in the first surgery, and a mucoperiosteal flap was elevated to visualize the site. The augmented site showed partial resorption of the originally augmented site at the crestal area (k); however, the width of the crest was significantly improved (l).

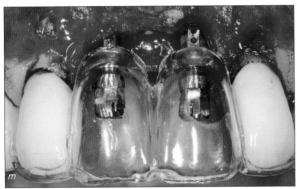

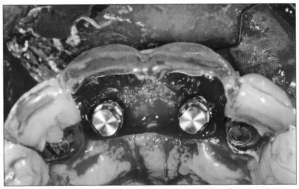

Figs 8m-n   Two bone-level narrow implants were inserted by a prosthetically driven placement protocol using a surgical stent (BL, diameter 4.1 mm, length 10 mm; Institut Straumann AG). The implant shoulder was placed 3 mm below the suture and 1 mm palatally of the incisal edge, for 3 mm of interimplant distance.

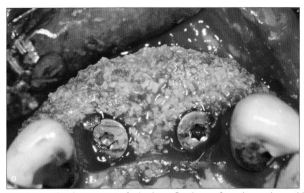 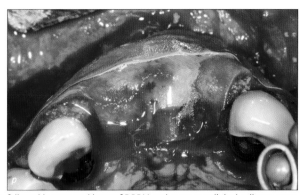

Figs 8o-p   The site was re-grafted using a first layer of autologous bone chips, followed by a second layer of DBBM and a non-crosslinked collagen membrane (Bio-Oss/Bio-Gide; Geistlich Pharma).

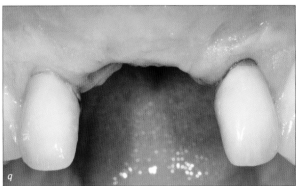 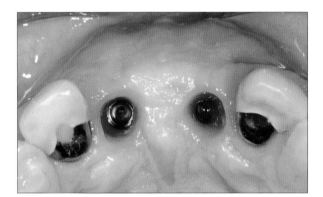

Figs 8q-r   After twelve weeks of healing, the abutment was connected.

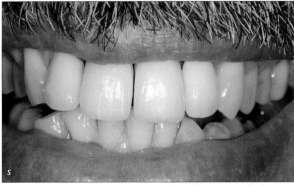 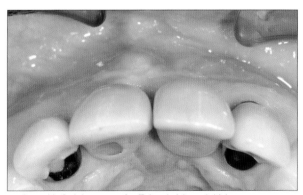

Figs 8s-t   Two-year follow-up. Good esthetics with a nice prosthetic restoration and a stable facial contour of sufficient height and thickness.

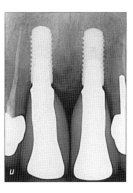

Fig 8u   Radiograph. Stable peri-implant bone levels.

4.2.3 Xenografts

Particulate xenografts. A multitude of xenografts consisting of minerals derived from animals, corals, or algae are commercially available. The best-documented bone substitute material in the field of oral surgery and implant dentistry is deproteinized bovine bone mineral (DBBM) (Jensen and Terheyden 2009). Xenografts, especially those derived from natural bone, have been extensively studied. The organic component may be removed by means of heat or chemical action to ensure that the material is inert and still biocompatible. However, deproteinization may have an impact on the osteogenic behavior of the biomaterial. Two bovine xenografts of identical origin deproteinized by chemical methods vs. high temperatures showed highly different osteoconductive capacities when implanted in rabbit tibiae (Jensen and coworkers 1996). The resorption of xenografts is less pronounced than that of autografts or allografts (Buser and coworkers 1998; Jensen and Terheyden 2009). Whether DBBM is truly bioresorbable remains controversial (Berglundh and Lindhe 1997; Busenlechner and coworkers 2012). Even though osteoclast-like cells can be observed on DBBM particles after grafting (Piattelli and coworkers 1999; Jensen and coworkers 2014; Jensen and coworkers 2015), in daily practice, some xenografts can be considered close to non-resorbable once bone integration has been successfully accomplished.

Xenograft blocks. Xenograft blocks were developed for horizontal ridge augmentation. Preclinical data comparing autologous bone blocks and xenograft blocks yielded a similar increase in ridge width. But histologically, xenograft blocks are mainly embedded in connective tissue, with only limited amounts of new bone ingrowth at the base of the xenograft block (Araújo and coworkers 2002; Schwarz and coworkers 2008). Implants inserted in xenograft blocks following second-stage surgery did not promote osseointegration, although the installed implants were stable owing to the osseointegration at the sites of the parent bone (De Santis and coworkers 2012).

4.2.4 Alloplastic Bone Substitutes

Alloplastic bone substitutes represent a large group of chemically diverse biomaterials made of different materials, most commonly calcium phosphate (tricalcium phosphate, hydroxyapatite, calcium phosphate cements), bioactive glass, or polymers. Alloplastic materials are highly biocompatible and support bone formation; they have variable rates of resorption (Jensen and coworkers 2007). Nevertheless, their bone-inducing properties remain inferior to autologous bone grafts (Jensen and coworkers 2007).

Hydroxyapatite (HA) is the main inorganic component of natural bone and the least soluble of the naturally occurring calcium phosphates, which makes it generally resistant to physiologic resorption. β-tricalcium phosphate (β-TCP), on the other hand, also demonstrates osteoconductive properties, but resorbs rapidly (Jensen and coworkers 2006; Jensen and coworkers 2007). In clinically challenging bone-defect morphologies, such as lateral ridge augmentation, the resorption rate of β-TCP is too fast, so the space-making capacity is limited to allowing new bone formation to stabilize the augmented volume (von Arx and coworkers 2001).

HA and β-TCP have been combined in biphasic calcium phosphates. Biphasic calcium phosphates benefit from the stable space-maintaining properties of HA and the degradation properties of β-TCP (LeGeros and coworkers 2003). A randomized controlled trial found that biphasic calcium phosphate performed similarly to DBBM in the regeneration of peri-implant dehiscence-type defects with respect to vertical bone-defect reduction (Van Assche and coworkers 2013). Even though the results have been promising, further long-term clinical studies are necessary to demonstrate its equivalence to DBBM.

 For more in-depth information on biomaterials, please check out the ITI Online Academy's congress lecture "Biomaterials for Bone Augmentation" by Dr. Simon S. Jensen (charges apply). See what else the Online Academy has to offer at **academy.iti.org**

4.3 Biologics

4.3.1 Growth Factors

Research has been directed to identify potential growths factors in order to reduce the need for harvesting major autologous bone grafts. Growth factors are able to regulate cell proliferation, cell activity, chemotaxis, and/or cell differentiation and have been tested in animal experiments for dental applications (Schliephake 2002; Bosshardt 2008; Jung and coworkers 2008a).

The complex sequence of molecular and cellular events that are carefully orchestrated during wound healing is difficult to emulate and remains a challenge in tissue engineering strategies. Although in-vitro studies increasingly reveal the roles of the individual growth factors, their complex positive and negative feedback loops often make them unpredictable when placed in a biologic environment. In addition, the regenerative potential of growth factors also depends on the carrier material that serves as a delivery system and as a scaffold for cellular ingrowth (Chen and coworkers 2010).

Identification of the most effective individual (BMPs, TGF-β) or combinations of growth factors (BMP/VEGF, BMP-2/BMP-7) and their release profiles in different defects has the potential to improve the osteoinductive efficacy in vivo (Sigurdsson and coworkers 1996). Although further investigation is needed in the optimization of material and growth factor combinations, controlled delivery of bioactive factors via biomaterial carriers shows great potential for optimizing bone repair (Schwarz and coworkers 2008; Sigurdsson and coworkers 1996). The identification and production of recombinant morphogens and growth factors that play key roles in tissue regeneration have generated much enthusiasm and numerous clinical trials, but the results of many of these trials have been largely disappointing (Vo and coworkers 2012). Recent progress highlights the importance of materials science and engineering in growth-factor delivery within regenerative medicine (Lee and coworkers 2011).

4.3.2 Enamel Matrix Derivative

Enamel matrix derivative (EMD), composed of amelogenins with metalloendoprotease and serine protease activity and other enamel proteins, appears to promote periodontal regeneration by mimicking the specific events occurring during the development of the periodontium (Giannobile and Somerman 2003; Mao and coworkers 2006). Although the precise role of EMD in these complex epithelial/mesenchymal interactions has yet to be delineated, EMD has been shown to promote periodontal regeneration in several controlled human clinical trials (Pontoriero and coworkers 1999; Tonetti and coworkers 2002; Sculean and coworkers 1999). There is evidence that EMD supports wound healing and periodontal regeneration (Bosshardt 2008). EMD might result in more bone formation in supporting defects than in non-supporting defects (Rathe and coworkers 2009). In suprabony defects, the effect of EMD appears to be limited (Graziani and coworkers 2014). Some studies suggest that EMD increases the initial growth of trabecular bone around endosseous implants by inducing the formation of new bone, but this needs to be confirmed by additional research (Rathe and coworkers 2009).

4.3.3   Autologous Platelet Concentrates

Platelets are known to contain many of the growth factors involved in bone healing (Khan and coworkers 2000). Several techniques have been used to easily and inexpensively obtain these autologous growth factors in physiological proportions from the patient's whole blood (Marx and coworkers 1998; Roffi and coworkers 2013). Even though many scientists and clinicians have employed platelet concentrates in orthopedic and oral surgery, their effect on bone regeneration remains controversial—some authors observed favorable effects, while others concluded that their use was irrelevant (Jensen and coworkers 2005; Intini 2009).

A recent systematic review revealed that our understanding is still preliminary and that many aspects have yet to be clarified, such as the best protocol for platelet concentrate production and the application method (Roffi and coworkers 2013). Autologous plasma concentrates have also been used for socket grafting and ridge preservation. It appears that plasma concentrates accelerate healing and soft-tissue epithelialization in extraction sockets and reduce postoperative pain and discomfort. However, so far there has been no evidence to confirm that plasma concentrates improve hard-tissue regeneration (Moraschini and Barboza 2015).

4.4 Membranes

The principle of guided bone regeneration (GBR) using barrier membranes was developed in the late 1980s for the treatment of peri-implant bone defects and bone augmentation with preclinical studies (Dahlin and coworkers 1990; Schenk and coworkers 1994). Different types of membranes have been used to prevent the ingrowth of non-osteogenic connective-tissue cells into the regenerating bone defect. Over the last 27 years, a variety of barrier membranes have been developed for use in GBR. The criteria for selecting the appropriate barrier membranes include biocompatibility, cell occlusion, tissue integration, space-making capacity, adequate clinical manageability, and susceptibility to complications (Bornstein and coworkers 2009c). Membranes are classified into resorbable/bioabsorbable and non-resorbable bioinert membranes (Table 3).

Table 3   Classification of barrier membranes

	Advantages	**Disadvantages**
Non-resorbable membranes • PTFE • ePTFE • ePTFE, titanium-reinforced	+ Prolonged barrier function	– Second surgical procedure to remove the membrane – Technique-sensitive – Membrane exposure and infection – Need for mechanical fixation
Bioresorbable membranes • Natural polymers (collagen) • Synthetic polymers (polyglycolic acid, polylactic acid, polyethylene glycol, etc.)	+ No need for secondary surgery + Decreased morbidity + Simplified surgical procedure	– May elicit unfavorable tissue reactions – Uncontrolled duration of barrier function – Need for mechanical support to avoid membrane collapse

4.4.1 Non-resorbable Membranes

Non-resorbable, bioinert membranes maintain their barrier function until they are removed. Expanded polytetrafluoroethylene (ePTFE) membranes are clinically well documented for GBR procedures (Dahlin and coworkers 1990; Buser and coworkers 1990; Jovanovic and coworkers 1992; Simion and coworkers 1994b; Buser and coworkers 1996). ePTFE is a synthetic polymer with a porous structure that does not induce an immune reaction and resists enzymatic degradation by hosts cells and microbes. The integration of reinforcing titanium within ePTFE membranes increases their space-making capacity and allows the membrane to be individually shaped (Simion and coworkers 1998). A favorable correlation has been observed between space maintenance and the level of new bone formation (Polimeni and coworkers 2005). The titanium-reinforced high-density PTFE membrane revealed superior regenerative capacity when compared to the traditional expanded PTFE due to improved mechanical support against the compressive forces of the overlaying soft tissue (Jovanovic and coworkers 1995; Carbonell and coworkers 2014).

The major drawback of these ePTFE membranes was the susceptibility of soft-tissue complications in case of a premature membrane exposure, showing much higher complication rates than resorbable membranes (Augthun and coworkers; Chiapasco and Zaniboni 2009) (Figs 9a-b). Another disadvantage is the need for membrane removal at a second surgical procedure, which increases morbidity.

To avoid these drawbacks, dense PTFE (dPTFE) membranes have been developed. Like ePTFE membranes, they are bioinert, cell-occlusive, and may be Ti-reinforced. Unlike ePTFE membranes, they are less prone to infections when exposed during healing and are easier to remove. However, so far the clinical scientific documentation is very limited (Carbonell and coworkers 2014).

4.4.2 Resorbable Membranes

Resorbable membranes were developed to eliminate the second surgical intervention where membranes are removed, which may reduce morbidity. Nevertheless, resorbable membranes have some drawbacks. First, the duration of the barrier function for an appropriate period may vary considerably (Gielkens and coworkers 2008). Second, the degradation process could possibly interfere with the wound healing process. Finally, the duration of barrier function is a critical issue, because these membranes should be maintained for at least four to six weeks to allow successful tissue regeneration (Piattelli and coworkers 1996; Milella and coworkers 2001). Due to the risk of risk for membrane collapse and early degradation, resorbable membranes should be supported by a bone filler with a low substitution rate to avoid early collapse and to maintain the augmented bone volume (Hürzeler and coworkers 1997). Thus, degradable membranes eliminate the removal surgery and exhibit better biocompatibility. But there are still challenges, such as external tissue invasion if the membranes degrade rapidly and unfavorable mechanical properties during surgery and the subsequent healing phase (Fujihara and coworkers 2005; Bottino and coworkers 2012).

Collagen membranes. Collagen is a major component of the extracellular matrix. Most commercially available collagen membranes were developed from type I collagen or from a combination of types I and III, originating from bovine tendon, bovine dermis, calf skin, or porcine dermis (Bunyaratavej and Wang 2001). Collagen membranes are valuable alternatives to synthetic polymers in GBR procedures due their excellent cell affinity and biocompatibility (Hürzeler and coworkers 1998). The advantages of collagen membranes have been described as hemostasis and fast vascularization, chemotaxis for periodontal and gingival fibroblasts, low immunogenicity, and easy surgical handling (Schlegel and coworkers 1997).

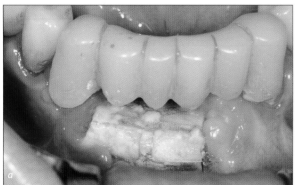 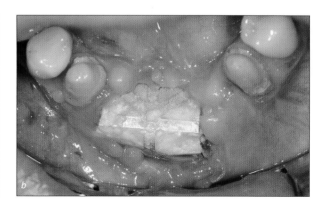

Figs 9a-b   Severe dehiscence of a titanium-reinforced ePTFE membrane.

While collagen membranes appear to be more tissue-friendly, they also have been reported to have unfavorable mechanical properties and variable degradation profiles (Hürzeler and coworkers 1998; Strietzel and coworkers 2006; Rothamel and coworkers 2012). By cross-linking the collagen fibrils, the barrier function can be prolonged, but the cross-linking process is still associated with poorer tissue integration, delayed vascularization and an increased invasion by inflammatory cells (Rothamel and coworkers 2005; Bornstein and coworkers 2009b).

Polymeric membranes. Synthetic resorbable membranes are polyesters such a polyglycolides (PGA), polylactides (PLA), trimethyl carbonates (TMC), or their copolymers; they have been reported to be effective (Simion and coworkers 1997), However, these membranes may present disadvantages related to their degradation products (von Arx and coworkers 2005).

Polylactic acid/polyglycolic acid copolymer (PLGA) membranes have shown promising results in preclinical and clinical studies (Miguel and coworkers 2009; Zwahlen and coworkers 2009). A commercially available polyester-based membrane revealed high initial tensile strength, but the structural and mechanical properties were lost after four weeks of incubation (Milella and coworkers 2001). A recent study compared a modified PLGA membrane with to an ePTFE control. No statistical evidence in favor of one membrane was found. Soft-tissue complications leading to membrane exposure were observed in both groups and can alter the amount of regenerated bone volume (Schneider and coworkers 2014). More clinical studies are need to improve the validity of these membranes.

Poly(ethylene glycol)- (PEG-) based hydrogels can serve as an in-situ formative matrix for optimal cell ingrowth and the retention of bioactive proteins (Lutolf and coworkers 2003). PEG hydrogels are known for their biocompatibility and are currently used in several medical devices (Boogaarts and coworkers 2005; Wallace and coworkers 2001). An attempt to further simplify the clinical handling using in-situ polymerization from polyethylene glycol was shown to trigger a foreign-body reaction in the surrounding tissues (Wechsler and coworkers 2008). As for the mechanical properties, the hydrogel alone may provide insufficient stability. A combination of particulated bone substitutes and the hydrogel used

to reinforce the mechanical strength enabled efficient and localized bone regeneration (Jung and coworkers 2007a; Thoma and coworkers 2012; Thoma and coworkers 2015). However, the formation and application of synthetic materials in contact with biological matter still presents a substantial challenge to today's biomedical materials research (Lutolf and Hubbell 2005).

4.4.3 New Development in Membranes with a Functionally Graded Structure

The critical disadvantages of PTFE-based membranes (such as the need for second-stage surgery) and resorbable membranes (such as the risk for membrane collapse and early degradation) have fostered research into alternative membrane materials (Bottino and coworkers 2012).

Advances in the technology of nanomaterials have led to an increased interest in approaches such as electrospinning, which has been recognized as an efficient technique for the fabrication of nanofibrous scaffolds or membranes (Huang and coworkers 2003). These electrospun nanofibrous materials mimic the extracellular matrix proteins more closely and have been used as controlled-release reservoirs for drug delivery and as artificial matrices for tissue engineering (Goldberg and coworkers 2007). Sequential spinning has been employed to fabricate tubular scaffolds with a different layered structure to increase mechanical properties and to allow a tailored degradation (Thomas and coworkers 2009; McClure and coworkers 2010).

Several research groups have investigated the possibility of using membranes with a functionally graded structure to maintain sufficient mechanical properties during healing, predictable degradation rates, and bioactive properties (Bottino and coworkers 2012; Giannobile and Somerman 2003; Liao and coworkers 2005; Chen and coworkers 2011; Erisken and coworkers 2008). With these membranes, bone formation would be stimulated by calcium phosphate-based nanoparticles or growth factors on the bone/membrane interface, and bacterial colonialization would be inhibited by antibacterial drugs delivered at the soft tissue/membrane interface (Bottino and coworkers 2012).

For more in-depth information on bone grafting, please check out the ITI Online Academy's learning module "Biological Principles of Bone Grafting" by Dr. Andreas Stavropoulos (charges apply). See what else the Online Academy has to offer at **academy.iti.org**

For more in-depth information on guided bone regeneration, please check out the ITI Online Academy's congress lecture "Guided Bone Regeneration: Factors for Success" by Dr. Nikolaos Donos (charges apply). See what else the Online Academy has to offer at **academy.iti.org**

For more in-depth information on the use of GBR, please check out the ITI Online Academy's congress lecture "How to Use GBR in Implant Patients" by Dr. Daniel Buser (charges apply). See what else the Online Academy has to offer at **academy.iti.org**

For more in-depth information on bone regenerative materials, please check out the ITI Online Academy's congress lecture "Advances in Bone Regenerative Materials" by Dr. Nikos Mardas (charges apply). See what else the Online Academy has to offer at **academy.iti.org**

For more in-depth information on contour augmentation, please check out the ITI Online Academy's congress lecture "Current Approaches of Horizontal or Contour Augmentation" by Dr. Simon S. Jensen (charges apply). See what else the Online Academy has to offer at **academy.iti.org**

5 Surgical Considerations for Optimal Esthetic Outcomes

V. Chappuis, S. Chen, D. Buser

As dentistry evolves into the modern era, research has focused on a better understanding of the biological processes underlying alveolar bone healing, osseointegration, and tissue regeneration (Berglundh and Giannobile 2013). These aspects are critical to further promote the development of predictable and successful implant treatment protocols, with the ultimate goal of providing high-quality patient care (Berglundh and Giannobile 2013). The increasing demand for esthetics in implant dentistry remains a challenge in clinical practice and has become critical for successful implant-supported prostheses in the anterior maxilla (Belser and coworkers 2009).

A strict assessment of medical, dental, esthetic, and anatomical risk factors is the key to selecting the most suitable treatment approach, providing successful outcomes with a high predictability and a low risk of complications (Chen and Buser 2009).

For the clinician it is important to understand that all these treatment options have specific characteristics with associated advantages and disadvantages. The aim of this chapter is to explain the differences between these options to support the clinician's decision-making process based on the evidence of the available literature.

5.1 Post-extraction Dimensional Ridge Alterations in the Esthetic Zone

To achieve esthetic success, regenerating of the natural hard- and soft-tissue architecture of the natural dentition is a primary concern. In current dental research, the healing process following tooth extraction and its related dimensional- hard and soft-tissue alterations have become an important research topic (Araújo and coworkers 2015a).

A key prerequisite for esthetic outcomes in the anterior maxilla is an adequate three-dimensional (3D) osseous volume of the alveolar ridge, including an intact facial bone wall of sufficient thickness and height in combination with correct restoration-driven implant positions (Buser and coworkers 2004a; Grunder and coworkers 2005). Deficiencies of the facial bone anatomy have a negative impact on esthetics and are a critical causative factor for complications and failures (Chen and Buser 2009). Clinicians need to understand these physiological dimensional alterations of the ridge that occur following tooth extraction and implant placement in the anterior maxilla. Based on this knowledge, the clinician will be able to select the most suitable protocol and the most appropriate biomaterials.

5.1.1 Flapless Low-trauma Tooth Extraction to Reduce Dimensional Alterations

Even though tooth extraction has been considered a simple and straightforward procedure, it should be performed with care and with the understanding that dimensional ridge alterations will follow (Araújo and coworkers 2015b). Tooth extractions are invasive procedures since they disrupt vascular structures and cause damage to the soft tissue and the associated periodontal ligament (Cardaropoli and coworkers 2003).

Therefore, a low-trauma tooth extraction with minimal invasiveness should be applied that includes a flapless approach whenever possible. Flapless tooth extraction has been shown to reduce the amount of bone loss in the early healing phase (four to eight weeks post-extraction) compared to a full-thickness flap (Fickl and coworkers 2008). However, no differences in bone loss were observed after six months of healing with or without flap elevation (Araújo and Lindhe 2009a). Therefore, a flapless extraction should always be considered when early implant the early placement protocol is selected (Buser and coworkers 2008b).

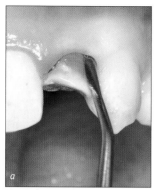
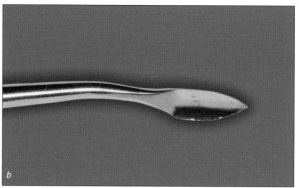

Figs 1a-b   A periotome is used to carefully mobilize the root by gently cutting the periodontal ligament fibers.

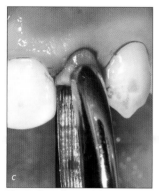
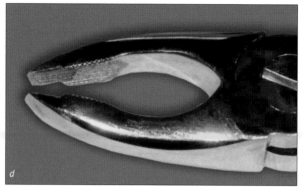

Figs 1c-d   A diamond-tipped extraction forceps helps prevent injuries of the delicate gingival tissues when removing the tooth remnant.

The extraction itself should be performed without applying force to the thin facial bone wall. Several new surgical instruments are available to facilitate low-trauma tooth extraction, such as periotomes (Figs 1a-d; Dr. V. Chappuis), piezosurgery (Figs 2a-h; Dr. V. Chappuis), and vertical tooth extraction devices (Figs 3a-f; Dr. V. Chappuis).

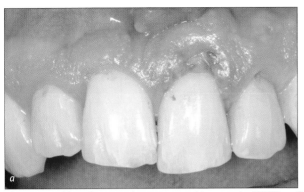
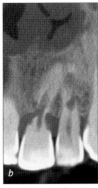
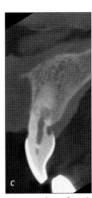
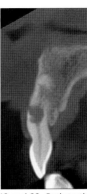

Figs 2a-c   In this patient, cone-beam computed tomography (CBCT) confirmed post-traumatic external root resorption of teeth 12 and 22. Both teeth were hopeless and needed to be extracted. Since the roots were ankylosed and fractured inside the bone, a low-trauma, minimally invasive extraction was performed by piezosurgery.

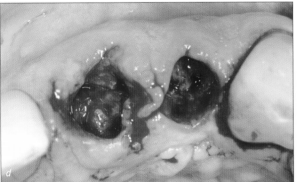
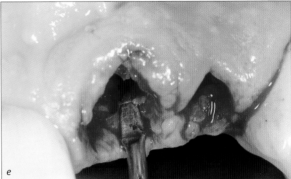

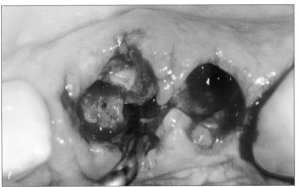
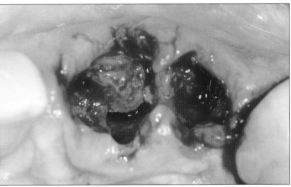

Figs 2d-g   The fibers of the periodontal ligament were piezosurgically cut to facilitate low-trauma, flapless removal of the tooth roots.

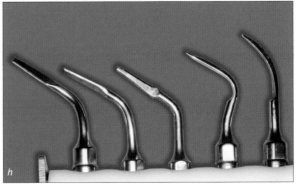

Fig 2h   Different piezosurgical instruments that can be used for low-trauma tooth extraction.

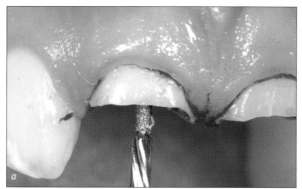

Fig 3a   Preparation of a slot after removal of the crown.

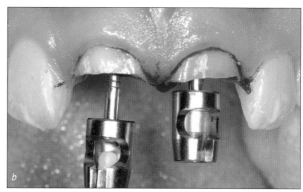

Fig 3b   A screw-insertion adapter was placed using a screwdriver.

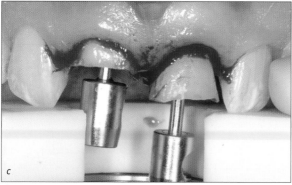

Fig 3c   A Benex device was applied and the pull rope hooked into the screw adapter.

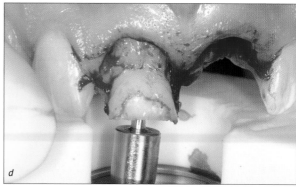

Fig 3d   Using an axial alignment and providing robust support for the Benex device, both roots were extracted vertically with minimal forces acting on the facial bone wall.

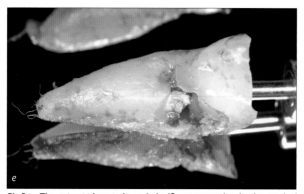

Fig 3e   The extracted root showed significant resorption in the cervical area.

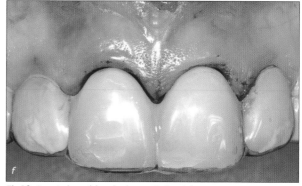

Fig 3f   Inserted provisional using an Essix retainer.

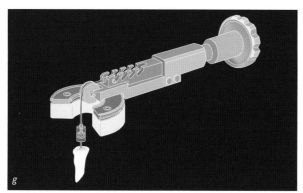

Fig 3g   Benex device (Hager & Meisinger, Neuss, Germany; Helmut Zepf Medizintechnik, Tuttlingen, Germany).

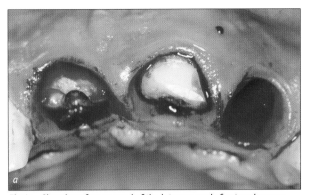

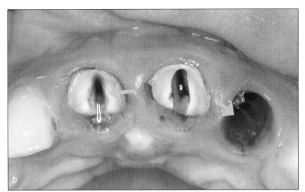

Fig 4a Situation after removal of the intraosseously fractured crowns.

Fig 4b Situation after sectioning the roots along their longitudinal axis. In this way, forces acting on the thin facial bone wall can be reduced, since most of the forces are directed toward the mesial and distal bone structures.

If these techniques cannot be applied in a given situation, sectioning the roots orofacially along the longitudinal axis is recommended to minimize pressure on the facial bone wall and to remove the root fragments separately (Figs 4a-b; Dr. V. Chappuis).

For more in-depth information on minimally traumatic extraction techniques, please check out the ITI Online Academy's learning module "Minimally Traumatic Extraction Techniques" by Dr. Eduardo R. Lorenzana (charges apply). See what else the Online Academy has to offer at **academy.iti.org**

For more in-depth information on post-extraction healing, please check out the ITI Online Academy's congress lecture "Post-Extraction Healing - Implications for Implant Treatment and Ridge Maintenance" by Dr. Stephen Chen (charges apply). See what else the Online Academy has to offer at **academy.iti.org**

For more in-depth information on post-extraction ridge alterations, please check out the ITI Online Academy's congress lecture "Post-Extraction Ridge Alteration, A Risk for Esthetics" by Dr. Stephen Chen (charges apply). See what else the Online Academy has to offer at **academy.iti.org**

5.1.2 Post-extraction Dimensional Alterations of the Hard Tissues

Dimensional alterations in animal studies. The dimensional and structural alterations following tooth extractions have been examined in mandibular premolar sites of beagle dogs (Cardaropoli and coworkers 2003; Araújo and Lindhe 2005). These catabolic changes are initiated by the resorption of the bundle bone that lines the extraction socket. They are correlated with the disruption of blood supply from the periodontal ligament, subsequently initiating significant osteoclastic activity (Cardaropoli and coworkers 2003; Araújo and Lindhe 2005).

As the bundle bone is a tooth-dependent structure, it is gradually resorbed following the extraction, leading to a vertical bone loss of 2.2 mm on the facial aspects in mandibular premolar sites in dogs (Araújo and Lindhe 2005). In contrast, minimal bone resorption was observed on the lingual aspect. This phenomenon has been attributed to the thickness of the thinner facial bone-wall dimensions.

Full maintenance of facial bone wall has been observed for a facial bone wall thickness of 2 mm in an experimental dog study (Qahash and coworkers 2008). However, dimensional alterations after the extraction appear to be related to several additional factors, including surgical trauma, a lack of functional stimuli to the remaining bone walls, the absence of a periodontal ligament, and genetic information (Araújo and coworkers 2015b).

Dimensional alterations in clinical studies. In patients, the facial bone wall is less than 1 mm thick in 90% of clinical situations, and even less than 0.5 mm in almost 50% of cases (Huynh-Ba and coworkers 2010; Braut and coworkers 2011; Januário and coworkers 2011; Vera and coworkers 2012). These thin bone-wall phenotypes, with a facial bone-wall thickness of 1 mm or less, exhibited progressive bone resorption after eight weeks of healing with a median vertical bone loss of 7.5 mm, or 62% of the former facial bone height (Chappuis and coworkers 2013b). By contrast, patients with a thick bone-wall phenotype with a thickness of more than 1 mm revealed a median vertical bone loss of only 1.1 mm or 9% of the former bone-wall height.

In single extraction sites with healthy neighboring dentition, these changes occur mainly in the central area of the socket wall, whereas the proximal areas remain nearly unchanged after flapless tooth extraction. This minimal bone loss in proximal areas after eight weeks of socket healing provides a two-wall defect morphology at sites where the facial bone wall has been resorbed, or even a three-wall morphology in sites with an intact thick facial bone wall. This two or even three wall defect morphology is considered relevant for predictable regenerative outcomes of single implant sites (Buser and coworkers 2009). These two- or three-wall bone defects have a high regenerative potential, which has been attributed to the ratio between the area of exposed bone marrow and the defect volume to be regenerated (Schenk and coworkers 1994) (Figs 5a-h).

5.1.3 Post-extraction Dimensional Alterations of the Soft Tissues

Although the facial soft-tissue appearance plays a pivotal role in achieving esthetic success in the anterior maxilla (Belser and coworkers 1998), the impact of dimensional alterations of the soft tissues in post-extraction sites has received little attention in clinical research (Sculean and coworkers 2014).

Wound healing is a complex process that requires a spatially and temporarily regulated expression as well as a coordinated interplay between many different types of tissues and cells (Gurtner and coworkers 2008). As a consequence, wound healing of extraction sockets results not only in dimensional alterations of the underlying bone, but also of the overlying soft tissues. Dimensional alterations of the overlying facial soft tissues and their contribution to post-extraction bone remodeling are little-known and poorly understood (Chappuis and coworkers 2016a).

The facial soft-tissue thickness in the anterior maxilla by nature is thin in most patients, ranging from 0.5 to 1 mm (Müller and coworkers 2000; Fu and coworkers 2010). Free gingival grafts and subepithelial connective-tissue grafts have been proposed to increase the band of keratinization and the soft-tissue volume (Thoma and coworkers 2014b). Thicker soft tissues not only have a higher volume of extracellular matrix and collagen, but also exhibit increased vascularity, which enhances the clearance of toxic products and favors the immune response (Hwang and Wang 2006; Nauta and coworkers 2011). Therefore, thicker soft tissue has been shown to respond favorably to wound healing, flap management, and restorative trauma, not only in periodontal (Hwang and Wang 2006), but also in implant surgery (Evans and Chen 2008; Vervaeke and coworkers 2014).

Soft-tissue thickness in thick and thin bone-wall phenotypes is similar in the anterior maxilla (Chappuis and coworkers 2016a). Interestingly, thin bone-wall phenotypes revealed a sevenfold increase in soft-tissue thickness after an eight-week healing period post-extraction, whereas the soft-tissue dimensions remained unchanged in thick bone-wall phenotypes (Chappuis and coworkers 2016a).

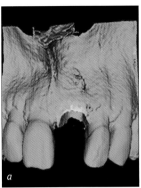
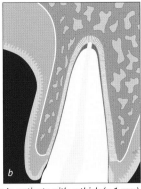
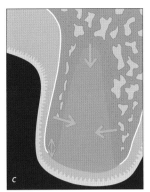
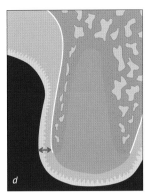

Figs 5a-d   Thick bone-wall phenotype: In patients with a thick (> 1 mm) facial bone wall, minimal dimensional alterations occur in the central aspect (a; yellow color showing minimal bone loss). A minimal vertical bone loss of 1.1 mm is observed (b-c). The facial soft-tissue thickness remains unchanged over an 8-week healing period post-extraction (d, red arrow). (Fig 5a reprinted from Chappuis and coworkers 2013b with permission from Sage Journals; © International & American Associations for Dental Research.)

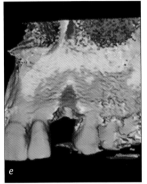
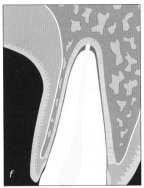
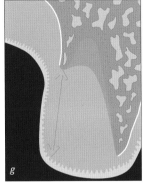
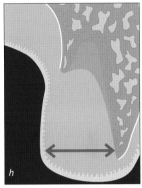

Figs 5e-h   Thin bone-wall phenotype: In patients with a thin (≤ 1 mm) facial bone wall, progressive dimensional alterations occur in the central aspect, whereas the proximal areas remain nearly unchanged (e; red color showing significant bone loss). A significant vertical bone loss of 7.5 mm is observed (f-g). This is in contrast to the facial soft-tissue thickness. The facial soft tissue shows spontaneous thickening, with a median increase of 4.8 mm over an 8-week healing period post-extraction (h, red arrow). (Fig 5e reprinted from Chappuis and coworkers 2013b with permission from Sage Journals; © International & American Associations for Dental Research.)

It may be hypothesized that the rapidly resorbed thin facial bone wall favors facial soft-tissue ingrowth because of their high proliferative rate. These soft-tissue cells occupy the majority of the available space in extraction-socket defects, favoring spontaneous soft-tissue thickening in thin bone wall phenotypes. This is in contrast to thick bone-wall phenotypes, where the alveolus provides a self-contained bony defect, which in turn favors the ingrowth of cells from the bony socket walls and the surrounding bone-marrow space. In sites with minimal bone resorption on the facial aspect, soft-tissue ingrowth will take place only crestally.

A trend toward soft-tissue thickening following tooth extraction has also been shown in other studies. One study described post-extraction sites alone or treated with bone substitute material and a collagen membrane (Iasella and coworkers 2003). After four and six months of healing, the authors reported a significant increase in soft-tissue thickness (0.4 mm) in sites with extraction alone, compared with a significant decrease (– 0.1 mm) in sites treated with barrier membranes to protect the grafting material (Iasella and coworkers 2003).

A recent report on ridge preservation revealed less bone loss in grafted sites compared to extraction alone (Jung and coworkers 2013). However, no significant soft-tissue contour changes were observed, which implies thicker soft tissues in non-grafted sites (Schneider and coworkers 2014) (Figs 5a-h; Dr. V. Chappuis).

5.2   Indications for Post-extraction Ridge Preservation

Since dimensional alterations following tooth extractions are an irreversible and inevitable process, attempts have been made to preserve the facial bone wall by immediate implant placement (Araújo and coworkers 2005), by immediate socket grafting (Araújo and coworkers 2015a), or by augmenting the facial bone plate (Favero and coworkers 2013). Even though these attempts have failed to arrest the inevitable biological process of dimensional alterations, in particular with respect to the preservation of the alveolar bone volume, grafting of extraction sockets by different biomaterials and using barrier membranes can reduce the degree of dimensional alterations (Avila-Ortiz and coworkers 2014).

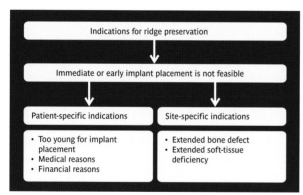

Fig 6   Decision tree for post-extraction ridge preservation.

Ridge preservation is indicated whenever immediate or early implant placement is not feasible. Indications can be can be patient-specific or site-specific. Patient-specific indications for ridge preservation are patients too young for implant placement or patients where implant placement has to be postponed for medical or economic reasons. Site-specific indications are related to extended bone defects at the extraction site. Such large lesions require partial bone healing to achieve sufficient primary stability of the implant in a correct 3D implant position. Sites associated with extended soft-tissue defects may require soft-tissue grafting to improve keratinization or tissue volume prior to implant placement (Fig 6).

5.2.1   Ridge Preservation by Root Maintenance

First attempts to prevent alveolar-ridge resorption were made by root retention, with the primary goal of maximizing the stability of removable prostheses (Osburn 1974). Clinical studies have tested the hypothesis that root retention by decoronation of the former crown to the bone level can reduce ridge alterations and help maintain the existing bone volume (Filippi and coworkers 2001; Andersson and coworkers 2003) (Figs 7a-h; Dr. V. Chappuis).

Other authors even suggested to maintain a facial shield of a root remnant simultaneous with implant placement with the aim to preserve the facial bone architecture (Hürzeler and coworkers 2010). However, root retention with simultaneous implant placement is rarely feasible due to fracture, decay, or strategic reasons related to the affected tooth. If compromised roots are maintained in close contact with an implant, they may cause severe damage to the neighboring implants (Langer and coworkers 2015).

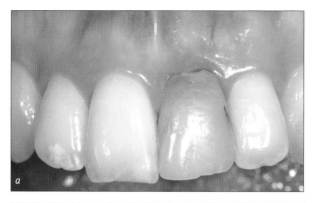

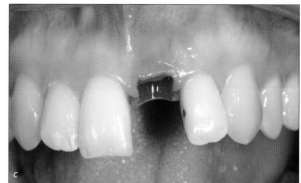

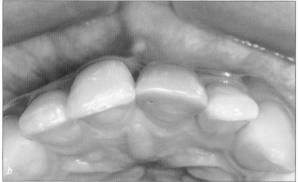

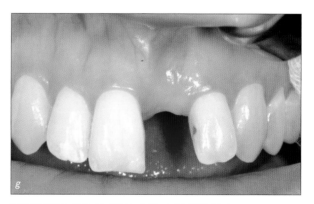

Figs 7a-b   Ridge preservation by root retention: Clinical situation revealed a pink spot on the facial aspect of the crown with inflammation-related root resorption. Since the patient was traveling and therefore not available for treatment, a ridge-preservation approach by root maintenance was chosen.

Figs 7c-d   The former crown was reduced to the level of the bone by decoronation. The soft tissue was left to heal by secondary intention.

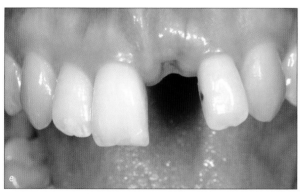

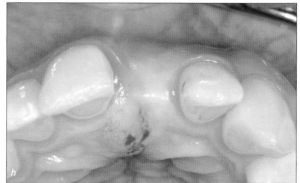

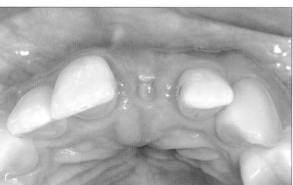

Figs 7e-f   Uneventful wound healing after two weeks.

Figs 7g-h   One year after decoronation: the ridge was well preserved.

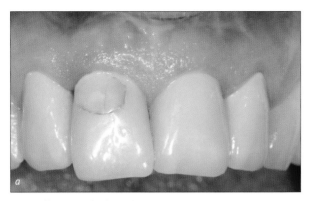

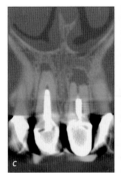
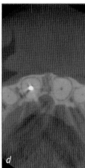
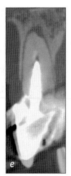
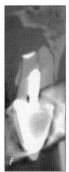
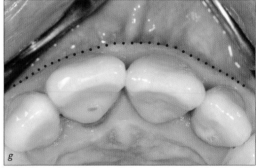

Figs 8a-b   The patient suffered from recurrent infection at sites 11 and 21.

5.2.2 Ridge Preservation by Socket Grafting

Socket grafting has gained popularity in recent years due to its conceptual attractiveness and technical simplicity (Christensen 1996). A large variety of biomaterials have been employed and tested in several studies, including autologous bone, bone substitutes (allografts, xenografts, and alloplasts), autologous blood-derived products, and bioactive agents (Darby and coworkers 2009).

At the Osteology Consensus Conference in 2012, the majority of studies and systematic reviews did not reveal any significant differences between the various biomaterials and treatment approaches. Although primary wound closure was considered an important factor, the literature did not allow a meaningful comparison of different techniques (Hämmerle and coworkers 2012).

A recent systematic review has shown that wound closure, the use of a membrane, and the application of a xenograft or allograft are associated with superior outcomes, particularly concerning the mid-buccal and mid-lingual height preservation (Avila-Ortiz and coworkers 2014) (Figs 8a-r; Dr. V. Chappuis).

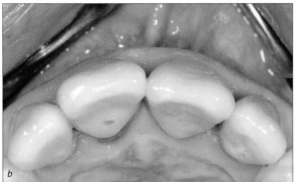

Figs 8c-g   CBCT scans (frontal, horizontal, and sagittal views) of the anterior portion of the maxillary alveolar ridge and the contour of the alveolar ridge before the extraction of teeth 11 and 21 showing periapical lesions with insufficient endodontic treatment and poorly fitting crowns.

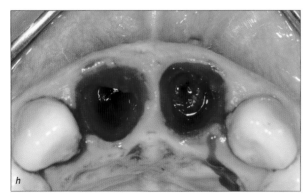
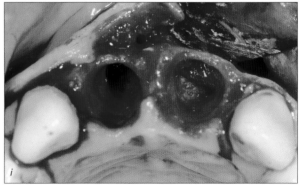

Figs 8h-i   After the minimally invasive low-trauma extraction of teeth 11 and 21. A small flap had to be raised to allow for removal of a cyst associated with tooth 21, whose removal would not have been possible transalveolarly.

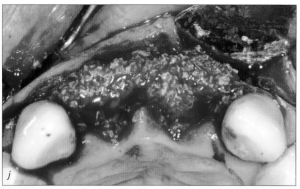

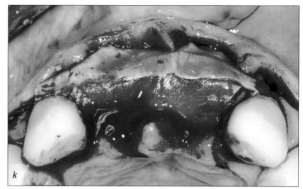

Figs 8j-k   After application of grafting material (Bio-Oss; Geistlich Pharma, Wolhusen, Switzerland) and coverage of the grafted site with a resorbable collagen membrane (Bio-Gide; Geistlich Pharma).

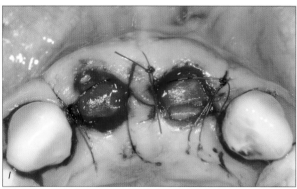

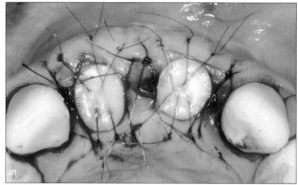

Figs 8l-m   To facilitate tension-free wound closure but to avoid periosteal relieving incisions, keratinized free gingival grafts from the palate were used to augment the post-extraction soft-tissue defects. This approach establishes functional and biological stability around the future implants by increasing the band of keratinized mucosa.

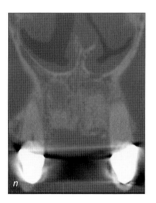

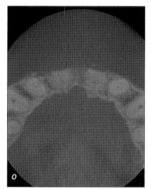

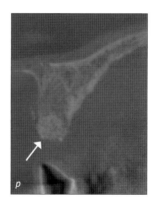

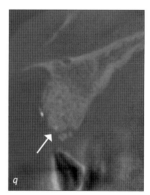

Figs 8n-r   CBCT scans (n-q; frontal, horizontal, and sagittal views) of the anterior portion of the maxilla and the contour of the alveolar ridge six months after socket grafting. Sufficient bone volume was gained apically, but due to the resorption of the bundle bone, a significant part of the augmented volume was lost in the crestal area of the augmented ridge. Dimensional alterations were significant despite socket grafting visualized by superimposing the ridge contour prior to extraction (r; blue dotted line) to the site six months after socket grafting (green dotted line).

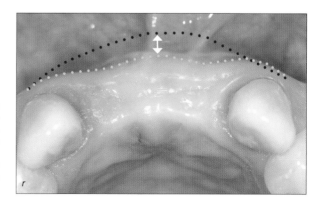

For more in-depth information on socket preservation, please check out the ITI Online Academy's congress lecture "Socket Preservation - When and How is it Evidence-based" by Dr. Simon S. Jensen (charges apply). See what else the Online Academy has to offer at **academy.iti.org**

For more in-depth information on post-extraction ridge maintenance, please check out the ITI Online Academy's congress lecture "Maintenance of the Ridge Post-extraction" by Dr. Stephen Chen (charges apply). See what else the Online Academy has to offer at **academy.iti.org**

5.3 Indications for Soft-tissue Grafting

In the esthetic zone, reconstructing a harmonious soft-tissue appearance is important for a successful outcome. Soft-tissue grafting has been proposed to establish functional and biological stability around teeth and implants by increasing the band of keratinized mucosa or by augmenting the soft-tissue volume (Cairo and coworkers 2008; Thoma and coworkers 2009). Although there is some controversy regarding some of these interventions, several parameters may indicate the need for soft-tissue enhancement around implants (Thoma and coworkers 2009; Wennström and Derks 2012).

5.3.1 Increasing the Band of Keratinized Mucosa

In the 1990s, clinical evidence suggested that a lack of keratinized mucosa (KM) around dental implants may not be crucial for maintaining the health of the peri-implant soft tissue (Wennström and coworkers 1994) and may not be associated with additional bone loss (Chung and coworkers 2006). However, recent clinical studies have indicated that a wider zone of KM may preserve the soft and hard tissues better (Bouri and coworkers 2008) and may be more favorable for the long-term maintenance of dental implants (Kim and coworkers 2009b). In addition, the lack of KM could result in poorer oral hygiene and more extensive soft-tissue recession (Schrott and coworkers 2009; Lin and coworkers 2013a). These observations resulted in a clinical recommendation of 2 mm for the width of KM (Adibrad and coworkers 2009).

Free gingival grafts are considered a reliable technique for augmenting peri-implant soft-tissue defects and are the method most often used to increase the band of KM. The most common donor site for a free gingival graft is the keratinized palate, whose color and shade do not always blend in naturally with the adjacent soft tissue and can compromise the esthetic result. Plastic procedures to augment the keratinized mucosa include an apically positioned flap or a vestibuloplasty (Palacci and Nowzari 2008). This can be performed prior to implant placement, simultaneously with second stage surgery or after delivery of the final reconstruction.

A recent systematic review has revealed that various methods and materials can be successfully used. All techniques applied were based on an apically positioned flap or a vestibuloplasty in combination with autologous soft tissue (connective-tissue graft), a free gingival graft, or a soft-tissue substitute (acellular dermal matrix/collagen matrix). These techniques resulted in a gain in keratinized mucosa over an observation period up to 48 months (Thoma and coworkers 2009). This review paper, however, demonstrated some shrinkage with all grafting materials applied, which can result in a decrease in the width of the keratinized mucosa of more than 50% within a couple of months (Figs 9a-h; Dr. V. Chappuis).

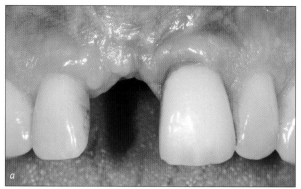
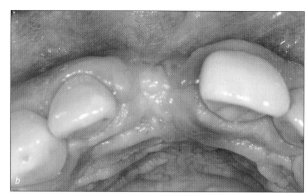

Figs 9a-b   Future implant site 11 showing no keratinized mucosa with scar tissue formation due to previous surgeries, labial and incisal view. The aim was to increase the band of keratinization and to reduce the scar tissue using a free gingival graft from the palate.

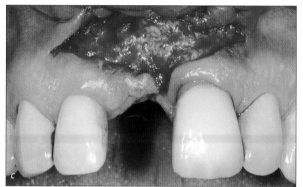
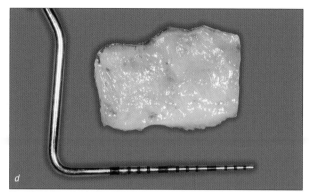

Fig 9c   Preparing the recipient area by a vestibuloplasty.

Fig 9d   A free gingival graft was harvested from the palate.

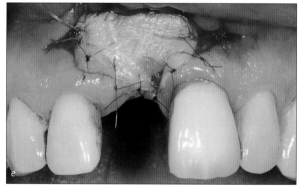
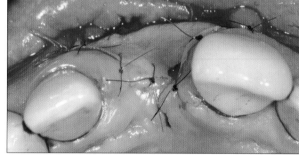

Figs 9e-f   Situation after suturing of the graft with simple interrupted sutures, labial and incisal view.

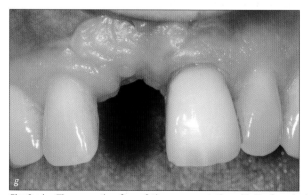
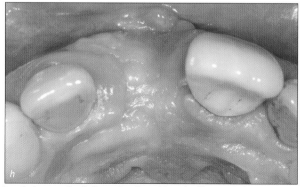

Figs 9 g-h   Three months after soft-tissue augmentation with the free gingival graft. Improved soft-tissue situation with a significant gain in keratinized mucosa and reduction around the future implant site.

5.3.2 Improving the Soft-tissue Volume

In conjunction with dental implants, plastic augmentative procedures have been recommended to enhance the thickness of the soft tissues simultaneously with implant placement or during the healing phase of the implants (Schneider and coworkers 2011).

Connective-tissue grafts or connective-tissue pedicle grafts have been used for the management of recessions and for augmenting ridge contours. Several surgical techniques have been developed to improve soft-tissue integration and potentially reduce patient discomfort associated with the free gingival graft. In order to avoid morbidity, soft-tissue substitute materials such as acellular dermal allografts (acellular dermal matrix) or xenograft materials (collagen matrix) have been tested as a potential substitute for the palatal donor tissue (Yan and coworkers 2006; Sanz and coworkers 2009).

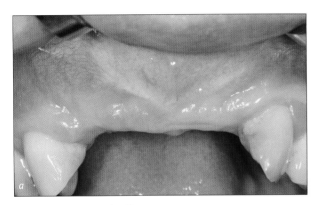

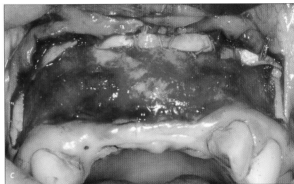

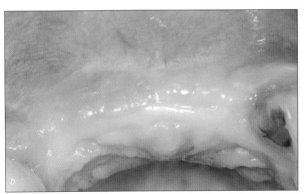

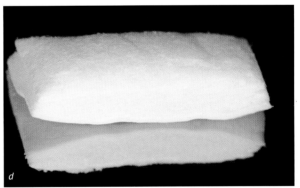

Figs 10a-b   Following implant placement at sites 12 und 21. Only a small band of keratinization was available.

Figs 10c-d   A vestibuloplasty in combination with a strip gingival graft from the palate and a xenogeneic collagen matrix was performed according to Urban and coworkers (2015b).

Four studies reported two-dimensional changes in soft-tissue volume applying autologous tissue and soft-tissue substitutes (the mentioned acellular dermal matrix and collagen matrix) (Batista and coworkers 2001; Speroni and coworkers 2010; Wiesner and coworkers 2010; Simion and coworkers 2012). For soft-tissue augmentation, autologous tissue has to be considered as treatment of choice resulting in an increase in soft-tissue thickness at implant sites, even though some soft-tissue shrinkage

has to be expected (Thoma and coworkers 2014a). There is still a lack of scientific evidence whether thicker peri-implant soft tissues result in better long-term success and survival rates of dental implants (Thoma and coworkers 2009) (Figs 10a-h; Dr. V. Chappuis; soft-tissue conditioning and provisional restoration by Dr. Fiona Forrer, Department of Reconstructive Dentistry and Gerodontology, University of Bern, Switzerland).

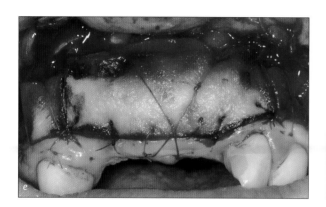

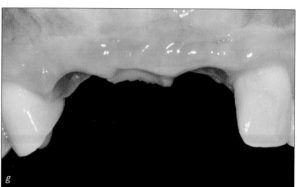

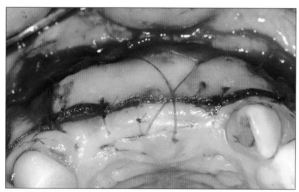

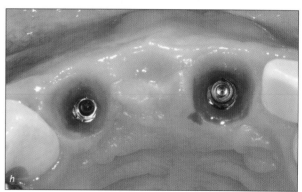

Figs 10e-f   The xenogeneic collagen matrix (Mucograft, Geistlich, Switzerland) was sutured to the surgical site.

Figs 10 g-h   The implant sites showed improved keratinization and soft-tissue volume in the soft-tissue conditioning phase.

5.4 Flap Design and Suture Techniques

5.4.1 Flapless Approach

The concept of flapless implant surgery has been advocated to reduce postoperative discomfort for patients (Komiyama and coworkers 2008). Flapless implant surgery is defined as a surgical procedure to prepare the implant osteotomy and to place the implant without elevating a mucoperiosteal flap in sites providing sufficient keratinized mucosa and bone volume.

A flapless surgical approach offers many advantages, such as improved patient comfort, less pain, less bleeding, less swelling, no need for sutures, shorter procedures, and shorter healing periods (Becker and coworkers 2005). Despite these many potential advantages, flapless implant surgery has generally been regarded as a "blind" procedure because of the difficulty in evaluating alveolar bone contours and angulations. In addition, with regard to the implant site and inclination of the implants, the surgeon will be guided only by the anatomy of the patient if not using any navigation system (Sclar 2007).

Due to the increased risk of malpositioned implants and the decreased ability for bone augmenation procedures to compensate for the inevitable post-extraction ridge alterations, the flapless approach is considered a niche procedure for ideal anatomic sites with a thick facial bone-wall phenotype (Morton and coworkers 2014). In such sites, a 3D CBCT analysis is indicated and computer-guided surgery is recommended to optimize the 3D position of the implants (Morton and coworkers 2014) (Figs 11a-j; Dr. V. Chappuis; prosthetic restoration by Dr. D. Cornioley, Bern, Switzerland).

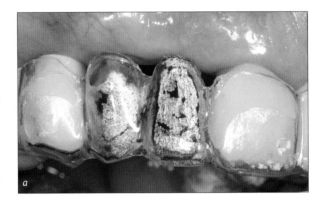

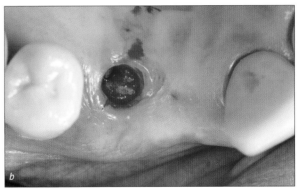

Figs 11a-b   Mucosa punched under stent guidance. The patient was on phenprocoumon (Marcumar; MEDA Pharma, Bad Homburg, Germany), an anticoagulant. On the day of surgery, the INR (International Normalized Ratio) was measured at 2.5. Flapless implant placement was performed as a minimally invasive therapy.

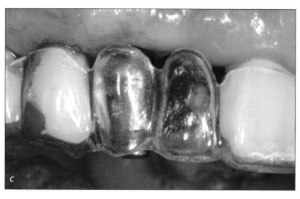

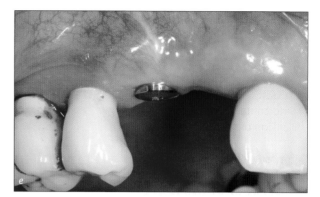

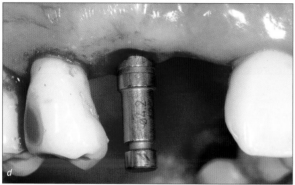

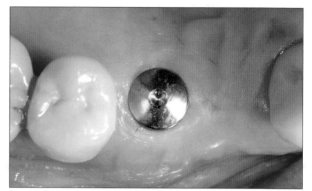

Figs 11c-d   The implant bed was prepared accordingly.

Figs 11e-f   A 3-mm healing cap was inserted.

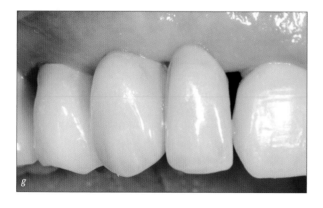

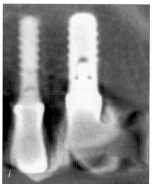

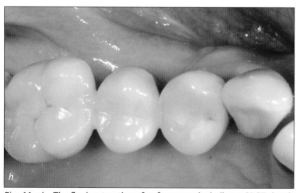

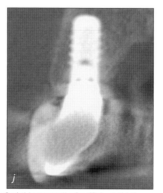

Figs 11 g-j   The final restoration after four years including a CBCT showing a facial bone wall of sufficient thickness and height.

5.4.2 Elevation of a Mucoperiosteal Flap

Soft-tissue management is a critical aspect for regenerative procedures. Primary wound closure in association with GBR techniques is desirable in order to achieve intimate contact of the wound margins without any signs of tension or pressure.

Soft-tissue dehiscences, however, can occur and may lead to infection and premature degradation of the membrane, which can compromise the amount of regenerated bone (Simion and coworkers 1994a; Zitzmann and coworkers 1999; Nemcovsky and Artzi 2002; Machtei 2001). As a basic surgical rule, the flap design should be planned in advance. In addition, incisions, flap elevation, and manipulation should be planned to optimize blood supply and wound closure (Greenstein and coworkers 2009). Delicate instruments and sutures ensure optimized wound healing (Cortellini and Tonetti 2001; Burkhardt and coworkers 2008) (Figs 12a-d; Dr. V. Chappuis).

The following surgical procedures are recommended to avoid soft-tissue complications:

Flap design

In procedures involving the esthetic zone, it is desirable to utilize only one vertical incision outside the esthetic zone—distally of the canine or even the first premolar (Grunder 2015). A triangular flap design with one releasing incision in the distal aspect provides sufficient access and increased vascularity compared to a trapezoidal flap using two vertical releasing incisions (Kleinheinz and coworkers 2005). In single-tooth cases, a triangular flap will be is sufficient in most cases, whereas in extended edentulous sites with multiple missing teeth or ridge augmentation using block grafts and GBR, two vertical releasing incisions are often needed to permit tension-free flap closure.

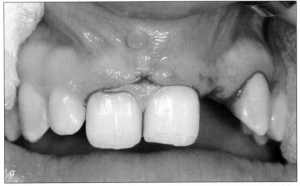
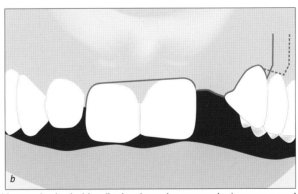

Figs 12a-b   A papilla-base incision in combination with a sulcular incision (with one releasing incision distal to the canine or premolars) ensures a good blood supply and wound closure.

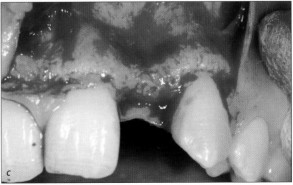

Fig 12c   A mucoperiosteal flap provides sufficient access to the surgical site for simultaneous or even for staged GBR procedures.

Incision design

For the incision, sharp blades in a rounded scalpel are recommended to cut the tissue in one stroke. In most sites, an appropriate surgical access is provided by a midcrestal or a slightly palatally located incision in the edentulous space, combined with a sulcular or papilla-base incisions (Velvart and coworkers 2004; von Arx and Salvi 2008). The incision should normally be extended at least one tooth beyond the edge of the bone defect. The vertical incision is located at the distal line angle in a paramedian position. The initial portion of the vertical incision is placed perpendicular to the marginal course of the gingiva, and gradually turning the incision parallel to the tooth axis. A full mucoperiosteal flap is usually raised to gain sufficient surgical and visual access to the implant site.

Wound closure

For wound closure, a releasing incision in the periosteum is essential to give the flap elasticity and to permit tension-free flap closure (Park and coworkers 2012). As a short-term disadvantage, the releasing incision will cause a postsurgical swelling in the upper lip that lasts two to five days. Wound closure is achieved with interrupted single sutures, if needed in combination with horizontal or vertical mattress sutures to approximate the connective tissue and to adapt the wound edges. The suturing technique depends on the grafting volume and the extent of flap mobilization. Removable provisional prostheses should be sufficiently shortened to avoid direct contact with the soft-tissue surface. In GBR cases, a first follow-up after two to three days is recommended to examine postsurgical swelling, hematoma formation and soft-tissue status. Suture removal is suggested after ten days to two weeks.

For more in-depth information on flap design, please check out the ITI Online Academy's learning module "Flap Design" by Dr. Merete Aaboe (charges apply). See what else the Online Academy has to offer at **academy.iti.org**

5.5 Implant Selection

New developments in implant design and surface technology have emerged in the past twenty years to minimize crestal bone-level changes (Wenneberg and Albrektsson 2009; Strietzel and coworkers 2014; Gittens and coworkers 2014). These new elements were integrated in the bone-level implant design (BL), with the aim to preserve more bone at the implant shoulder compared to the soft-tissue-level implant design (STL) (Fig 13). Other efforts have been directed at developing stronger titanium alloys for narrow-diameter implants (NDI) in order to reduce the risk of implant fracture. The appropriate implant type (implant diameter and length) depends on clinical parameters such as crest width, bone height at the recipient site, and the planned prosthetic reconstructions (Buser and coworkers 2000). In the esthetics zone, recreating a harmonious soft-tissue outline and balanced relative tooth dimensions are a primary concern (Belser and coworkers 2009). Therefore, the implant surgeon should not sacrifice implant length or diameter unless this is not required from an anatomical or restorative point of view (Figs 13a-c).

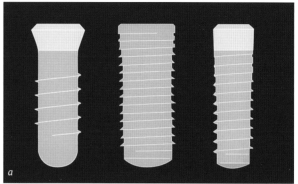

Fig 13a   Soft-tissue-level implants (left and right) and bone-level implant (middle) (Institut Straumann AG, Basel, Switzerland).

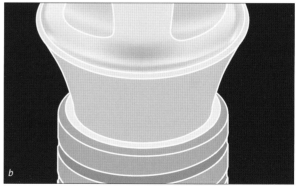

Fig 13b   Platform-switching interface with a microrough collar design.

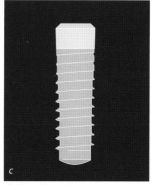

Fig 13c   Butt-joint interface with a machined collar design.

5.5.1 Selection Criteria for Soft-tissue-level (STL) vs. Bone-level (BL) Implants in the Anterior Maxilla

A first concept that has arisen from these new developments is a microrough implant-surface topography up to the implant shoulder level (Le Guéhennec and coworkers 2007; Wenneberg and Albrektsson 2009; Svanborg and coworkers 2010). There is some evidence that surface characteristics at the implant neck influence the preservation of marginal soft and hard tissue (Schwarz and coworkers 2007). Even though a smooth neck design is accompanied by the lowest accumulation of plaque (Teughels and coworkers 2006), several clinical studies in posterior sites have shown more marginal bone remodeling for these implants compared to microrough surfaces at the neck portion (Shin and coworkers 2006; Bratu and coworkers 2009; Nickenig and coworkers 2009). A recent study that included anterior sites revealed that regenerative procedures on the facial aspect of smooth-neck designs were less successful, even though bone graft material or barrier membranes were utilized over cover screw (Fu and coworkers 2014). This is in contrast to the findings by den Hartog and coworkers, who observed no significant differences in proximal sites between a smooth and a rough neck design after eighteen months in the esthetic zone (den Hartog and coworkers 2011). The reason for this conflicting evidence is not clear.

A second concept follows the principle of platform switching, which had coincidentally revealed a better long-term preservation of crestal bone levels around wide-diameter implants connected with a standard abutment (Lazzara and Porter 2006). Efforts have been made to reduce microleakage caused by microgaps at the implant/abutment interface. Regarding the concept of platform switching, the horizontal offset of the implant/abutment interface not only reduces the inflammatory cell infiltrate (Broggini and coworkers 2006), but it also decreases the area of maximum biomechanical stress at the marginal bone level (Maeda and coworkers 2007). A recent meta-analysis has confirmed that an implant/abutment offset of ≥ 0.4 mm was associated with a more favorable bone response (Atieh and coworkers 2010). To date, the effect of platform switching remains inconclusive, particularly with respect to long-term data and also due to the multifactorial causes of peri-implant bone loss (Abrahamsson and Berglundh 2009; Atieh and coworkers 2010; Annibali and coworkers 2012a; Cumbo and coworkers 2013; Striezel and coworkers 2014; Romanos and Javed 2014).

In single-tooth sites with intact adjacent natural teeth, pleasing esthetics can be achieved with both STL and BL designs (Jung and coworkers 2012; Buser and coworkers 2013a; Buser and coworkers 2013b; Morton and coworkers 2014). However, in single-tooth sites the BL design appears to preserve more bone at the facial aspect of the implant shoulder (Chappuis and coworkers 2015). In some cases, the BL design allowed the reconstruction of the facial bone wall coronal to the implant abutment junction, which supports the soft tissues mid-facially. Thus, the BL implant design is favored for single-tooth replacement in the esthetic zone (Fig 13d).

Evidence that these findings also apply to multiple edentulous sites is limited. However, an STL implant in the esthetic zone remains a valuable option in sites with a vertical deficiency. In such sites, the microrough implant surface is located below the bone crest, whereas the STL implant shoulder can be positioned 1.8 mm or even 2.8 mm further coronally, compensating for the vertical deficiency.

V. Chappuis, S. Chen, D. Buser

A: Soft-tissue-level implants (STL)   **B: Bone-level implants (BL)**

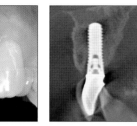
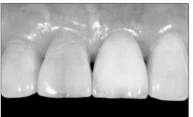
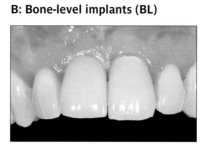
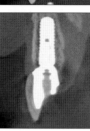
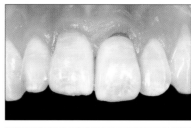
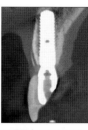

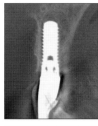
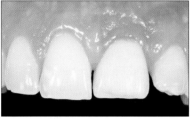
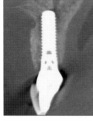
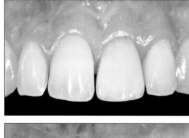
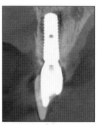

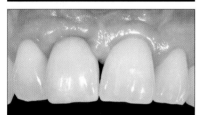
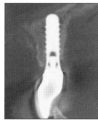
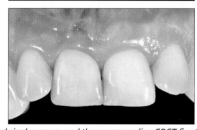
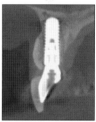

Fig 13d   Clinical and radiographic cases: Clinical images of implant-supported single crowns and the corresponding CBCT five to nine years after contour augmentation. (Reprinted from Chappuis and coworkers 2016a with permission from John Wiley & Sons Ltd; © 2015 John Wiley & Sons A/S.)

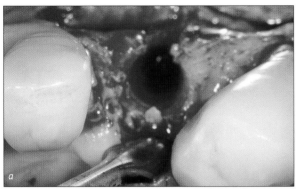

Fig 14a   A narrow-diameter implant (NDI) made of Ti-Zr alloy was used to replace a maxillary left canine in a 68-year-old patient with a complex medical history. Following flap reflection, the ridge revealed a reduced oro-facial width. The osteotomy was prepared to a diameter of 2.8 mm. There is a dehiscence of the facial bone.

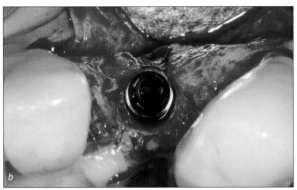

Fig 14b   A 3.3-mm implant (NC Bone Level Roxolid with a SLActive surface, diameter 3.3 mm, length 10 mm; Institut Straumann AG) in place. The implant is located entirely within the bone envelope. The defect on the facial side has two bone walls, which is conducive to simultaneous bone augmentation. If an implant with a greater diameter had been selected, there would have been a risk that the resultant facial defect would have had no bone walls.

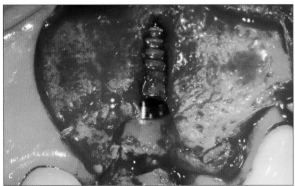

Fig 14c   The dehiscence in the facial bone after implant placement.

5.5.2   Implant Diameters in the Anterior Maxilla

The appropriate implant diameter depends on the width of the alveolar crest and the size of the tooth to be restored. It is recommended to preserve a palatal bone wall of at least 1 to 2 mm in thickness, resulting in a minimal crest width of 5.5 to 6 mm for narrow-diameter implants (NDI) with simultaneous GBR (Buser and coworkers 2000).

In recent years, NDI have been recommended for the following indications (Klein and coworkers 2014): NDI of 3.3 to 3.5 mm in diameter are well documented for all indications, including load-bearing posterior regions. Smaller implants 3.0 to 3.25 mm in diameter are well documented only for single-tooth replacements in non-load-bearing regions. For clinicians it is important to know when these NDI should be used in the anterior maxilla. In the esthetics zone, the regeneration of a harmonious soft-tissue appearance and a natural anatomy is the treatment of choice. However, bone augmentation especially in staged protocols is more invasive and the associated morbidity should be kept to a minimum to increase patient acceptance of implants therapy through pleasing esthetics. NDIs may thus reduce the need for staged grafting procedures in borderline cases with ridge atrophy, allowing simultaneous GBR.

Nevertheless, NDI are associated with certain risks. First, NDI present a smaller area for osseointegration. NDI should therefore only be used with a length of at least 10 mm (Sohrabi and coworkers 2012), combined with a high-quality surface to compensate for the smaller bone-to-implant contact area (Oates and coworkers 2007). Second, the reduced diameter leads to distortion of the implant body and may imply a certain risk of mechanical and technical complications, such as an increased fracture rate of 0.67% (Zinsli and coworkers 2004; Karl and coworkers 2014). To reduce the risk of NDI fracture, it is recommended to use reinforced titanium such as TiZr (Chiapasco and coworkers 2012). Finally, the greater horizontal distance between the implant and the neighboring teeth may result in a poor emergence profile and poor access for oral hygiene.

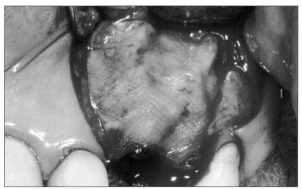

Fig 14d *Simultaneous bone augmentation using the principles of GBR was performed. Autologous bone chips were placed directly on the implant surface, and a DBBM graft was used to convert the facial aspect of the ridge for contour augmentation. A resorbable collagen membrane was placed over the graft.*

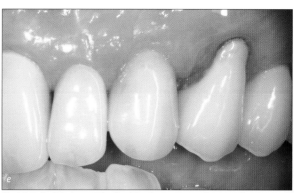

Fig 14e *Facial view of the final implant-supported restoration for tooth 23. The NDI had eliminated the need for staged augmentation for this patient.*

NDI in the esthetic zone can be considered for three different clinical situations (Figs 14a-e; clinical case courtesy of Dr. Stephen Chen, Melbourne, Australia):

1 Single-tooth sites with a narrow gap, such as lateral incisors, where BL NDI are most often used.
2 Implant sites with a borderline crest width of 5 to 6 mm, where NDI allow a simultaneous GBR procedure to avoid staged ridge augmentation.
3 Central incisor sites with an extended nasopalatine foramen, forcing the clinician to place a standard-diameter implant (diameter 4.1 mm) in a more facial position to maintain an intact palatal bone wall.

In these situations, NDI should be utilized to avoid facial malpositioning of a standard-diameter implant shoulder. NDI should not be used if a correct 3D prosthetically driven implant position is not achievable. These cases require bone augmentation. Despite the enhanced mechanical properties of titanium alloy compared to commercially pure titanium, NDI should be used with caution in borderline cases and adhere to the ITI Consensus Conference recommendations (Klein and coworkers 2014).

Unlike NDI, wide-platform implants should not be used in the anterior maxilla. They bear a high risk of facial malpositioning due to their increased diameter (Chapter 8.1.2). Wide-diameter implants in the esthetic zone most often cause facial recession of the peri-implant mucosa, leading to esthetic complications or failures (Chen and Buser 2009).

For more in-depth information on reduced diameter implants, please check out the ITI Online Academy's congress lecture "The Challenges of Reduced-Diameter Implants" by Dr. Stephen Chen (charges apply). See what else the Online Academy has to offer at **academy.iti.org**

For more in-depth information on reduced diameter implants, please check out the ITI Online Academy's congress lecture "Is the Dogma of Using the Largest Diameter Still Valid?" by Dr. Bilal Al-Nawas (charges apply). See what else the Online Academy has to offer at **academy.iti.org**

5.5.3   Implant Lengths in the Anterior Maxilla

The appropriate implant length depends on the vertical bone height at the recipient site. In standard sites, an implant length of 10 or 12 mm will be adequate. Longer implants (14 mm) may be indicated in special circumstances, such as in lateral incisor sites with extended apical lesions that may compromise the primary stability of NDI.

A recent systematic review has evaluated short implants with a length of < 10 mm (Annibali and coworkers 2012b). Although short implants have historically been considered less reliable due to a greater crown-to-implant ratio and a smaller surface area available for osseointegration, that review reported successful results with a pooled survival rate of 99.1% and a low incidence of complications after a mean follow-up period of 3.2 ± 1.7 years.

Positive results have been reported for short implants (6 to 8 mm) for single crowns and short-span fixed and removable prostheses, with survival rates between 98.1% and 99.7%, but they were recommended to be used only "under strict clinical protocols" (Fugazzotto 2008; Anitua and Orive 2010). However, the survival rate of implants with a length of only 6 mm was lower in the maxilla (94.7%) than in the mandible (98.6%), with 76% early implant failures (Srinivasan and coworkers 2014). Therefore, an implant length of 6 mm cannot be recommended in single-tooth implant sites in the anterior maxilla, whereas 8-mm implants with a standard diameter of 4.1 mm seem to be applicable in certain situations.

5.6 Correct Three-dimensional Implant Positioning

One critical aspect of an esthetically successful outcome of implant treatment is the correct restoration-driven 3D implant position, to replace the tooth in a natural position and to emulate a natural emergence profile (Garber and Belser 1995; Buser and coworkers 2004a; Grunder and coworkers 2005). It is important to note that the CEJ of adjacent teeth may vary depending on the position of the tooth to be replaced and on any existing recessions (Belser 1980).

The concept of "comfort" and "danger" zones was established at the 3rd ITI Consensus Conference to help achieve correct 3D implant positioning in esthetic sites (Buser and coworkers 2004a) (Figs 15a-k).

In complex cases, a diagnostic wax-up can help fabricate a surgical template to achieve correct 3D implant positions. The template should provide two important parameters: (a) the outline of the future implant crown, indicating the desired future soft-tissue margin mid-facially; and (b) the location of the incisal edge.

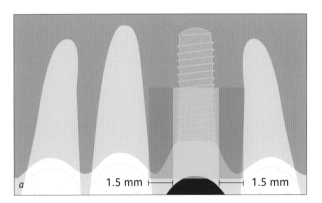

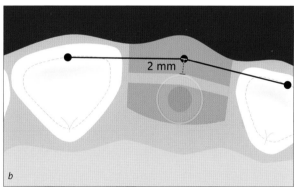

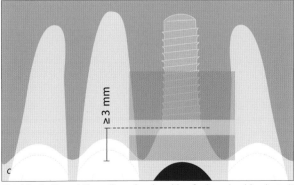

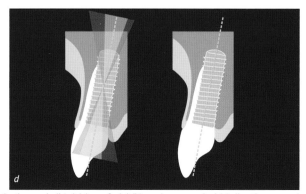

Figs 15a-d   Correct three-dimensional position for bone-level implants (BL) in the mesiodistal (a), orofacial (b), and coronoapical (c) direction; correct implant angulation (d).

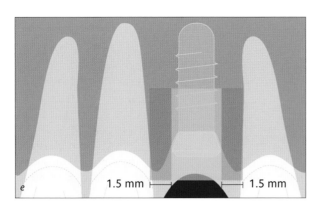

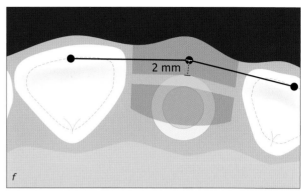

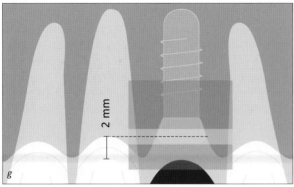

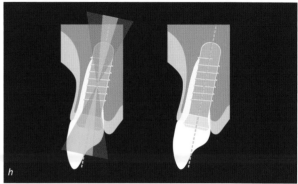

Figs 15e-h   Correct three-dimensional positioning for soft-tissue-level implants (STL) in the mesiodistal (e), orofacial (f), and coronoapical (g) direction; correct implant angulation (h).

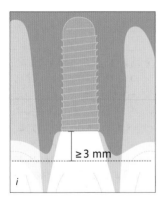

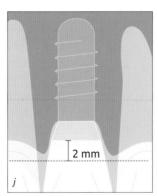

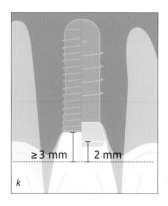

Figs 15i-k   The coronoapical implant placement differs between bone-level and soft-tissue-level implants.

5.6.1   Mesiodistal Dimensions

Selecting the correct implant relative to the mesiodistal dimensions of the tooth to be replaced is critical. It is important to consider the horizontal biologic width around the implant (Tarnow and coworkers 2000). Implant placement too close to the neighboring teeth will lead to bone loss and reduced papillary height. An interproximal distance of at least 1 to 1.5 mm should be respected between the implant neck and the periodontal attachment of the adjacent tooth, irrespective of implant design (Krennmair and coworkers 2003; Buser and coworkers 2004a; Grunder and coworkers 2005; Figs 15a and e).

5.6.2   Orofacial Dimensions

The orofacial position of the implant shoulder should be located 1.5 to 2 mm palatally of the point of emergence of the future implant crown (Buser and coworkers 2004a; Figs 15b and f). A severe facial malposition of the implant leads to soft-tissue recession and implant exposure. It can be caused by the utilization of a wide-platform implant (Chen and Buser 2009). Wide-diameter implants should be used with caution due to the risk associated with placing implants too far facially, favoring facial recession.

Comparisons of a bone-level implant design with a neck diameter of 4.1 mm to a soft-tissue-level design with a neck diameter of 4.8 mm have revealed that the orofacial positioning of the STL design was more critical and significantly influenced the facial bone crest dimensions (Chappuis and coworkers 2016a). A palatal malposition can affect the ideal emergence profile of the future restoration.

5.6.3   Coronoapical Dimensions

The ideal coronoapical position is slightly different between STL and BL implants. Whereas for an STL implant, the implant shoulder is positioned about 2 mm below the future mucosal margin of the implant-supported crown, in the BL design, the implant shoulder is placed at a distance of about 3 mm (Buser and coworkers 2004a; Buser and coworkers 2013b; Figs 15c, g, i, j, and k). If implants are inserted too deep in an apical malposition, more pronounced vertical bone resorption will occur with a subsequent soft-tissue loss. This mechanism has been observed in experimental studies (Hermann and coworkers 1997; Piattelli and coworkers 2003).

The coronoapical position is also dependent on the gap size (width of the edentulous space). If a larger central incisor (gap size: 9 to 11 mm) is replaced by a standard implant (diameter 4.1 mm), the coronoapical position needs to be adapted, locating the implant shoulder slightly deeper (3 to 4 mm below the future crown margin). For a small lateral incisor (gap size: 5.5 mm) utilizing an NDI (diameter 3.3 mm), the implant shoulder is placed in a shallower coronoapical position (2 to 3 mm below the future crown margin in order to obtain a good emergence profile).

5.6.4   Implant Angulation

A correctly planned implant angle will help optimize the emergence profile and simplifies the prosthetic restoration. An implant angle leaning too far facially will lead to facial hard- and soft-tissue loss. The correct implant axis should be located roughly 1 mm palatally of the future incisal edge, allowing transocclusal screw retention of the implant restoration in the cingulum area (Figs 15d and h). In the esthetic zone, a screw-retained restoration is clearly desirable and offers different clinical advantages, which will be discussed in Chapter 6.

5.7 Surgical Approach: Simultaneous vs. Staged GBR

Guided bone regeneration (GBR) has become a standard of care that provides predictable treatment outcomes over the long-term perspective (Aghaloo and Moy 2007). The combination of barrier membranes, autologous bone, and bone fillers with a low substitution rate offers long-term stability of the regenerated volume (Buser and coworkers 2013b). Ridge augmentation by GBR can be performed either simultaneously with implant insertion or as a staged procedure prior to implant placement. Both the simultaneous and the staged GBR approach are well documented and considered predictable (Jung and coworkers 2013a; Chen and Buser 2014; Kuchler and von Arx 2014; Sanz-Sánchez and coworkers 2015; Chappuis and coworkers 2017).

The decision whether a simultaneous approach is feasible or a staged approach should be based on three decision criteria (Buser and coworkers 1993; Kan and coworkers 2007):

1 The implant can be inserted with primary stability.
2 The implant can be inserted in a correct prosthetically driven 3D position.
3 The local bone defect shows a favorable defect morphology for a simultaneous approach (Figs 16a-c).

5.7.1 Simultaneous GBR

Simultaneous GBR has clear advantages, since bone augmentation and implant placement are performed in one surgery. It causes less morbidity, is less time-consuming and less costly than a staged GBR approach.

A simultaneous approach can be recommended when the local bone defect shows a favorable morphology. The following two anatomical conditions should be satisfied to allow a simultaneous GBR protocol: First, a sufficient crest width is needed at the future implant site, to allow a circumferential bone anchorage of the implant following bone healing. At the 2nd ITI Consensus Conference, the minimum crest width was defined as the implant diameter plus 2 mm (Buser and coworkers 2000). Second, a favorable defect morphology is needed that provides sufficient stability for the grafted site. As a rule of thumb, a localized two-wall defect with the exposed implant surface within the "bony envelope" is required for a highly predictable successful regenerative outcome. Therefore, the crest width in the proximal areas of the future implant site is most critical and should be assessed prior to implant surgery (Figs 16a-f and Fig 17).

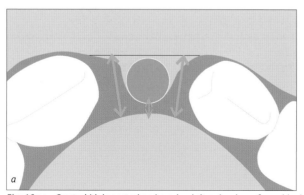
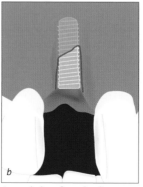
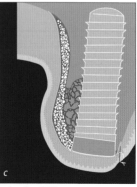

Figs 16a-c   Crest width in central and proximal sites showing a favorable defect morphology for a simultaneous approach using GBR.

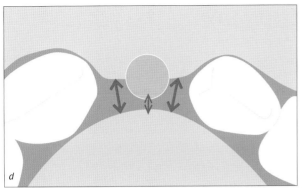
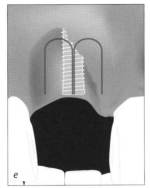
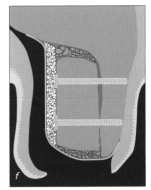

Figs 16d-f Crest width in central and proximal sites showing an unfavorable defect morphology. In such sites, a staged approach is recommended.

In order to assist the clinician's decisions in implant sites with limited bone volume, cone-beam computed tomography (CBCT) is indicated. In the past fifteen years, significant progress in digital 3D diagnostic radiology has been made with CBCT, which provides better images and significantly lower radiation exposure for patients than conventional computed tomography (Bornstein and coworkers 2014a).

5.7.2   Staged GBR

Staged GBR is indicated in implant sites with advanced horizontal atrophy resulting in an unfavorable one-wall defect morphology with a planned implant position outside the bony envelope (Jovanovic and coworkers 1992; Buser and coworkers 1993; Garber and Belser 1995; Chiapasco and coworkers 2006; Sanz-Sánchez and coworkers 2015). In such sites, implant-bed preparation and a correct 3D implant position are not only difficult to obtain but also reduce the potential for a successful regenerative outcome if simultaneous GBR would have been selected. In sites with advanced horizontal atrophy, a staged GBR approach is therefore recommended (Fig 16a-f).

A well-documented staged surgical protocol for the reconstruction of large horizontal defects is the use of autologous corticocancellous block grafts from intraoral harvesting sites such as the ramus or the symphysis, an approach often termed onlay grafting (Widmark and coworkers 1997; Antoun and coworkers 2001; Cordaro and coworkers 2002; Maiorana and coworkers 2005; Cordaro and coworkers 2011). This technique provides successful outcomes but exhibits great variation in bone resorption, between 22% and 60% of the inserted block grafts, as demonstrated by the above-mentioned clinical

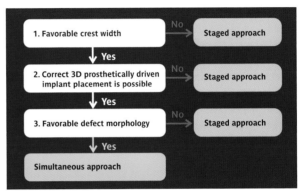

Fig 17   Decision tree: simultaneous versus staged-approach GBR.

studies. In the 1990s, barrier membranes or bone fillers with a low substitution rate were used to protect autologous block grafts against resorption. Several clinical studies revealed a better maintenance of the augmented bone volume with a reduced resorption rate of only 6% to 12% (Antoun and coworkers 2001; Maiorana and coworkers 2005; von Arx and Buser 2006; Cordaro and coworkers 2011; Chappuis and coworkers 2017). Ridge augmentation using a staged approach was discussed in detail in Volume 7 of the ITI Treatment Guide (Cordaro and Terheyden 2014) (Figs 16d-f and 17).

5.8 Surgical Approach: Immediate vs. Early vs. Late Implant Placement

Immediate post-extraction placement has gained considerably ground in the past twenty years. Preclinical and clinical research has demonstrated that the timing of implant placement plays an important role for treatment outcomes (Chen and Buser 2009). The clinician has four different treatment options as defined by the 3rd, 4th and 5th ITI Consensus Conferences (Hämmerle and coworkers 2004; Chen and coworkers 2009; Morton and coworkers 2014).

In the 1980s, the concept of late implant placement was the standard of care, allowing the site to heal at least six months prior to implant insertion (Schroeder and coworkers 1991). In order to reduce the treatment time, the concept of immediate implant placement was first proposed in the 1970s (Schulte and coworkers 1978) and reintroduced in the late 1980s in combination with GBR (Lazzara 1989). In the mid-1990s, the early implant placement protocol or immediate delayed procedure was proposed by several authors (Ashman 1990; Gelb 1993; Grunder and coworkers 1999; Attard and Zarb 2005).

The 3rd ITI Consensus Conference undertook to sort out the various treatment options and defined four protocols for clinicians (Hämmerle and coworkers 2004):

Type	Description
1	Immediate implant placement
2	Early implant placement with soft-tissue healing (four to six weeks)
3	Early implant placement with partial bone healing (twelve to sixteen weeks)
4	Late implant placement in healed sites (six months or more)

5.8.1 Immediate Implant Placement (Type 1)

Immediate implant placement at the time of tooth extraction is considered a complex surgical procedure (Morton and coworkers 2014). Immediate implant placement with or without immediate restoration has often been proposed to enhance esthetic outcomes (Kan and coworkers 2003). However, implant-bed preparation requires surgical skills and diligence to prepare the implant bed to the correct 3D position. The difficulty for the clinician is the discrepancy between the correct restoration-driven 3D implant position (Chapter 6.6) and the more facially located extraction socket.

Clinical studies have demonstrated that mucosal recession around immediate implants is often caused by facial malpositioning (Evans and Chen 2008). In addition, the lack of soft-tissue integrity may require soft-tissue grafting, which increases complexity, morbidity, and cost. Root-shaped implant designs have been proposed for reducing the gap between the implant surface and the former socket walls, aimed at supporting the facial socket wall to prevent bone loss.

Recent animal studies evaluated the effect of different implant designs on facial bone-wall resorption. They revealed that implant design has no effect in limiting the facial bone-wall resorption in immediate implant placement protocols (Vignoletti and coworkers 2009; Alharbi and coworkers 2015).

By contrast, wide root-shaped implants occupying most of the socket caused more pronounced alveolar bone resorption (Caneva and coworkers 2010). Two recent clinical studies using consecutive CBCTs at implant placement and at one year have confirmed significant mid-facial vertical bone loss in immediate implant cases (Roe and coworkers 2012; Vera and coworkers 2012). Recent systematic reviews have shown that predictable results are difficult to obtain and that these techniques carry an increased risk of significant mucosal recessions if this approach is not applied with strict inclusion criteria (Kan and coworkers 2011; Cosyn and coworkers 2012; Chen and Buser 2014).

Following immediate implant placement, mid-facial recession greater than 1 mm occurs in 9% to 41% of sites between one year and three years (Chen and Buser 2009). Other surgical factors, such as the use of a flapless technique, immediate provisional restorations, the applications of soft-tissue grafts, or the use of implant/abutment connections with a platform-switching concept are still controversial because there is still no clear evidence of any added value, which is why these factors should be further investigated in well-designed clinical trials (Vignoletti and Sanz 2014).

Immediate implant placement can be recommended in ideal sites with a thick bone-wall phenotype (> 1 mm) and a thick gingival phenotype, as recommended by the 4th ITI Consensus Conference (Morton and coworkers 2014). If ideal conditions are not present, other protocols are preferred to achieve predictable esthetic outcomes (Morton and coworkers 2014; Vignoletti and Sanz 2014) (Figs 18a-o; clinical case courtesy of Dr. Stephen Chen, Melbourne, Australia).

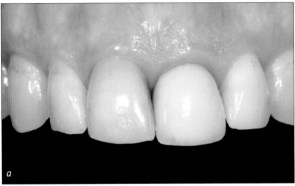

Fig 18a Tooth 21 had experienced repeated loosening of the post-retained crown. The tissue phenotype was thick and the mid-facial gingival margin of the tooth was coronal to that of the adjacent tooth 11. There was an excess of soft-tissue height. Probing pockets around the tooth were in the range of 2 to 3 mm.

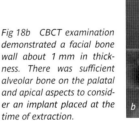

Fig 18b CBCT examination demonstrated a facial bone wall about 1 mm in thickness. There was sufficient alveolar bone on the palatal and apical aspects to consider an implant placed at the time of extraction.

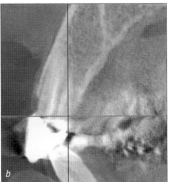

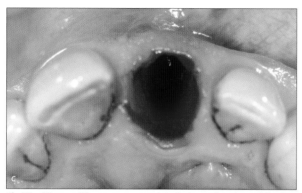

Fig 18c   The conditions were appropriate for immediate (type 1) implant placement. This is an occlusal view of the site after flapless extraction of the tooth. The facial bone wall was undamaged.

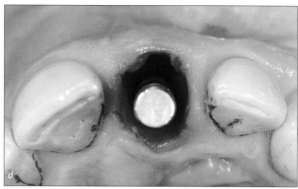

Fig 18d   The implant (RC Bone Level with a SLActive surface, diameter 4.1 mm, length 12 mm; Institut Straumann AG) was placed in the correct 3D position.

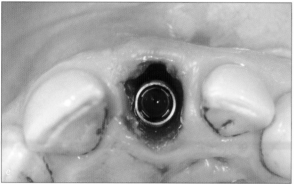

Fig 18e   There was a distance of 2 mm between the implant shoulder and the internal aspect of the facial socket wall.

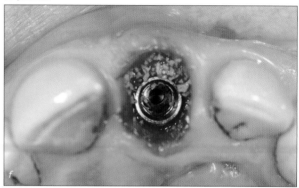

Fig 18f   The facial gap was grafted with DBBM particles (Bio-Oss; Geistlich Pharma AG).

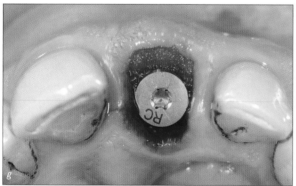

Fig 18 g   A collagen membrane created a barrier to protect the graft.

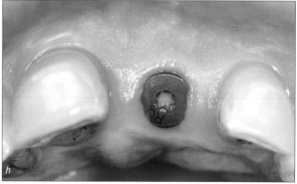

Fig 18h   Ten weeks later. The healing process had progressed uneventfully with good soft-tissue healing.

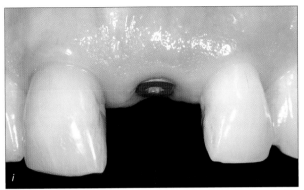

Fig 18i   Facial view of implant 21, sixteen weeks after placement. The patient subsequently returned to the referring prosthodontist to commence prosthodontic procedures.

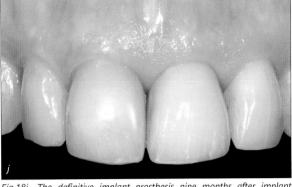

Fig 18j   The definitive implant prosthesis nine months after implant placement.

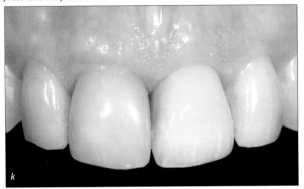

Fig 18k   Two years after implant placement, the peri-implant tissues were healthy and stable.

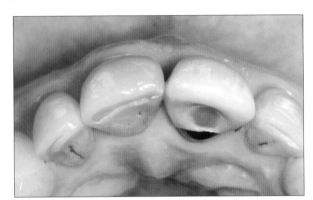

Fig 18l   Occlusal view two years after implant placement.

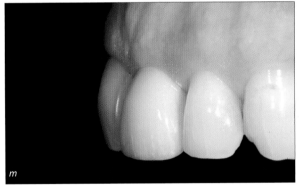

Fig 18m   Lateral view of the implant-supported restoration two years after implant placement.

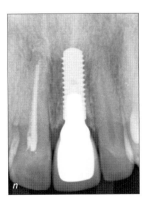

Fig 18n   Radiographic control two years after implant surgery.

Fig 18o   The CBCT of the implant two years after placement shows maintenance of a thick facial bone wall.

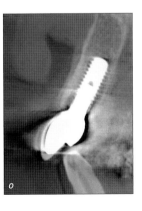

5.8.2 Early Implant Placement (Type 2 and 3)

In an early implant placement protocol with soft-tissue healing (type 2), the implant is normally placed four to eight weeks after the extraction. This protocol offers several advantages from a clinical point of view.

First, the complete soft-tissue coverage after healing provides an increased amount of keratinized mucosa, which facilitates flap closure and favors bone regeneration (Zitzmann and coworkers 1999; Nemcovsky and Artzi 2002; Buser and coworkers 2008a).

Second, several animal studies have shown a boost of osteoclastic activity during the initial healing phase for the resorption of the bundle bone (Cardaropoli and coworkers 2003; Araújo and Lindhe 2005). In early placement, this initial osteoclastic phase is completed at the time of implant insertion. This provides a more stable environment for bone regeneration to occur, which is most often needed in esthetic implant sites to compensate for the dimensional ridge alterations on the facial aspect (Buser and coworkers 2008a, Sanz and coworkers 2012; Chappuis and coworkers 2013). This protocol has therefore been recommended as the treatment of choice in sites exhibiting a pronounced bone resorption pattern, as it occurs in thin bone-wall phenotypes or thin gingival phenotypes (Morton and coworkers 2014). As demonstrated by several CBCT studies, these thin bone-wall phenotypes dominate in the esthetic zone, with a prevalence of more than 90% (Braut and coworkers 2011; Januario and coworkers 2011; Vera and coworkers 2012).

Third, early implant placement provides spontaneous soft-tissue thickening in the former socket (see Chapter 6.1) (Chappuis and coworkers 2016a). Utilizing a palatal incision technique on the crestal aspect, this spontaneously thickened soft tissue inside the socket can be mobilized as part of the mucoperiosteal flap, providing a soft-tissue thickness of roughly 5 mm with high vascularity and a good healing potential. In addition, such a thick soft-tissue flap does not require additional connective-tissue grafting in routine cases, reducing the morbidity of surgical interventions. Finally, early placement also offers the advantage that acute or chronic infections, sometimes in combination with a fistula, will be resolved during the post-extraction healing phase, since the cause of infection will have been treated by tooth removal.

A drawback of early implant placement is that it requires two surgical interventions such the extraction and the subsequent implant surgery. To limit morbidity, the first intervention is performed in a flapless manner to avoid an open-flap procedure. Flapless tooth extraction is of importance in this approach to avoid additional bone resorption from the bony surface related to the elevation of the mucoperiosteal flap (Wood and coworkers 1972; Fickl and coworkers 2008). This minimizes ridge alterations in proximal areas of the extraction socket at eight weeks of healing, as shown in a CBCT study, leading to a favorable two- or three-walled defect morphology (Chappuis and coworkers 2013).

After implant placement in a correct 3D position, simultaneous contour augmentation is routinely performed to overcontour the local bone anatomy on the facial aspect. Contour augmentation uses two bone fillers with synergistic properties. First, autologous bone chips, providing a high osteogenic potential, are harvested locally to cover the exposed implant surface. Second, a superficial layer of deproteinized bovine bone mineral (DBBM) particles is applied to serve as a scaffold for bone ingrowth and to support the collagen membrane.

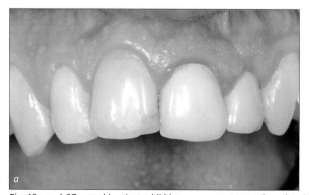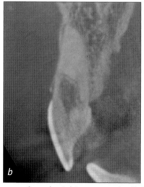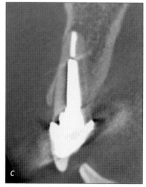

Figs 19a-c   A 37-year-old patient exhibiting a severe root resorption related to a previous dental trauma on tooth 11 and a chronic periapical endodontic lesion on tooth 22.

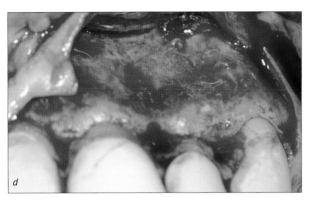

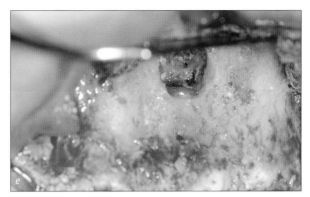

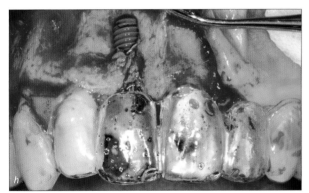

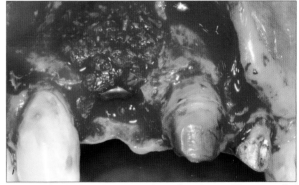

Figs 19d-g   Following endodontic revision of tooth 22, apical surgery was performed. The apical end was sealed with mineral trioxide aggregate (MTA). Root 11 was extracted during the same surgical session. A collagen sponge was applied to stabilize the blood clot and to promote soft-tissue healing. The healing period was uneventful.

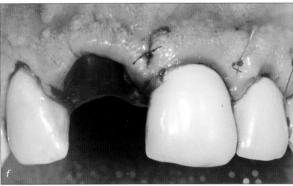

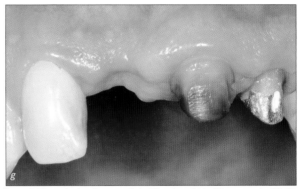

Fig 19h   After the elevation of a mucoperiosteal flap, a surgical stent was used for correct 3D implant positioning.

Fig 19i   After implant placement, a layer of autologous chips was applied on the hydrophilic microrough implant surface.

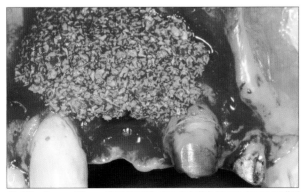

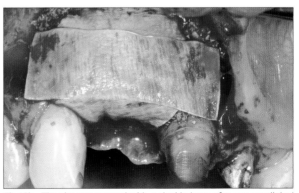

Fig 19j   A second layer of DBBM (Bio-Oss; Geistlich Pharma) was applied to achieve an optimal contour if the facial bone.

Fig 19k   The site was covered with a double layer of a non-crosslinked collagen membrane (Bio-Gide; Geistlich Pharma).

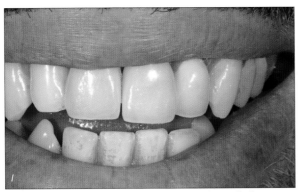

Fig 19l   Four-year follow-up with the patient's medium smile line.

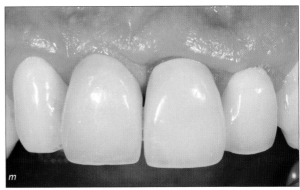

Fig 19m   Implant-supported crown 11.

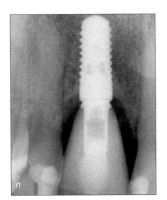

Fig 19n   Periapical radiograph. Stable peri-implant bone levels after four years.

This synergistic combination of composite grafts, consisting of autologous bone chips and DBBM, fosters the formation of new bone in the defect area, mainly due to the osteogenic potential of the autologous bone chips. Whereas the DBBM particles provide for the long-term stability of the augmented volume due to their low substitution rate (Buser and coworkers 2008b). Bone augmentation is attempted up to the top of the implant healing cap at a height of 1.5 to 2 mm above the implant shoulder level. The augmented site is covered with a non-crosslinked collagen membrane using a double-layer technique, followed by tension-free wound closure. The reentry procedure is performed after eight weeks of healing using a semilunar incision, applied slightly palatal to the healing cap (Figs 19a-n; Dr. V. Chappuis; prosthetic restoration by Dr. S. Ramseier, Bern, Switzerland).

Early implant placement with partial bone healing (type 3) is rarely used. It is indicated in sites with an extended periapical bone lesion that does not allow implant placement with sufficient primary stability after type 2 implant placement. In these sites, a prolonged healing period of twelve to sixteen weeks is advisable (Morton and coworkers 2014).

5.8.3   Late Implant Placement (Type 4)

Late implant placement includes implant insertion into a fully healed ridge with a post-extraction healing phase of at least six months. In most cases, late placement is not intentional, such as when patients seek implant therapy years after tooth extraction. In such sites, the edentulous area often presents with significant facial bone loss, requiring ridge augmentation with a staged approach.

In patients where the timing of tooth extraction and implant placement can be controlled by the clinician, late placement (type 4) should therefore be avoided whenever possible. When late implant placement is the treatment of choice, socket grafting for ridge preservation is advisable to minimize ridge alterations during the healing phase. These clinical situations can be divided into patient-specific or site-specific indications and have been described in Chapter 5.2 (Figs 4 to 6). Socket grafting is a well-documented technique today and helps maintain ridge volume in post-extraction sites (Darby and coworkers 2009; Avila-Ortiz and coworkers 2014).

However, socket grafting has not been able to fully prevent the loss of bone volume in the crestal area in clinical and preclinical studies (Araújo and Lindhe 2009b; Araújo and coworkers 2015a). As a consequence, the goal of ridge preservation is to avoid a staged ridge augmentation procedure after completion of the healing period. Nevertheless, most patients require simultaneous GBR to optimize the esthetic outcome once an implant has been inserted (Figs 20a-aa; Dr. V. Chappuis; prosthetic restoration by Dr. F. Jeger-Kissling, Bern, Switzerland).

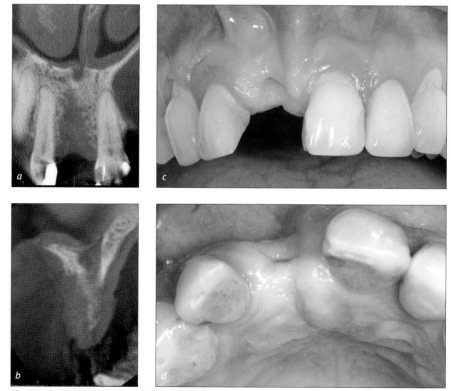

Figs 20a-d   Situation after loss of tooth 11. The CBCT reveals an unfavorable one-wall defect morphology with an insufficient crest width of 2 mm).

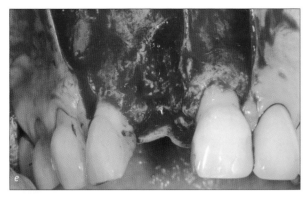

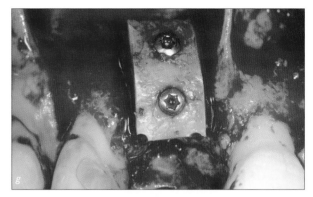

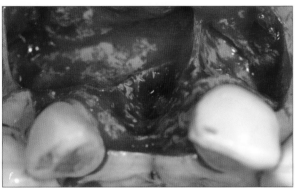

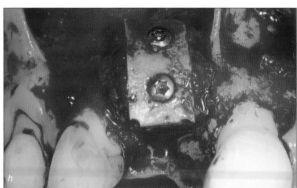

Figs 20e-f   A staged ridge augmentation was necessary. Following muco-periosteal flap elevation, an autologous block graft was harvested from the chin area.

Figs 20g-h   The autologous graft was adapted to the surgical site and stabilized using two fixation screws (Medartis, Basel, Switzerland) (g). The voids around the block were filled with autologous bone chips (h).

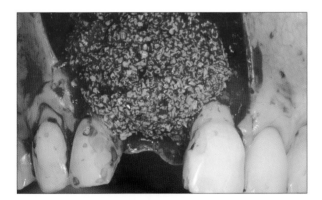

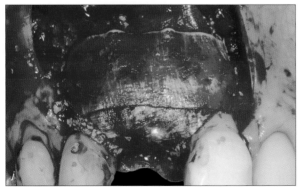

Figs 20i-j   The autologous bone block was then covered with DBBM (Bio-Oss; Geistlich Pharma) and a collagen membrane (Bio-Gide; Geistlich Pharma) to protect it from resorption during healing.

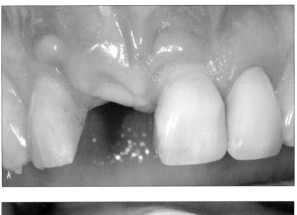

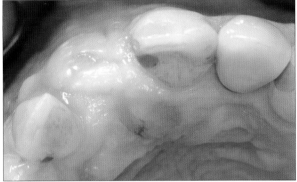

Figs 20k-l   After the six-month healing period.

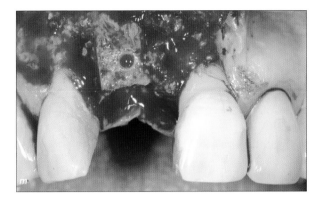

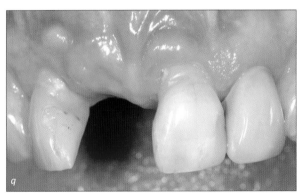

Figs 20m-n   The site was reentered, the fixation screws were removed, and a bone-level implant (Bone Level, diameter 4.1 mm, length 10 mm; Institut Straumann AG) was placed with good primary stability.

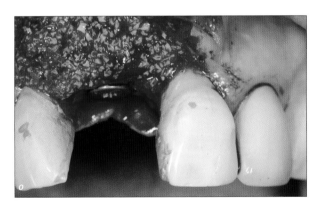

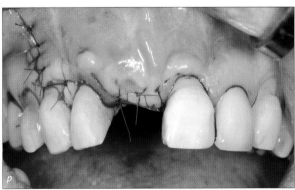

Figs 20o-p   An additional contour augmentation was performed using DBBM and a collagen membrane (Geistlich Pharma, Wolhusen, Switzerland) and the wound closed by sutures.

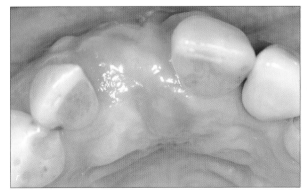

Figs 20q-r   After a twelve-week period, the site had nicely healed.

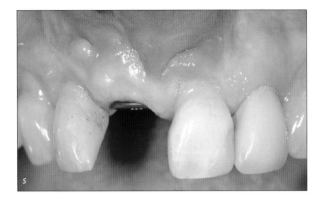

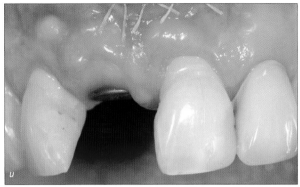

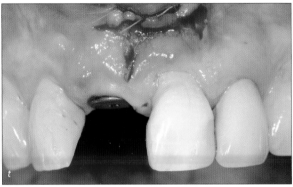

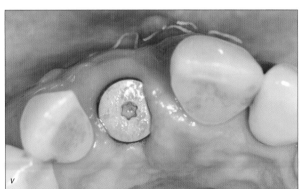

Figs 20s-t   The abutment was connected and the soft tissues were corrected. The implant exhibited an ISQ of 80 (Implant Stability Quotient; Ostell).

Figs 20u-v   After two weeks, the soft tissues had nicely healed and the patient was referred to the restorative dentist.

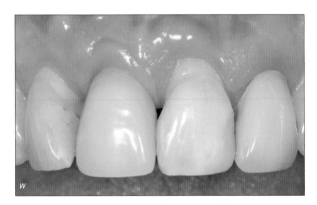

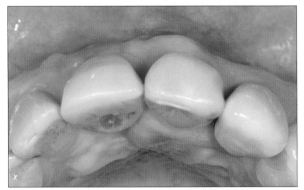

Figs 20w-x   A provisional restoration was provided for soft-tissue conditioning.

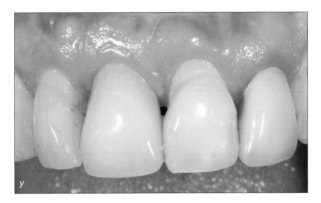

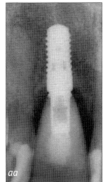

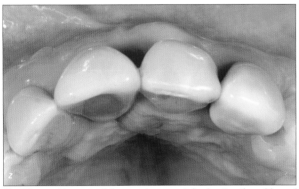

Figs 20y-aa Three-year follow-up. A screw-retained restoration with good esthetics and a nice soft-tissue contour. The periapical radiograph reveals stable peri-implant bone levels.

In the case of a 32-year-old female patient, late implant placement (type 4) was necessary due to a large cystic lesion at site 21 (Figs 21a-z; Prof. D. Buser, prosthetic restoration: Dr. Julia Wittneben, Department of Reconstructive Dentistry and Gerodontology, University of Bern, Switzerland).

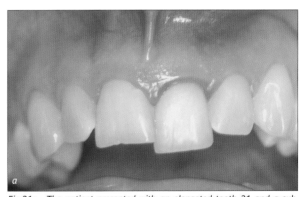

Fig 21a The patient presented with an elongated tooth 21 and a sub-acute infection in this area. Tooth 21 was hypermobile and caused pain on palpation.

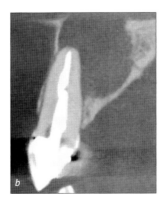

Fig 21b The CBCT scan showed a large cystic lesion (radicular cyst) apically to the root of tooth 21 with nasal floor resorption.

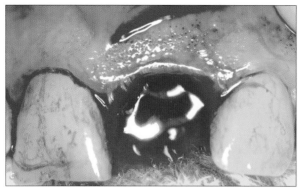

Fig 21c   Status after extraction of tooth 21 and drainage of the cystic fluid.

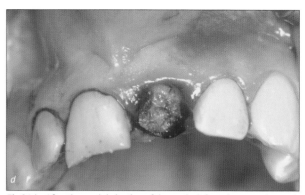

Fig 21d   After thorough irrigation of the cystic defect, the extraction socket was filled with a drainage.

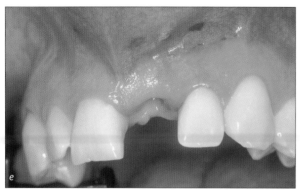

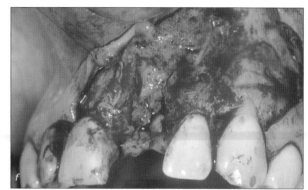

Figs 21e-f   Two months later, a cystectomy was performed to remove the radicular cyst.

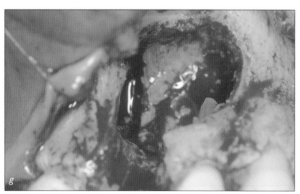

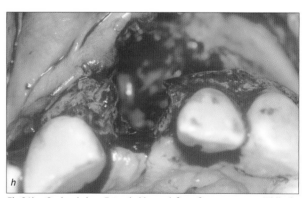

Fig 21g   Simultaneously, an apicoectomy of the tooth 22 with a retrograde root-end filling was done.

Fig 21h   Occlusal view. Extended bone defect after cystectomy. While the facial bone wall of the extraction socket was resorbed during the eight-week healing period, the width of the crest was excellent.

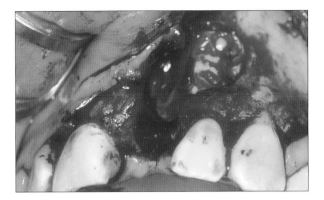

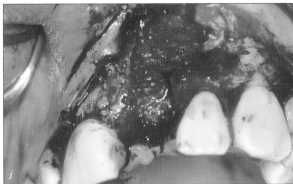

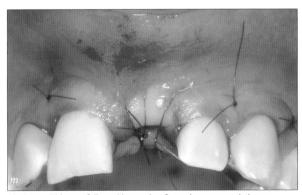

Figs 21i-k   To restore and maintain the ridge volume for later implant placement, the ridge was preserved with autologous bone chips and deproteinized bovine bone mineral particles (Bio-Oss; Geistlich Pharma).

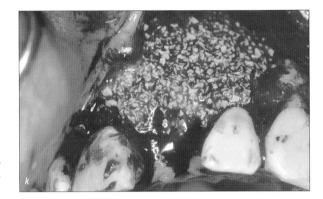

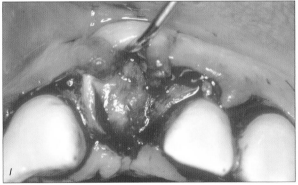

Fig 21l   The augmentation material was covered with a collagen membrane (Bio-Gide, Geistlich Pharma).

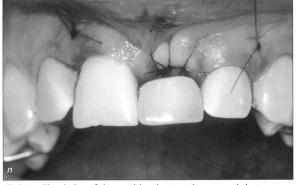

Fig 21m   This was followed by tension-free primary wound closure.

Fig 21n   The design of the provisional restoration ensured that no pressure was applied to the surgical site.

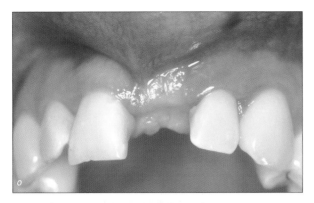

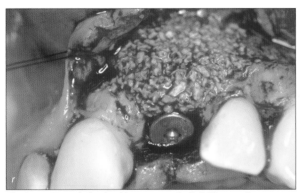

Figs 21o-p   Six months following an uneventful healing, the site was re-opened and presented nicely healed and with sufficient volume for late (Type 4) implant placement (figs 21o-p).

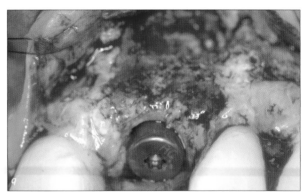

Fig 21q   A Bone Level implant (diameter 4.1 mm, length 10 mm; Institut Straumann AG) was inserted. In addition, a 2-mm healing cap (Institut Straumann AG) was connected.

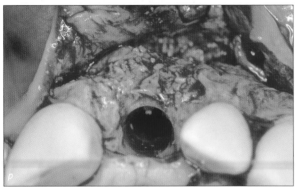

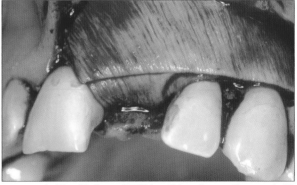

Figs 21r-s   To optimize the ridge contour, the facial bone wall was once more augmented with a thin layer of DBBM particles subsequently covered with a collagen membrane (Bio-Gide; Geistlich Pharma) applied using the double-layer technique.

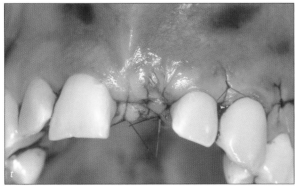

Fig 21t   This was followed by tension-free would closure.

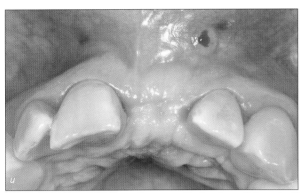

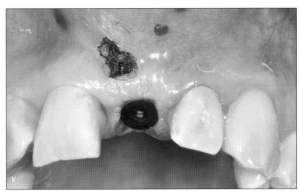

Figs 21u-v   Two months later, after a complication-free soft-tissue healing phase, the single-tooth gap presented with excellent volume. The site was reentered using a punch technique, and a longer healing cap (Institut Straumann) was inserted. The frenulum was cut with a CO_2 laser to prevent tension on the peri-implant mucosa.

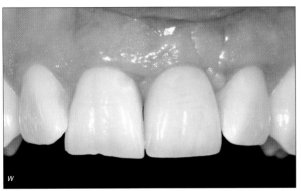

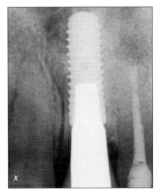

Fig 21x   Six-year periapical radiograph. Stable bone crest levels around the bone level implant.

Fig 21w   Six-year follow-up. A pleasing esthetic outcome with harmonious mucosal margins.

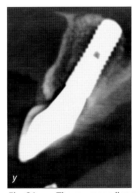

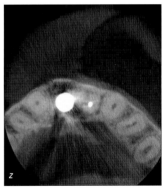

Figs 21y-z   The corresponding sagittal and horizontal CBCT sections show a thick facial bone wall extending far beyond the implant shoulder.

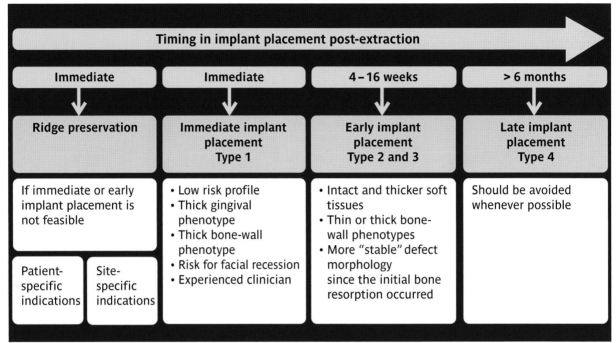

Fig 22   Decision tree for post-extraction implant placement.

Figure 22 gives an overview of the decision-making process as to determining the appropriate timing for implant placement.

For more in-depth information on the timing of implant placement, please check out the ITI Online Academy's congress lecture "Implant Placement after Tooth Extraction—Selecting the Optimal Time" by Dr. Stephen Chen (charges apply). See what else the Online Academy has to offer at **academy.iti.org**

For more in-depth information on the timing of implant placement, please check out the ITI Online Academy's learning module "Timing of Implant Placement After Tooth Extraction" by Dr. Stephen Chen (charges apply). See what else the Online Academy has to offer at **academy.iti.org**

6 Prosthetic Management for Optimal Esthetic Outcomes

W. Martin, A. Hamilton

6.1   Evaluation of Esthetic Outcomes in Single-tooth Replacement

The restoration of single-tooth implants in the esthetic zone is a demanding procedure that requires attention to peri-implant tissue, the surrounding dentition, implant positions, and the materials used to restore them. Compromises in any of these areas may require modifications to the prosthetic approach in order to create an acceptable clinical outcome. The esthetic success or failure of an implant restoration should be evaluated by objective and subjective parameters (Gallucci and coworkers 2011; Fuentealba and Jofré 2015).

Objective esthetic indices have been created to evaluate treatment outcomes with regard to the peri-implant tissues (*pink esthetic score*, PES) and the restoration (*white esthetic score*, WES) (Fürhauser and coworkers 2005; Belser and coworkers 2009).

The PES by Belser and coworkers (2009) evaluates the following variables:

1   Mesial papilla
2   Distal papilla
3   Curvature of the facial mucosa
4   Level of the facial mucosa
5   Root convexity/soft-tissue color and texture

These variables are scored on a scale from 0 to 2, for an ideal PES result of 10 (Fig 1).

The WES focuses on the visible part of the implant-supported restoration and is based on the following parameters:

1   General tooth shape
2   Outline and volume of the clinical crown
3   Shade (including hue and value)
4   Surface texture
5   Translucency and characterization

These parameters are also scored on a scale from 0 to 2, for an ideal WES result of 10 (Fig 2).

While clinicians strive for a PES/WES score close to 20, several publications have reported that laypeople find a score of 12 or greater to be acceptable in most clinical situations (Jones and Martin 2014; Fava and coworkers 2014; Tettamanti and coworkers 2015). It has also been reported that persons without dental training can be more sensitive to WES than PES scores with single-tooth implants in the esthetic zone, which may influence the choice of abutment material and design in the definitive prosthesis (Jones and Martin 2014; Sailer and coworkers

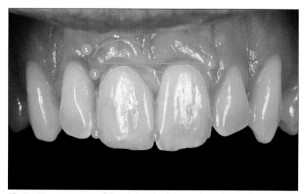

Fig 1   Measurements of the pink esthetic score (PES) (according to Belser and coworkers 2009).

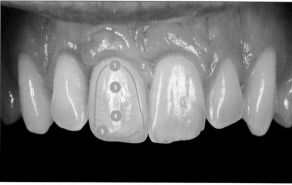

Fig 2   Measurements of the white esthetic score (WES) (according to Belser and coworkers 2009).

2014). These findings can depend on the thickness of the facial mucosa and its ability to mask the underlying abutment and emerging restoration; a threshold value for thickness of 2 mm has been reported (Jung and coworkers 2008b; Van Brakel and coworkers 2011).

If the clinical scenario is ideal (implant position allowing for an adequate prosthetic volume), the restorative materials for single-tooth implant restorations (metal-ceramics vs. all-ceramics) may have little influence on the esthetic outcomes from both an objective and subjective viewpoint (Gallucci and coworkers 2011). In addition, the survival rates of abutments (zirconia vs. titanium) supporting restorations in the anterior region show similar five-year survival rates, suggesting that the choice of the abutment should depend on to the clinical situation and not on the material (Sailer and coworkers 2009a; Zembic and coworkers 2013). In clinical situations where the facial mucosa is thin, the choice of abutment can have a negative influence on PES scores in the form of tissue graying if metal abutments are used and tissue

lightening if zirconia abutments are employed (Jung and coworkers 2008b; Park and coworkers 2007; Zembic and coworkers 2009; Ishikawa-Nagai and coworkers 2007). In these situations, modifying a zirconia abutment underlying the tissues with pink ceramics should be considered to minimize the brightness of the mucosa (Thoma and coworkers 2015).

A similar consideration should be given to the WES component of the restoration. If the prosthetic volume is compromised in the orofacial dimension, the underlying support for the restoration could have significant influence on the translucency of the restoration. If the substructure is metal or zirconia in these situations, the technician will find it difficult to create translucency and the restoration will appear more opaque than the adjacent tooth (Figs 3a-b). A titanium bonding base with a restoration made of a more translucent material (lithium disilicate) will provide more technical flexibility in achieving an esthetic outcome (Figs 4a-b).

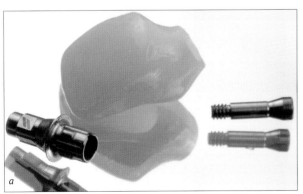
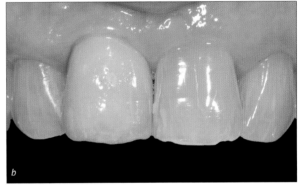

Figs 3a-b   Zirconia abutment (CARES Zirconia; Institut Straumann AG, Basel, Switzerland) and veneering ceramics at site 11 (Vita VM9; Vita North America, Yorba Linda, CA, USA).

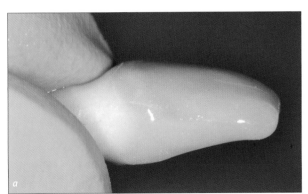
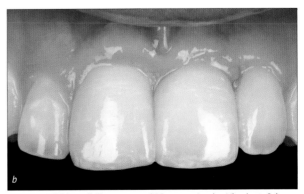

Figs 4a-b   Titanium bonding base (Variobase; Institut Straumann AG) with a cemented lithium disilicate crown (IPS e.max; Ivoclar Vivadent, Schaan, Liechtenstein) replacing tooth 21. The final restoration was screw-retained.

In an effort to maximize the PES/WES outcomes, clinicians must focus on several key areas during the restorative phase of the treatment. The process is initiated directly after implant placement by interim restorations to maintain contours and space and to shape the peri-implant tissues during the run-up to the final restorative phase. This is followed with detailed laboratory communication:

- Photographs depicting the contours, shade, and surface texture of the adjacent teeth to be matched in addition to a full smile and contours of the provisional restoration.
- Accurate impressions capturing not only the implant position but the emergence profile of the tissue, from the implant shoulder to the mucosal margin (transition zone) and the surrounding peri-implant mucosa, extending as far vestibularly as possible.
- Information about the materials used in adjacent restorations, if present.

This information is then utilized by the clinician and technician to determine the ideal abutment and restorative material and design for an optimized PES/WES outcome.

6.2 Interim Prostheses

The treatment of failing or missing teeth in the esthetic zone is often met with the need to utilize interim (provisional) prostheses either prior to or after the placement of the dental implant(s). This section will highlight the various types of interim prostheses and their advantages and disadvantages for use during the rehabilitation process in areas of esthetic importance.

6.2.1 Before Implant Placement

The treatment of edentulous spaces in the esthetic zone that will require delayed placement (types II, III, IV) of the implant due to deficits of the soft or hard tissues, pathology, or compromises in the restorative space will require the use of an interim restoration in preparation for implant placement. A well-designed interim prosthesis should provide esthetic and functional use while protecting the tissues during their healing phase (Markus 1999).

Interim prostheses can be fixed or removable. Both options can provide benefits for the patient, but certain key principles should be followed to prevent deleterious effects on the tissue in the edentulous space (Buser and coworkers 2004a). The interim prosthesis should do the following:

- Provide acceptable esthetic and functional use
- Prevent intermittent pressure on grafted areas
- Maintain restorative space
- Be durable and be easily repaired when needed
- Provide diagnostic value in implant position planning

When vertical site enhancement is performed, it is necessary to design an interim prosthesis that prevents intermittent pressure on the grafted site. Fixed interim prostheses are desirable in this situation, but when a removable prosthesis is the only option, selective pressure should be confined to areas distant from the grafted site.

Options for an ideal interim prosthesis include:

- *Fixed dental prosthesis (FDP).* If teeth adjacent to the edentulous site are planned for full-coverage restorations, incorporating them as abutments to retain an interim prosthesis will provide the ideal result. Interim fixed retention with controlled and selective pressure to the grafted area will allow for optimized healing and esthetics (Figs 5a-c).
- *Resin-fiber reinforced fixed dental prosthesis (RRF-DP).* If teeth adjacent to the site are not planned for restoration but reduced vertical overlap is present, a denture tooth with fiber wings can be bonded to the palatal (or lingual) surfaces of the adjacent teeth, providing an esthetic fixed alternative (Figs 6a-c). A drawback to this procedure lies in the retention of the prosthesis, which needs to be removed and re-bonded on multiple occasions throughout the course of treatment.
- *Orthodontic retention.* In patients undergoing orthodontic treatment or in situations where excessive vertical overlap is present, pontics incorporated into a bracket-retained archwire can present a low-maintenance, easily retrievable fixed alternative (Fig 7).
- *Vacuform retainer (ESSIX).* If interocclusal space is limited and orthodontic treatment is not indicated, a vacuform retainer housing an ovate pontic can provide an interim prosthesis that will exert controllable pressure on the edentulous space (Moskowitz and coworkers 1997). In situations where a long healing period is anticipated, this interim prosthesis is contraindicated, as occlusal interference and excessive wear to the vacuform material must be expected. Here, consideration should be given to providing multiple retainers for the patient to reduce the number of return office visits (Figs 8a-b).

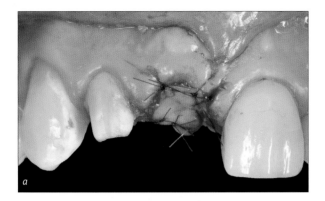
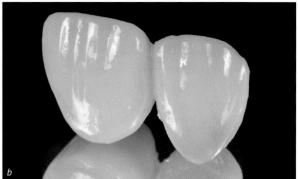

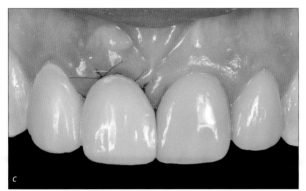

Figs 5a-c   A cantilevered interim fixed dental prosthesis (FDP) for sites 11 to 12.

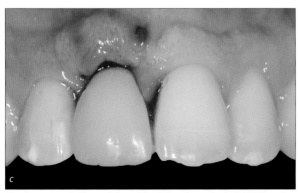
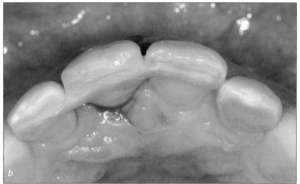

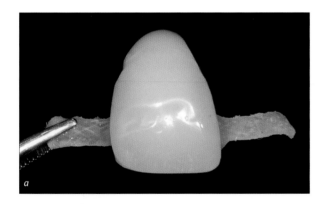

Figs 6a-c   A resin-fiber reinforced fixed dental prosthesis (RRFDP) replacing tooth 11.

- **Removable dental prosthesis (RDP).** If interocclusal space permits, patients can benefit from this prosthesis as the RDP gains its support from the palatal tissue and allows the pontic to be designed in ovate form for tissue shaping. This prosthesis is more durable than the vacuform retainer and should be considered if extended healing periods are expected and fixed alternatives are not an option (Figs 9a-c).

The selection of the type of interim prosthesis should be based on the esthetic demands, functional requirements, financial considerations, duration required, and ease of fabrication (Cho and coworkers 2007).

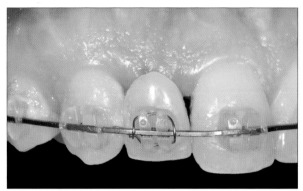

Fig 7   Orthodontic anchorage of a pontic at site 12.

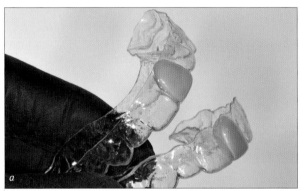
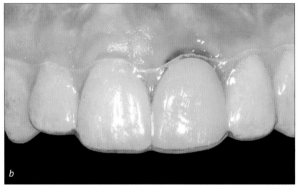

Figs 8a-b   A vacuform retainer (ESSIX) replacing tooth 21. Multiple ESSIX retainers made for long-term use due to wear.

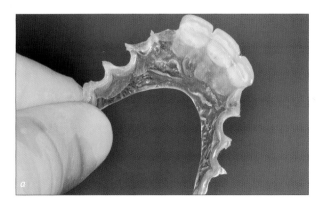
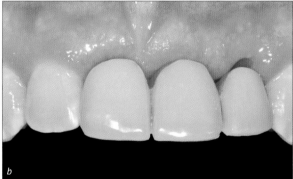
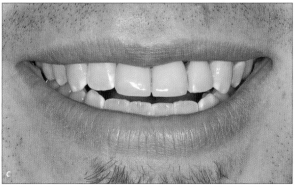

Figs 9a-c   A removable dental prosthesis replacing teeth 11 to 22.

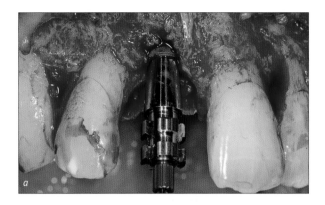

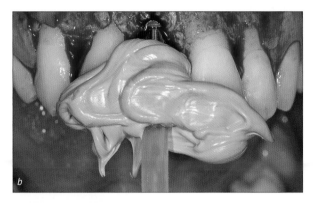

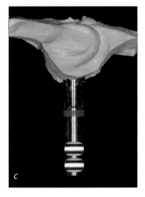

Figs 10a-c   *Surgical index of implant 11 with an impression coping and bite registration material.*

was to evaluate whether a provisional implant-supported crown provided an esthetic benefit on implants placed in the esthetic zone. Twenty single-tooth implants were inserted into consecutive patients and allowed to osseointegrate. At reentry, they were randomized into two groups: (1) provisional fabrication with tissue conditioning using the "dynamic compression technique" and (2) no provisional. All implants were restored with an all-ceramic crown. Follow-up evaluations were performed at 3 and 12 months. The two groups did not differ in terms of implant survival or bone levels, but did show a statistically significant difference in the mean values of combined modPES and WES (16.7 in group 1 vs. 10.5 in group 2). The study concluded that tissue conditioning with a provisional implant-supported restoration improved the final esthetic result. The International Team for Implantology also recommends their use in areas of esthetic demand based on the 5th ITI Consensus Conference (Morton and coworkers 2014).

Treatment guidelines
The use of provisional implant-retained restorations in the esthetic zone is recommended. Provisional restorations enhance communication between all members of the treatment team and the patient. They should be anatomically and functionally correct, and respect the emergence profile of the restoration apical to the planned mucosal margin (highest convexity) to allow for maximum tissue volume. Screw retention of the interim restoration is considered advantageous for multiple reasons (retrievability, tissue shaping, tissue health and maturation, ease of modification).

Provisional prostheses can be delivered at the time of implant placement (immediate) or after osseointegration (delayed). The immediate restoration of implants will require careful attention so as not to disturb the stability of the implant or to contaminate the submucosal tissue, bone grafts (if present), or implant body (if a horizontal defect is present).

6.2.2   After Implant Placement

At the time of implant placement or after osseointegration, the fabrication of an implant-supported provisional prosthesis can aid in developing ideal emergence profiles while initiating the shaping the peri-implant tissues, testing the contours of the final restoration and improving patient satisfaction.

Furze and coworkers (2016) conducted a randomized controlled trial on the esthetic outcomes of implant-supported crowns with and without peri-implant tissue conditioning using a fixed interim prosthesis. The objective

To prevent complications, the implant and temporary abutment can be carefully indexed by intraoral application of the provisional material, but any modification of the contours and final shaping (including occlusal adjustment) should be accomplished extraorally. Strong consideration should be given to screw retention in an effort to prevent the entrapment of cement in the submucosal tissues. In addition, screw retention will allow for "pulling" the restoration apically through the peri-implant tissues, as opposed to cementing, which will require "pushing" the prosthesis onto the abutment and implant, with cement easily getting trapped in the surgical site.

If immediate restoration is contraindicated, indexing the implant with an impression coping or with the implant mount will allow for retrofitting the working cast with accurate positioning of an implant analog for laboratory fabrication (Figs 10a-h). The provisional prosthesis can then be delivered at reentry or when the implant is ready for loading (Figs 11a-b). In delayed situations, the provisional can be fabricated intraorally or extraorally after an impression of the implant position has been made. Importantly, the emergence profile and contours of the provisional prosthesis should be designed such that they do not place excessive pressure on the peri-implant tissues, which could result in unwanted recession.

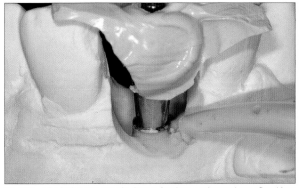

Fig 10d   The index was attached to an implant analog and retrofitted into a diagnostic cast with fast-setting stone.

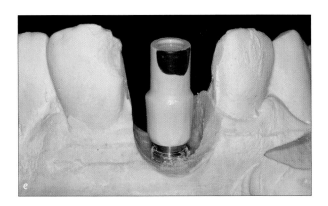

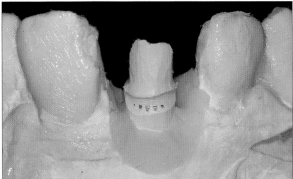

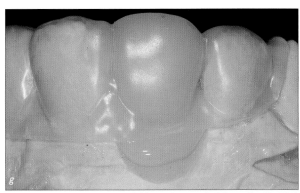

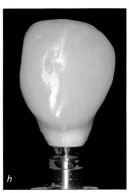

Figs 10e-h   A block-out material (Play-Doh; Mattel, El Segundo, CA, USA) was added to the undercuts around the analog to simulate peri-implant tissue. The provisional prosthesis was fabricated, shaped, and polished prior to delivery.

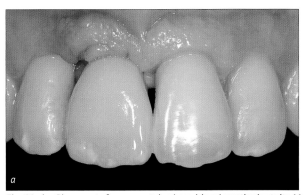

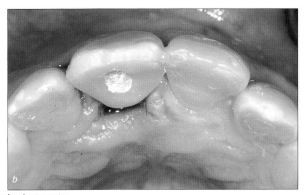

Figs 11a-b   Placement of a screw-retained provisional prosthesis at site 11 on implant reentry.

Wittneben and coworkers (2013) described a clinical procedure called the *dynamic compression technique* that consists of gradual conditioning of the soft tissues with a provisional restoration using selective pressure. This is accomplished through incremental adjustment of the contours of the restoration to establish an adequate emergence profile. Care is taken to recreate a balanced mucosal contour in harmony with the gingiva of the adjacent teeth, including papillary height/width, localization of the mucosal zenith, and the triangular shape of the tissue profile, as well as to establish an accurate proximal contact area with the adjacent tooth/implant crown.

A screw-retained interim prosthesis is best fabricated by using opaqued temporary titanium abutment picked up with a provisional material and contoured extraorally. Key components of this process focus on blocking out undercuts to allow for prosthesis removal, followed by careful contouring of the emergence profile in all dimensions to establish support for the peri-implant tissues through the interproximal contact points (Figs 12a-k). The contouring of the provisional restoration will be covered in Section 6.3.1.

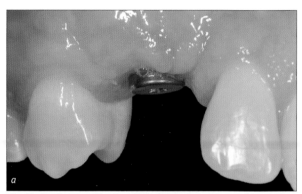
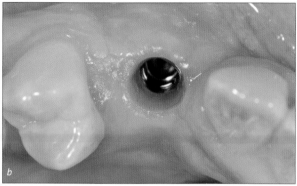

Figs 12a-b   Reentry of implant 13 for fabrication of the provisional. The transition zone was unshaped and contoured by the healing abutment.

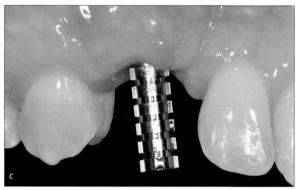
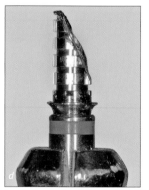
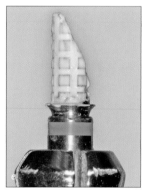

Figs 12c-e   Fabrication of a screw-retained provisional restoration is initiated by placing and reducing (extraorally) a temporary titanium coping based upon space requirements for the interim material. Once its proper reduction had been confirmed, the abutment was opaqued to minimize discoloration of the provisional material.

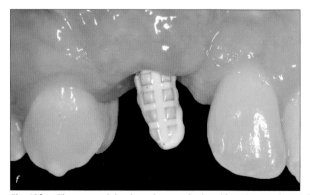
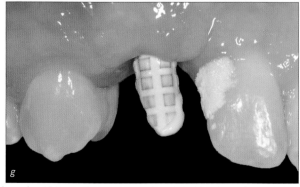

Figs 12f-g   The opaqued titanium abutment is placed into the mouth and tightened to 15 N·cm. The screw access is sealed with polytetrafluoroethylene (PTFE) tape and interproximal undercuts are blocked out.

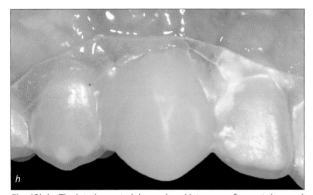
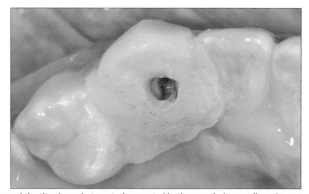

Figs 12h-i   The interim material was placed into a vacuform retainer and around the titanium abutment, then seated in the mouth. It was allowed to set according to the manufactures' instructions. Upon setting, the vacuform was removed and the screw access opened, allowing removal of the PTFE and loosening of the abutment screw.

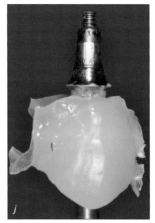
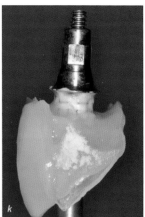

Figs 12j-k   The provisional prosthesis upon removal from the mouth showing a lack of material support in the transition zone. The addition of material is outlined in Figs 13a-f.

For more in-depth information on implant-supported provisional prostheses, please check out the ITI Online Academy's learning module "Provisional Implant Prostheses" by Dr. William Martin (charges apply). See what else the Online Academy has to offer at **academy.iti.org**

6.3 Management of Peri-implant Tissue

The peri-implant mucosa is composed of well-keratinized oral epithelium, sulcular epithelium, junctional epithelium, and underlying connective tissue. In natural teeth, the non-keratinized junctional epithelium attaches to the enamel surface via the internal basal lamina and desmosomes along the entire length of the junctional epithelium; however, the attachment of peri-implant epithelium to the implant surface is confined to the apical region (Dhir and coworkers 2013).

The orientation of the fibers in the transition zone runs parallel to the abutment. resulting in weak attachment to the abutment surface (Ericsson and Lindhe 1993), although the orientation of these fibers can also be dependent on the quality of the mucosa, and they tend to be more parallel in alveolar mucosa and perpendicularly in keratinized mucosa (Dhir and coworkers 2013).

Apart from the orientation of the fibers, the existence of connective tissue in the transition zone leads to poor mechanical resistance when compared to natural teeth (Hermann and coworkers 2001). Clinical implications include a transition zone that relies on structural support from the abutment and restoration to create the contours that mimic those of the surrounding gingival architecture. In order to achieve predictable esthetic results, proper management of the peri-implant tissues through contouring by the provisional restoration (or customized healing abutment) is critical to create mucosal contours that harmonize with the adjacent teeth.

6.3.1 Shaping the Transition Zone

The natural emergence profile of the tooth was first described by Croll in 1990 as a series of straight lines with curved transitions creating geometric patterns that facilitated the fabrication of natural-appearing restorations. These parameters have been carried to implant-supported restorations in an effort to recreate a natural-appearing restoration that supports the peri-implant mucosa and allows access for oral hygiene.

Several methods have been described for fabricating a provisional restoration with contours that achieve optimum esthetic results (Buser and coworkers 2004a; Shor and coworkers 2008; Wittneben and coworkers 2013). A key component common to them is that the provisional

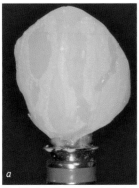 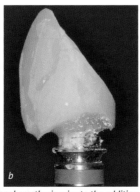 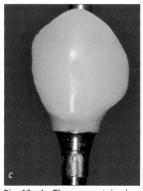 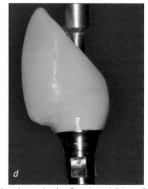

Figs 13a-b   The screw-retained provisional prosthesis prior to the addition of flowable composite resin in the transition zone for submucosal emergence.

Figs 13c-d   The screw-retained provisional prosthesis after the addition of flowable composite resin in the transition zone, creating ideal emergence profiles.

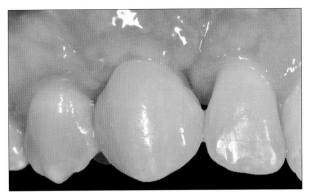

Fig 13e   Placement of the provisional on implant 13. Tissue blanching in the areas where shaping takes place.

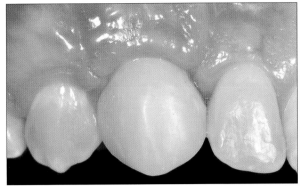

Fig 13f   Four weeks after placement of the provisional prosthesis on implant 13.

restoration emerges from the implant shoulder in the cylindrical form and is transformed to the trigonal shape of the tooth as it emerges at the mucosal margin on the facial and palatal aspects and contact points interproximally (Gallucci and coworkers 2004). These contours are best achieved with a screw-retained restoration, which will allow for full control over the emergence profile and easy retrievability and eliminate cement entrapments.

Careful attention should be given to the location and amount of tissue support applied in the transition zone, as over- or undercontouring will subtly influence mucosal and papillary levels (Grunder and coworkers 2005). A good starting point is to initiate the fabrication of the provisional by matching the clinical contours and contact points of the contralateral tooth (accomplished using a vacuform of the wax-up during planning), followed by careful addition of material in the transition zone starting at the implant shoulder and extending coronally (Figs 13a-f).

The emergence profile is contoured based upon the following principles:

- **Facial emergence.** Starting from the implant shoulder with a slightly flat/concave profile towards the height of convexity at the point where the mucosal margin will be established.
- **Interproximal emergence.** Starting from the implant shoulder with a straight emergence into slight convexity just apical to the contact area, providing support for the interproximal tissue.
- **Palatal emergence.** Starting from the implant shoulder with a straight to slightly convex emergence to the mucosal margin, focusing on matching the palatal contours of the adjacent teeth so there is a smooth transition between the two.

6.3.2   Capturing the Transition Zone

The shape of the transition zone successfully attained by the provisional restoration can be short-lived once the latter is removed for taking the impression. The poor structural support of the peri-implant mucosa will often lead to rapid collapse after removal of the provisional and in turn to inaccurate replication (analog and digital) of the transition zone on the master cast. This will result in the technician having to estimate and recreate the emergence profiles of the final restoration, potentially resulting in a variation of clinical outcomes by modifications in tissue support.

Several authors have reported on techniques to capture the shape of the provisional restoration and transfer it to the impression coping allowing for continue support of the transition zone during analog impression-taking (Zouras and coworkers 1995; Hinds 1997; Polack 2002; Spyropoulou and coworkers 2009; Schoenbaum and Han 2012; Patras and Martin 2016) (Figs 14a-l). This

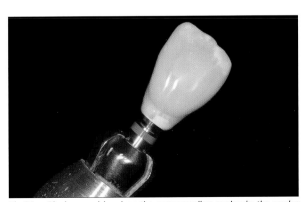

Fig 14a   Placing provisional on the corresponding analog in the analog holder (Institut Straumann AG).

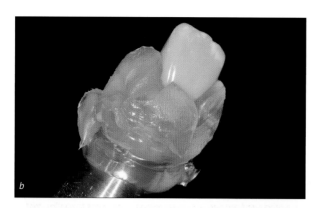

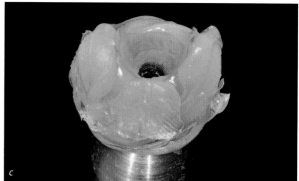

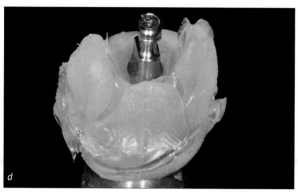

Figs 14b-d   Injecting clear bite registration material around the provisional prosthesis (b). Removing the provisional after setting (c). Placing an impression coping (d).

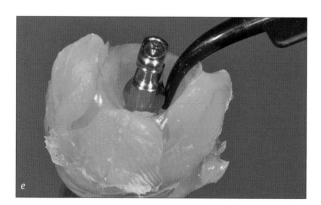

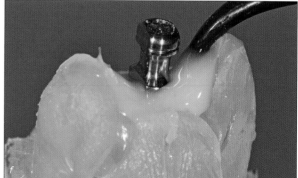

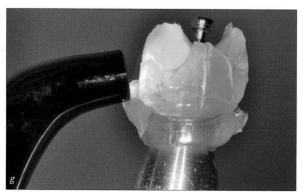

Figs 14e-g   Injection and light-curing of flowable composite resin around the impression coping.

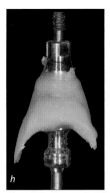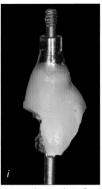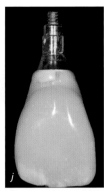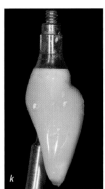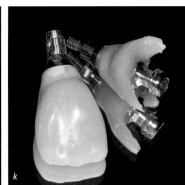

Figs 14h-l   Removal of the impression coping after setting, removing any blebs or artifacts and comparing to the provisional prosthesis to confirm that all submucosal contours have been matched.

technique is performed at chairside at the time of impression-taking and will add only a few minutes to the procedure, but will greatly enhance the communication of the ideal restoration contours to the laboratory (Figs 15a-g). Digital impressions require a slightly different approach that includes modification of the polyurethane cast after milling, which has been highlighted in recent publications (Hinds 2014; Joda and coworkers 2014; Lin and coworkers 2013b).

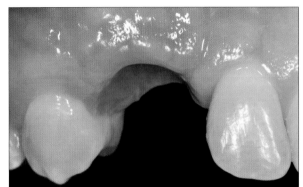

Fig 15a   Shaped transition zone of implant 13 after removing the provisional prosthesis.

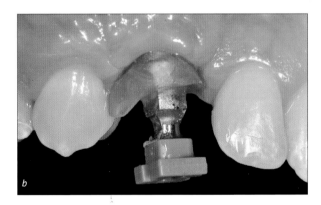

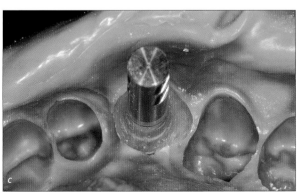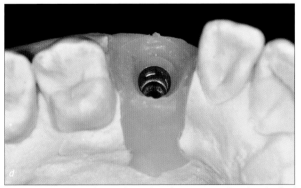

Figs 15b-d   A customized impression coping placed on implant 13. After the impression, the impression coping and analog were transferred to the final impression for fabrication of a tissue analog and a stone master cast. Upon setting, the master cast was removed from the impression, exposing the shaped transition zone in the tissue analog.

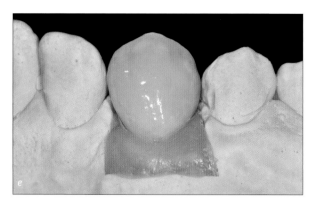

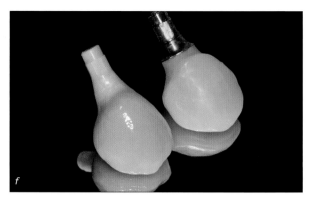

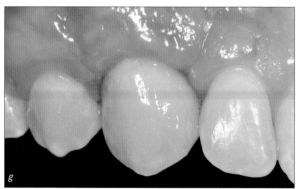

Figs 15e-g   The final screw-retained restoration 13 as delivered by the technician. The emergence profile of the restoration was created based upon the custom tissue analog on the master cast. The contours can be appreciated when the crown is placed next to the provisional prosthesis. At delivery, the peri-implant tissue was adequately supported for an ideal esthetic result.

6.4 Laboratory Communication

An important goal of the restorative phase in esthetic dentistry is the comprehensive communication of all clinical variables to the laboratory, providing the technician the opportunity to fabricate a restoration that mimics the missing dental unit(s) and blends in harmoniously with the surrounding dentition. Several key components are necessary to achieve this: photography, accurate records, and a detailed prescription.

6.4.1 Photography

The use of digital photography is an economical method to communicate key treatment variables in lieu of a patient's visit to the laboratory (Weston and Haupt 2011; Griffin 2009; Mendelson 2006). Using a dental camera that has features for macrophotography (macro lens and flash), the clinician can capture vital clinical information to complement the master casts and laboratory prescription (Lozano 2014; Lozano and Gonzaga 2015b).

The photos provided to the technician should include (Figs 16a-g):

- Frontal image at rest and full smile
- Retracted view showing the entire sextant surrounding the implant-supported restoration
- Close-up of the implant-supported restoration and adjacent teeth
- Slightly angled views showing the contour and texture of the teeth adjacent to the implant site

- View with the shade tab(s) placed in the same plane as the teeth to be matched, taken at multiple angles to minimize flash reflection. The goal for the shade tab is to communicate the translucencies, hue, chroma, and—most importantly—value of the surrounding dentition.
- When preparing teeth adjacent to the implant site, die shades with corresponding die tabs placed at the edge of the preparation
- Frontal and profile views of the provisional restoration

During shade communication, the standardization of white balance is important to assure that accurate color representation is achieved and implemented by the technician. This can be done before taking photos with through customized Kelvin settings in the camera, based upon the temperature of the macro flash and room lighting, or at the time of the photo, with a spectrally neutral gray card held within view of the image (Lozano 2015a). If a gray card is utilized, the color will be adjusted in the photo-editing software. If images are to be viewed on multiple monitors, calibration of the monitors is also critical to achieve consistent results. Several adjuncts have been developed to improve shade communication, including of shade colorimeters, polarizers, and digital shade-matching systems. The choice of instruments is often driven by the technician and should be embraced accordingly. In general, the more information that is provided to the technician through photography, the better the chance for an accurate adaptation of the implant-supported restoration to the adjacent teeth.

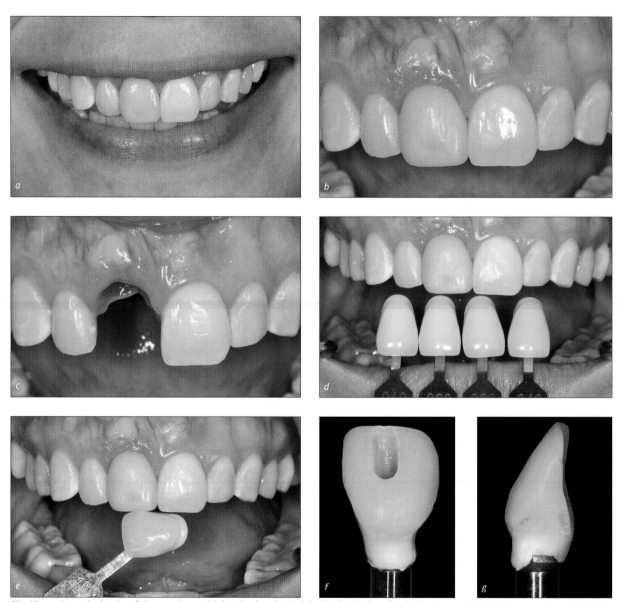

Figs 16a-g   *A standard series of photographs provided to the dental technician for fabrication of an implant-supported crown 11.*

For more in-depth information on dental photography, please check out the ITI Online Academy's learning module "Digital Clinical Photography" by Dr. Frank E. Lozano (charges apply). See what else the Online Academy has to offer at **academy.iti.org**

6.4.2   Records

In order to achieve optimum esthetic results, it is the restorative clinician's responsibility to provide the technician with accurate records for the fabrication of the implant-supported restoration. These records include: an impression (digital or analog) or master cast of the implant position related to the adjacent teeth, a recording of the shaped peri-implant tissues in the transition zone (customized impression coping), an impression with the provisional in place, and the interocclusal relationship to the opposing arch (jaw relation record and opposing cast).

When taking an impression of dental implants, overextending the impression material into the vestibule will capture the alveolar contours and provide valuable information for the technician when developing the emergence profile of the restoration. The use of photographic retractors held by the patient will assist in retracting the lips, allowing access to this area (Figs 17a-b).

6.4.3   Prescription

The prescription is an instruction written by the dental practitioner that authorizes the technician to manufacture a dental restoration. It is an integral component in the efficient communication between the clinician and technician and should contain information highlighting the key components in the design and fabrication of the restoration. A well-written prescription should not leave any areas left to interpretation by the technician to prevent delays in manufacturing or unexpected outcomes in restoration design or materials used.

A prescription for a single tooth anterior implant restoration should include:

- Dentist and patient demographics
- A return/due date
- Enclosures: impressions, casts, jaw relation records, photos, articulators, implant components (impression copings, screws, analogs, abutments), etc.
- Information on the implant system (implant connection type, platform, and diameter) with corresponding reference numbers.
- General description of the planned restoration (screw-retained or cemented), abutment design, and location in the mouth.
- Shade communication

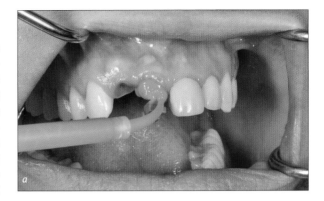

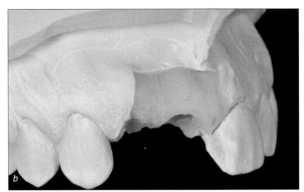

Figs 17a-b   Photographic retractors to assist in retracting the lips for overextension of the impression material into the vestibule. The master cast will provide valuable information for the technician to generate ideal emergence profiles in the definitive restoration.

- Desired restorative material and emergence profile design
- Desired abutment design and material and, if cemented restorations are planned, description of the location of the margin placement circumferentially
- Prescriber's signature and license information
- Point of origin: the dentist should be made aware of where all components of the restoration were fabricated (if outside the intended laboratory); this information should be reported back to the prescriber upon return of the laboratory work

6.5   Screw-retained vs. Cemented Restorations

The decision on the type of retention for the single-tooth implant-supported restoration is often influenced by several variables including: esthetic demands, cost, materials, retrievability and the implant location (depth and angulation).

In a recent systematic review on esthetic outcomes in implant dentistry, Martin and coworkers identified 24 studies (1 cohort study, 1 retrospective cross-sectional study, and 22 case series) where a cemented or screw-retained crown was defined in the protocol and esthetic outcomes were reported. No firm conclusions relating esthetic benefits based upon the mode of retention could be identified from the review. The limitations of this review could be due to the wide variation in crown and abutment materials and their diverse indications for use and the lack of their reporting in the literature. Future studies should focus on recording all aspects of the indications and use of materials, their combinations, and compatibility in diverse treatment indications as well as the mode of manufacture (Morton and coworkers 2014).

Wittneben and coworkers (2014) conducted a systematic review on the performance of screw-retained versus cemented prostheses, assessing the survival outcomes and reported complications. After extracting data from 73 articles fit for inclusion, they reported no statistical difference between cemented and screw-retained restorations in terms of survival or failure rates. They also reported that screw-retained restorations exhibited fewer technical and biological complications overall. In addition, no differences in failure rates were reported when evaluating different abutment materials (titanium, gold, ceramics). Given these results, the choice of retention—screw-retained or cemented—will provide an "equal opportunity" for an esthetic restoration, and decisions for either option can be based upon the clinician's preference (Morton and coworkers 2014).

**Treatment Guidelines
(5th ITI Consensus Conference)**
The abutment and prosthesis material are a patient- and site-specific choice for the clinician. Provided that the material chosen is of high quality and documented, the design of the abutment and/or prosthesis is more critical than the material chosen, for reasons including:

- Controlling emergence profile
- Material properties and strength
- Access to finish lines
- Retrievability

A key component of cemented restorations is the ability to remove excess cement at the time of crown placement. Residual cement is a common complication of cemented prostheses and has been linked to peri-implant disease. Removal of the residual cement may resolve the issue if addressed early, but is dependent on the ability to locate and adequately remove the foreign material (Wadhwani and coworkers 2012b; Sailer and coworkers 2012).

Clinical techniques have been reported in the literature as a way to reduce excess residual cement, ranging from cement application techniques to venting and abutment modification (Wadhwani and coworkers 2012a; Wadhwani and coworkers 2016; Wadhwani and Chung 2014; Wadhwani and coworkers 2011). The design of the custom abutment will have a profound effect on the ability to access the residual cement for removal.

Linkevicius and coworkers (2011) reported on the influence of the margin location on the amount of undetected residual cement after delivering cemented implant restorations. In their study, custom abutments were fabricated with cement margins ranging from 1 mm supramucosally to 3 mm submucosally, followed by a standardized delivery of a cemented and polished metal crown. They reported that all cement residue was removed only when the margin was visible; the greatest amount of residual cement was left when the crown margin was more than 2 mm below the mucosa. This finding underscores the need to carefully manage the peri-implant tissues through tissue shaping with provisional restorations and transferring the contours of the transition zone to the technician. This will allow for accurate fabrication of the custom abutment, with the cement lines positioned in a circumferentially accessible position for cement removal at the time of delivery.

Screw-retained restorations offer a distinct advantage over cemented restorations, as they eliminate the use of cement and offer improved control over emergence profiles and retrievability.

For more in-depth information on restoration retention, please check out the ITI Online Academy's congress lecture "Cement versus Screw Retention" by Dr. Julia G. Wittneben (charges apply). See what else the Online Academy has to offer at **academy.iti.org**

6.6 Material Selection for Abutments and Crowns

When designing a single-tooth implant-supported restoration, the clinician may choose from three main types of abutment designs on which to build the restoration: prefabricated (standard/stock), cast custom abutments, or CAD/CAM custom abutments.

The treatment of patients with esthetic demands requires careful consideration of the choice of the abutment and restorative material and should be based on the following factors: visibility of the region, tissue phenotype, color of the neighboring teeth, and the esthetic expectations of the patient (Sailer and coworkers 2007).

6.6.1 Prefabricated Abutments

A range of prefabricated abutments are manufactured by each implant manufacturer to provide clinicians with an off-the-shelf restorative option. Their indication is for cemented prostheses; however, they can also be modified to support a cross-pinned restoration. For implants that have been placed in an ideal position, suitable prefabricated abutments are available, with modification of the abutment thought to be a simpler and more economical procedure than fabricating a cast custom abutment. In situations where the implant position is not ideal or significantly aberrant, restoration with a prefabricated abutment may require compromise or might be impossible.

One of the major disadvantages of prefabricated abutments is related to their shape. The majority of prefabricated abutments are not anatomically designed for optimal submucosal contour support. They often exhibit flat or overcontoured emergence profiles, cylindrical configurations, and crown margins that do not follow the contours of the peri-implant mucosal margins. This may lead to problems with the management of soft tissue (especially in esthetically critical areas), difficulty in seating overcontoured restorations, or incomplete cement removal with deep submucosal margins, which may contribute to peri-implant disease (Agar and coworkers 1997; Pauletto and coworkers 1999; Weber and coworkers 2006; Gapski and coworkers 2008; Wilson Jr 2009; Linkevicius and coworkers 2011; Linkevicius and coworkers 2013).

Traditional laboratory techniques generally rely on choosing larger prefabricated abutments and milling the external contours to suit the clinical situation (Figs 18a-c). This can weaken the abutment walls and offers limited correction facilities for angulation change. The laboratory modification of the abutment is also a time-consuming and often costly process. This modification is also a contraindication for ceramic abutment materials (zirconia), where adjustments can lead to the formation of flaws and localized phase conversions, which may negatively affect the long-term performance of these abutments (Kelly and Denry 2008). Therefore, in the esthetic zone, stock abutments are often a compromise from the ideal.

Many of the problems associated with prefabricated abutments can be addressed using cast or CAD/CAM custom abutments.

Recent developments in the prefabricated abutment range have seen the introduction of the titanium-base (Ti-base) concept (Lin and coworkers 2014). This type of abutment is designed to allow for extraoral cementation of the restoration onto a prefabricated machined titanium implant/abutment connection, resulting in a customized emergence profile. This also permits several different restorative material combinations, maximizing the potential for esthetic results. The Ti-base abutment is suited for restorations with direct palatal/occlusal screw access or for individualized ceramic abutments and cemented all-ceramic crowns (Figs 19a-b). This abutment design can mitigate several concerns raised with all ceramic abutments, which can be prone to fracture within the implant/abutment connection, as well as address concerns arising from wear of the titanium implant interface by the ceramic abutment (Klotz and coworkers 2011; Stimmelmayr and coworkers 2012). Their design, however, can limit the customization of the emergence profile close to the implant and prevent proper seating of the restoration if there is bone present.

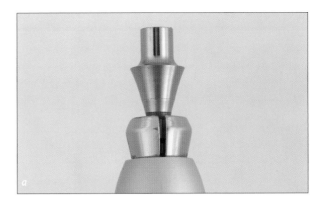

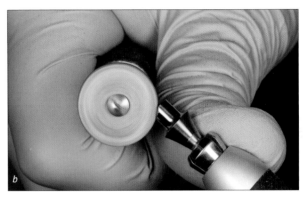

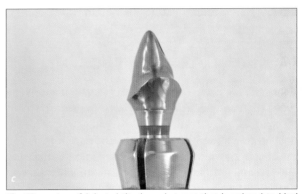

Figs 18a-c   A prefabricated titanium abutment that is reduced to ideal contours to support a cemented restoration.

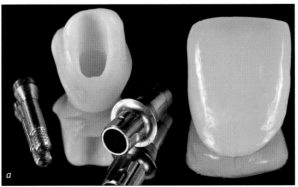

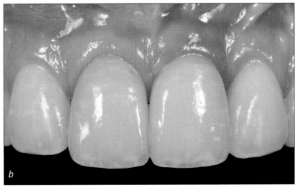

Figs 19a-b   Ti-base abutment (Variobase abutment; Institut Straumann AG) with a lithium disilicate custom abutment and crown 21.

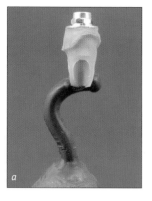
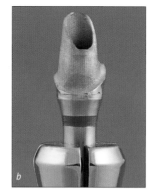
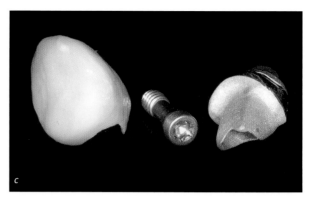
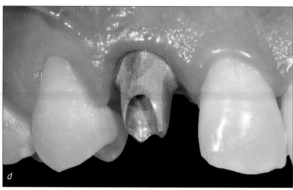
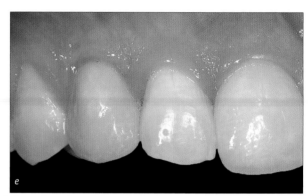

Figs 20a-e   Fabrication of a custom abutment using the lost-wax technique. Delivery of a custom abutment and a cemented metal-ceramic crown 13.

6.6.2   Cast Custom Abutments

Cast custom abutments enable the technician to design the abutment with ideal angulations, contours, and margin placement to facilitate adequate function, tissue health, and esthetics. These abutments were originally intended for application with ceramics in the fabrication of a single-piece abutment-crown complex, but cast custom abutments could also be shaped to support a cemented or cross-pin retained crown (Lewis and coworkers 1988).

Cast custom abutments are fabricated using the traditional lost-wax process, waxing up the desired abutment shape onto a plastic abutment burn-out pattern or by waxing and casting onto a pre-machined gold abutment (Figs 20a-e). The use of a cast-to abutments, where a pre-machined connection is waxed and cast onto, has been found to have a significantly superior fit than that of an entirely cast abutment fabricated from a burn-out coping (Byrne and coworkers 2008). However, it has been shown that during the processes of casting and finishing, "cast-to" abutments may be distorted and damaged reducing the accuracy of fit (Carr and coworkers 1996; Jaime and coworkers 2007). This technique is also limited to the high noble alloys that are compatible with machined cast-to abutments made from gold.

Due to the labor-intensive process of waxing, casting, milling, and finishing, as well as the rising cost of high-noble alloys, these abutments are often associated with high laboratory bills. Concerns have also been raised about the potential for galvanic reaction and corrosion between the gold abutment and titanium implant, as well as the biological response around gold and ceramics compared to the relatively biocompatible titanium (Linkevicius and Vaitelis 2015).

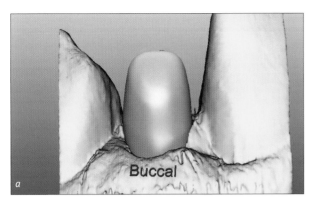
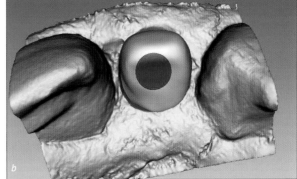
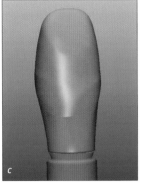
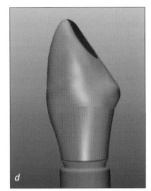
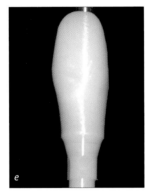
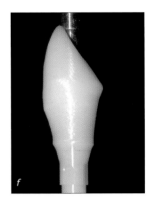

Figs 21a-f   CAD/CAM design and milling of a zirconia abutment for direct application of ceramics.

In order to reduce material costs and improve biocompatibility, titanium has also been used for cast custom abutments (Abduo and coworkers 2011). However, titanium and base-metal alloys are much more difficult to cast due to their higher reactivity, higher melting temperatures, and lower density, resulting in a poorer fit compared to gold, as well as alpha-case formation on the surface of the titanium following casting. The thickness of the alpha case has been reported as 50–450 µm, depending on the investment, casting machine, casting temperature, and the size/shape of the pattern (Miyakawa and coworkers 1989). The presence of this layer affects the surface finish, physical properties, and corrosion resistance of the titanium, and its removal can cause issues pertaining to restoration fit.

Due to the labor-intensive nature, rising gold costs, biocompatibility concerns, and casting problems associated with cast custom abutments, alternative fabrication methods for customized abutments have been developed that employ CAD/CAM technology.

6.6.3   CAD/CAM Custom Abutments

CAD/CAM custom abutments are virtually designed and then manufactured to the desired shape and form, based on a digital scan of the implant location and surrounding teeth (Figs 21a-f). This allows the creation of an ideally contoured emergence profile and margin location specifically designed for each patient, with consistent manufacturing quality and homogenous material properties. For these reasons, CAD/CAM abutments are perceived to be a better alternative to standard prefabricated abutments (Priest 2005; Strub and coworkers 2006). Manually-aided design MAD/CAM abutments can also be fabricated through a combination of conventional waxing techniques followed by scanning and milling resulting in a similar outcome to the CAD/CAM approach (Glauser and coworkers 2004) (Figs 22a-e).

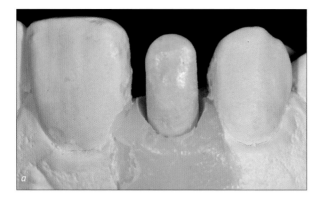

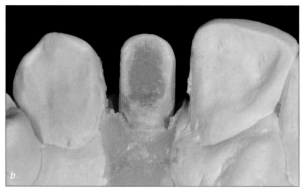

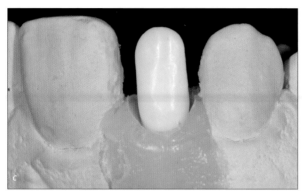

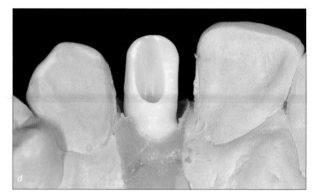

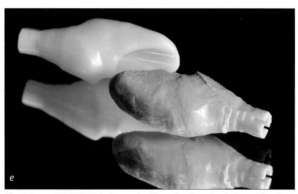

Figs 22a-e   MAD/CAM design and milling of a zirconia abutment for direct application of ceramics.

CAD/CAM abutments can be designed to support cemented or cross-pin-retained crowns. Alternatively, these abutments can also be designed for direct application of ceramics for a single-piece crown/abutment complex (Figs 23a-e).

The refining of ceramic bonding techniques for titanium, due to better control of the oxide layer, has led some authors to recommend ceramically veneered titanium crowns and fixed partial dentures for routine clinical use (Haag and Nilner 2010). But this option can be challenged, as ceramics compatible with titanium are limited in availability and often considered technique-sensitive.

Zirconia abutments and/or full contour crowns can also be milled in the "green" state, optimizing the physical properties of the material with very little monoclinic phase present (Denry and Kelly 2008).

In a five-year randomized controlled clinical trial by Zembic and coworkers (2013) comparing zirconia and titanium abutments supporting single-tooth implant-supported crowns, the authors reported no statistically or clinically relevant differences between survival rates or technical and biological complication rates between the two abutment materials.

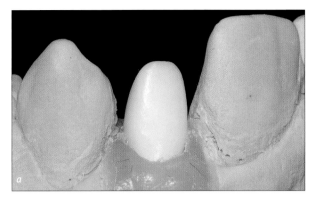
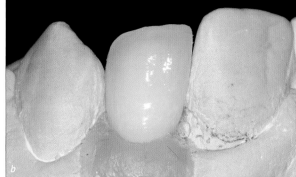

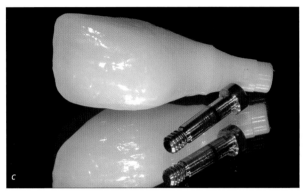
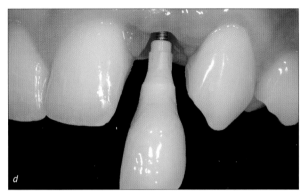

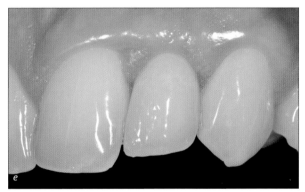

Figs 23a-e   A CAD/CAM zirconia abutment (Institut Straumann AG) ve-neered with feldspathic ceramics for restoring implant 22.

These findings support the increased use of CAD/CAM custom abutments to support individualized crowns and veneered-abutment restorations, as the abutment can be adequately contoured to provide porcelain support without additional cost. Preconceptions regarding CAD/CAM custom abutments have led them to be perceived as being of consistently higher quality and biologically more acceptable while costing less than cast custom abutments or customized prefabricated abutments (Kapos and Evans 2014; Priest 2005).

6.6.4 Original vs. Non-original

Many CAD/CAM systems are now available that produce abutments for a wide range of implants systems (open system). While this is convenient for laboratories, which may service customers utilizing many different implant systems, clinical and laboratory research has indicated that these third-party (non-original) abutments may not perform as well as proprietary (original) abutments made by the respective implant manufacturer (Figs 24a-d).

Implant/abutment connections have become very sophisticated and are specifically designed to minimize the mechanical risk of fracture, screw loosening, and biological complications such as early bone loss due to movement and microgaps at the implant/abutment interface. Non-original components often do not replicate the intended implant/abutment configuration designed by the implant manufacturer. During in-vitro testing, non-proprietary abutments have demonstrated substandard fit, decreased rotational stability, and inferior

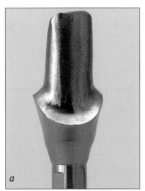
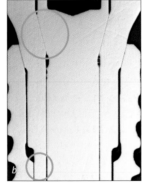

Figs 24a-b   *Original abutment manufactured by Institut Straumann AG for the bone level implant. Note the design of the abutment screw head and extension of the abutment within the connection.*

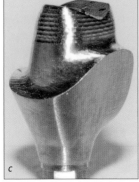
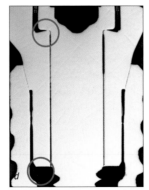

Figs 24c-d   *Non-original abutment made for the Straumann Bone Level implant. Note the variation in screw head design and the extension of the abutment within the implant connection.*

biomechanical performance of the implant/abutment connection and have the potential for increased risk of failures (Mattheos and Janda 2012; Hamilton and coworkers 2013; Berberi and coworkers 2014; Gigandet and coworkers 2014; Joda and coworkers 2015). For the best possible long-term biological and mechanical outcome, it is recommended that only proprietary componentry from the respective implant manufacturer should be utilized in prosthetic reconstructions that engage the internal connection within the implant.

6.6.5 Abutment Materials

When selecting appropriate materials for an implant abutment in the esthetic zone, consideration should be given to the material's physical properties and biocompatibility as well as esthetics. The current materials used for implant abutments include titanium, gold alloys, non-precious alloys, zirconia, alumina, and lithium disilicate. These materials are often used in various combinations and configurations based on the abutment design, and may also incorporate feldspathic ceramics that can be applied submucosally, as well as resin cements that may be used to join multiple components of an abutment assembly (Thoma and coworkers 2015).

Fenner and coworkers (2016) reported on the clinical performance of metal (titanium) and ceramic (alumina) abutments, showing similar results after a mean observation period of 7.2 years with regards to survival rate. Zembic and coworkers (2015) conducted an eleven-year follow-up of a prospective study evaluating zirconia abutments supporting single all-ceramic crowns in the anterior and premolar regions, reporting 100% survival of the abutments and restorations and cumulative success rates of 96.3% for abutments and 90.7% for crowns (2 cases of abutment screw loosening, 3 cases of minor crown chipping). There is currently no one ideal material that can be used universally for all abutments, and the advantages and limitations of each should be tailored to the clinical situation.

6.6.6 Biocompatibility

Biocompatibility is thought to be a key factor for long-term peri-implant tissue health. It is well known that titanium is an inert and highly biocompatible material, with a long history of use as a material for dental implants and prosthetic abutments. Due to its color and difficult customization and manufacturing with direct ceramic bonding, alternative materials to titanium such as gold alloys and various ceramics have been introduced. Of these materials, zirconia ceramics are comparable to titanium with regard to biocompatibility (Linkevicius and Vaitelis 2015).

Animal histological studies have suggested that the tissue response to gold alloys and dental feldspathic ceramics may not be as favorable as that of titanium or zirconia (Abrahamsson and coworkers 1998). However, this has yet to be validated in any robust clinical studies, with a systematic review finding no difference in peri-implant bone levels for gold alloy or zirconia abutments compared to titanium (Linkevicius and Apse 2008; Linkevicius and Vaitelis 2015).

6.6.7 Influence on Esthetics

Thin peri-implant mucosa can lead to discoloration of the mucosal margin around metallic abutments (Jung and coworkers 2008b). Mimicking the appearance of natural teeth and gingiva requires not only careful and skillful execution of the surgical phase of dental implant therapy, but appropriate prosthetic soft-tissue management and material selection. Ceramic abutments have been introduced to overcome the challenges associated with discoloration of the mucosal margin associated with thin peri-implant tissue when titanium abutments are utilized. However, both animal and clinical studies have demonstrated that when there is an adequate thickness of peri-implant mucosa, no difference in esthetic outcomes or pink esthetic scores (PES) is found between any of the available abutment materials (Jung and coworkers 2007b; Jung and coworkers 2008b; Zembic and coworkers 2009).

In situations where soft-tissue thickness is deficient, the peri-implant tissue around zirconia abutments displayed a better shade match to the soft tissue around adjacent natural teeth than titanium when measured spectrophotometrically (Linkevicius and Vaitelis 2015). In patients with thin tissues, a tissue-colored abutment emerging through the tissue can offer esthetic advantages and should be given consideration in situations where a high esthetic risk prevails (Thoma and coworkers 2015).

6.6.8 Physical Properties

Appropriate materials must be selected based on anticipated forces and the functional demands of each patient to minimize the risks of mechanical or technical complications.

Metallic titanium abutments have a well-documented history, with low rates of mechanical complications. The introduction of more esthetic ceramic abutment materials was originally associated with an increased risk of abutment fractures due to the poor mechanical properties of the ceramics. Zirconia has shown to be a more promising ceramic solution, with significantly improved mechanical strength and fracture resistance compared with other ceramic materials. In support, clinical studies have reported no difference in survival rates over five years between zirconia and titanium abutments (Sailer and coworkers 2015; Fenner and coworkers 2016), although some concerns have been raised as to the long-term behavior of this material and propensity for low temperature degradation/aging (Denry and Kelly 2008).

Laboratory studies and clinical observations of fractured zirconia abutments have shown that deep conical connections were particularly susceptible to the abutment fracturing within the connection, due to its thin cross-section in these areas (Foong and coworkers 2013). There have also been several reported incidences of zirconia abutments causing wear of the titanium implant at the implant/abutment interface (Klotz and coworkers 2011; Stimmelmayr and coworkers 2012). In several instances this resulted in titanium particles being deposited in the peri-implant mucosa, causing a "titanium tattoo" effect. Importantly, the use of a zirconia abutment requires a precise and stable match with the titanium implant connection designed for this use. Many studies evaluate zirconia abutments placed into implants developed prior to their availability, which may have had an influence on their performance under load.

For more in-depth information on restorative materials in esthetics, please check out the ITI Online Academy's congress lecture "Restorative Materials for Esthetic Restorations" by Dr. Irena Sailer (charges apply). See what else the Online Academy has to offer at **academy.iti.org**

For more in-depth information on abutment design for esthetic outcomes, please check out the ITI Online Academy's congress lecture "Abutment Design and Restorative Considerations for Esthetic Outcomes" by Dr. Konrad Meyenberg (charges apply). See what else the Online Academy has to offer at **academy.iti.org**

For more in-depth information on abutment selection, please check out the ITI Online Academy's learning module "Abutment Selection" by Dr. Julia G. Wittneben (charges apply). See what else the Online Academy has to offer at **academy.iti.org**

6.7 Prosthetic Design

The increasing number of restorative abutments and implant components has given the clinician many different options for restoring a single implant, with various different prosthetic designs. There is no one ideal design, each presenting some challenges associated with fabrication, delivery, or performance.

The general types of implant restoration designs in the esthetic zone include:

One-piece screw-retained crown/abutment complexes with either gold alloy or zirconia custom abutments and direct feldspathic ceramic application, with conventional direct screw access or – the more recently developed – angulated screw-channel abutments (Figs 25a-e).

Cement-retained metal-ceramic or all-ceramic crowns cemented onto a titanium custom abutment (CAD/CAM), ceramics/gold abutment, zirconia abutments (CAD/CAM), or customized prefabricated titanium or zirconia abutment (Figs 26a-e).

Cement-retained crowns with direct screw access, which incorporates a titanium abutment, such as the Ti-Base, onto which a conventional crown with an occlusal/palatal screw access hole is cemented extraorally (Figs 27a-f).

Transverse-screw or cross-pinned restorations, which utilize a titanium or gold abutment on which a metal-ceramic crown is retained with a lateral screw (Figs 28a-d).

6.7.1 Crown/Veneer Materials

In order to achieve a lifelike appearance of the restoration, it is important to understand the optical properties of different ceramic materials and abutment combinations in relation to the adjacent natural teeth. One of the most versatile and esthetic materials used is feldspathic ceramics, due to its ability to be individually layered and characterized to imitate the appearance of internal structures of natural teeth.

The ability to achieve excellent results heavily relies on the skill and artistic abilities of the dental technician. Due to its lower physical strength it needs to be veneered onto either a metallic (gold alloy, titanium, or non-precious) or stronger ceramic (zirconia, alumina, or lithium disilicate) core structure, which will significantly influence the optical properties and appearance of the restoration. Alternatively, stronger monolithic ceramic restorations can be fabricated from zirconia or lithium disilicate, which can be characterized by surface staining and have a reduced risk of ceramic chipping compared with layered feldspathic restorations (Kelly and Benetti 2011).

Ultimately, the choice of the crown/veneering material should be made based upon an evaluation of the surrounding dentition and restorations, characteristics of the individual teeth, and esthetic and functional requirements.

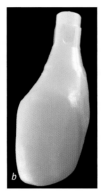
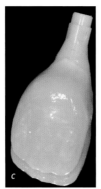
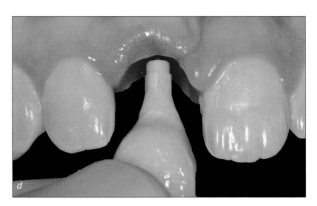

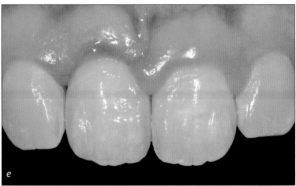

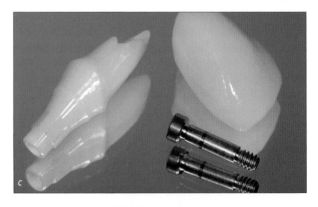

Figs 25a-e   A MAD/CAM zirconia abutment (Institut Straumann AG) designed for direct ceramic application, creating a screw-retained restoration.

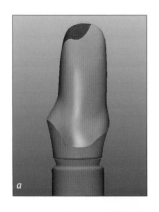
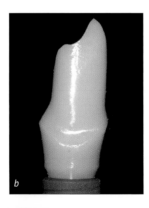

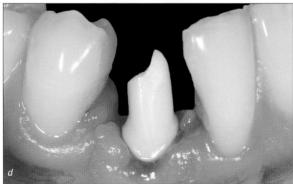
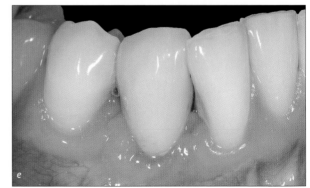

Figs 26a-e   A CAD/CAM zirconia abutment (Institut Straumann AG) created for a cemented lithium disilicate crown.

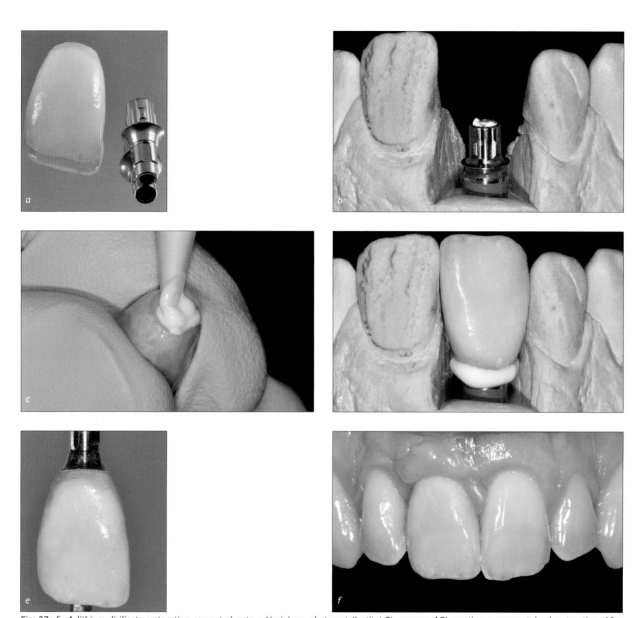

Figs 27a-f   A lithium disilicate restoration cemented onto a Variobase abutment (Institut Straumann AG) creating a screw-retained restoration. After confirmation of shade and fit, the restoration was cemented onto the abutment extraorally according to the manufacturer's instructions.

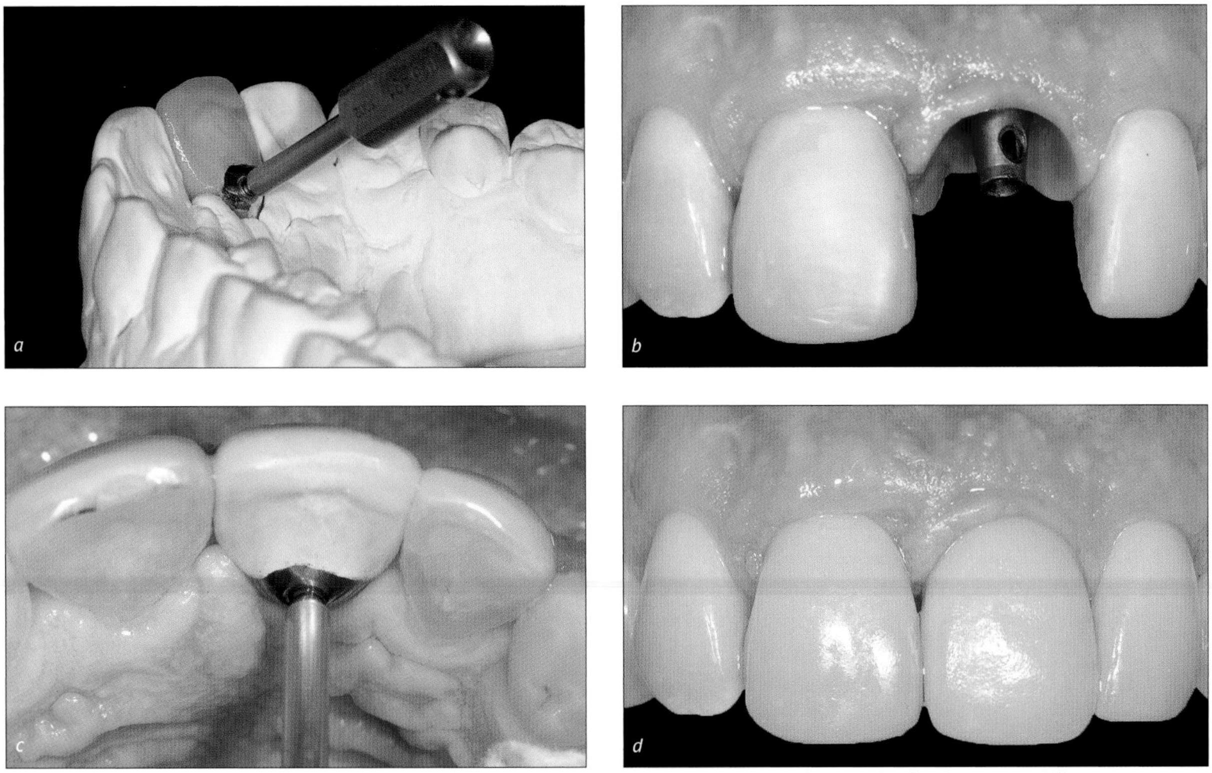

Figs 28a-d   Transverse screw-retained metal-ceramic restoration 21 placed onto a transverse screw abutment (Institut Straumann AG).

6.8 Handling of Abutments and Restorations

Any delivery of implant-supported restorations, whether screw-retained or cemented, begins with an understanding of the manufacturer's recommendations for handling and modifying of their respective materials. This includes the cement used to retain the restoration. With the wide array of available material options for crowns and abutments, specific protocols are in place for modifying, polishing, and cementing (where indicated) to achieve optimum strength, wear, and retention properties.

Upon receipt of the implant supported restoration from the laboratory, the fit of the abutment and crown should first be confirmed on the master cast. Preference should be given to a confirmation of fit on a solid cast, as this provides the highest accuracy in verifying interproximal contact points. Clinically, for cemented restorations, the abutment should be seated with light tightening to allow for expansion of the peri-implant tissue until fully seated. Radiographic confirmation should be performed in situations where clinical verification is unattainable. The restoration is then seated on the abutment adjusting and polishing interproximal contacts as needed.

With screw-retained restorations, the restoration is carefully seated by lightly tightening the abutment screw while simultaneously evaluating the interproximal contact points (adjusting and polishing as needed) until fully seated. Radiographic confirmation is also recommended if clinical verification is unattainable. If the patient experiences pain upon placement of the abutment or screw-retained crown, the submucosal contours in relation to proximal bone levels should be evaluated. Encroachment on this tissue can cause elevated pressure and pain, in which case a modification of the submucosal contours of the abutment/restoration will be needed to relieve pressure in these areas. In extreme situations, the removal of bone may be necessary. The use of a provisional restoration to shape the transition zone can isolate these problems and allow for correction prior to taking the impression.

When the restoration is successfully seated and the shade match is confirmed, abutment screws should be tightened to the manufacturer's recommendation. Attention should be given to the condition of the abutment screw, as repeated loosening and tightening can lead to decreased clamping force through elongation of the screw and subsequent increased leakage (Butkevica and coworkers 2016; Calcaterra and coworkers 2016; Haack and coworkers 1995; Winkler and coworkers 2003; Theoharidou and coworkers 2008; Yilmaz and coworkers 2015). The screw head should then be protected with polytetrafluoroethylene (PTFE) tape, as it is easy to manipulate, radiopaque, and associated with less malodor when retrieved (Morágues and Belser 2010). Improved access seals have been reported when using gutta-percha over PTFE, but the clinical advantages, such as ease of manipulation and retrieval, of the latter have led to its increased clinical use (Cavalcanti and coworkers 2016). The access hole should be closed with a composite resin material that creates a seal and allows for future removal if needed.

For cemented crowns, the preparation of the crown and the selection of the cement type used should be based upon the manufacturer's recommendations. The cementation of the restoration should focus on minimizing cement residue using techniques recommended in the literature: circumferential rim application, venting, or pre-seating on duplicated abutments (Santosa and coworkers 2010; Wadhwani and Piñeyro 2009; Wadhwani and coworkers 2016). A properly designed abutment with circumferential cement lines located less than 2 mm below the mucosal margin will minimize the potential for residual cement after cleaning (Linkevicius and coworkers 2011). The final occlusal adjustment should be followed with sequential polishing procedures with abrasive rubber cups/points or sandpaper disks, followed by diamond polishing pastes to minimize surface roughness and achieve a superficial smoothness (Silva and coworkers 2014). When polishing ceramics after occlusal adjustment, it is recommended to consult the manufacturer's recommendations, as not all ceramics polish in the same manner.

7 Clinical Case Presentations

7.1 Replacement of a Failing Upper Left Central Incisor: Immediate Placement of an RC Bone Level Implant and Provisionalization

E. R. Lorenzana, J. Gillespie

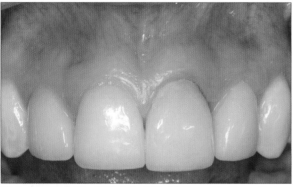

Fig 1   The patient presented with a medium to high lip line when smiling, exposing the papillae throughout the anterior sextant, but with the upper lip obscuring the gingival margins of the central incisors.

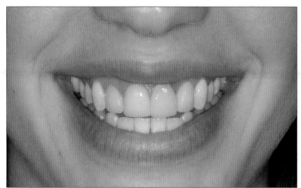

Fig 2   Retracted view. Medium to thick soft-tissue phenotype with symmetrical gingival margins.

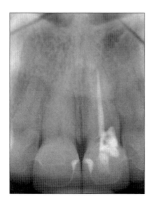

Fig 3   Periapical radiograph. Internal resorption defect coronally and result of previous endodontic treatment.

A healthy 23-year-old female patient was referred for a consultation on replacing tooth 21 with an implant-supported restoration. The patient had recently moved to the area and reported a history of endodontic and periodontal treatment for tooth 21. The tooth had been deemed non-restorable by her previous periodontist but since she was going to be moving, he recommended consulting to a dentist in her new city to continue her treatment. A review of her medical history yielded no significant findings and no known drug allergies.

The analysis of her smile revealed a medium to high symmetrical smile line and a slightly discolored tooth 21 (Fig 1).

Anterior retracted view revealed a medium to thick tissue phenotype and closely symmetrical gingival margins. A slight discoloration was noted at the cervical margin of tooth 21 (Fig 2). A wide band of attached gingiva was observed along the existing ceramic veneers on teeth 12 to 22.

The initial periapical radiograph was suggestive of internal root resorption with possible extension to the external aspect on the distal of tooth 21 (Fig 3). Postorthodontic root blunting was visible on teeth 12 and 22.

An esthetic risk assessment of the patient was completed and revealed a medium to high lip line and a medium scalloped phenotype. The adjacent teeth were restored and a horizontal bone deficiency was expected once the tooth was removed (Table 1).

Table 1   Esthetic Risk Assessment (ERA)

Esthetic risk factors	Level of risk		
	Low	Medium	High
Medical status	Healthy, uneventful healing		Compromised healing
Smoking habit	Non-smoker	Light smoker (≤ 10 cigs/day)	Heavy smoker (> 10 cigs/day)
Gingival display at full smile	Low	Medium	High
Width of edentulous span	1 tooth (≥ 7 mm)[1] 1 tooth (≥ 6 mm)[2]	1 tooth (< 7 mm)[1] 1 tooth (< 6 mm)[2]	2 teeth or more
Shape of tooth crowns	Rectangular		Triangular
Restorative status of neighboring teeth	Virgin		Restored
Gingival phenotype	Low-scalloped, thick	Medium-scalloped, medium-thick	High-scalloped, thin
Infection at implant site	None	Chronic	Acute
Soft-tissue anatomy	Soft tissue intact		Soft-tissue defects
Bone level at adjacent teeth	≤ 5 mm to contact point	5.5 to 6.5 mm to contact point	≥ 7 mm to contact point
Facial bone-wall phenotype*	Thick-wall phenotype ≥ 1 mm thickness		Thin-wall phenotype < 1 mm thickness
Bone anatomy of alveolar crest	No bone deficiency	Horizontal bone deficiency	Vertical bone deficiency
Patient's esthetic expectations	Realistic expectations	Moderate expectations	Unrealistic expectations

* If three-dimensional imaging is available with the tooth in place
[1] Standard-diameter implant, regular connection
[2] Narrow-diameter implant, narrow connection

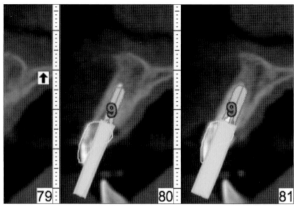

Fig 4 CBCT image with virtual implant placement showing the position of the natural tooth in relation to the proposed implant position. Adequate bone is available apically to support an immediately placed implant.

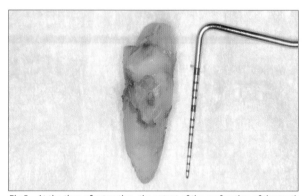

Fig 5 At the time of extraction, the extent of the perforation of the tooth root due to the internal resorption process became evident.

The patient was referred for a CBCT prior to the surgery. It documented adequate vertical bone height apically to allow engagement of the native alveolar bone by the implant following the extraction of the tooth. However, orthodontic extrusion was scheduled first, to be followed by immediate implant placement (Fig 4).

Unfortunately, the tooth became increasingly more uncomfortable, and it was decided that extrusion was not feasible, given the patient's level of discomfort. The revised treatment plan called for extraction, immediate implant placement and, if stability allowed, immediate provisionalization by the prosthodontist.

The tooth was carefully removed with a periotome without damaging the alveolar housing. Upon examination of the tooth, external root resorption was noticed on the distopalatal aspect of tooth 21. There was a concomitant probing depth at the location of the resorption, but it did not result in any significant bone loss that would have prevented treatment (Fig 5).

Figures 6 and 7 show the site following minimally traumatic extraction of tooth 21 (Figs 6 and 7). There was no incision, tissue trauma, or displacement following the extraction.

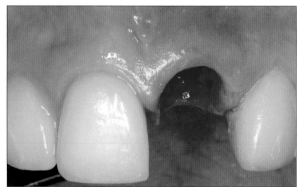
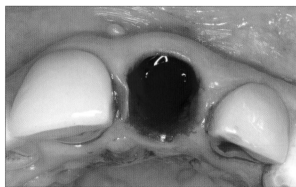

Figs 6 and 7 Soft-tissue contours following tooth removal and occlusal view of the socket following tooth removal.

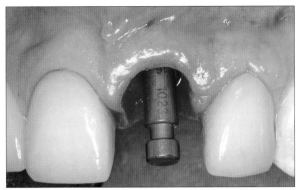

Fig 8 *3.5-mm depth gauge in position following preparation of the implant site.*

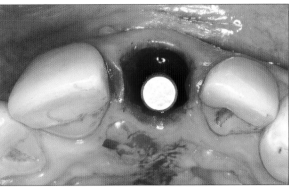

Fig 9 *Occlusal view following site preparation. Note the palatal position of the proposed implant site.*

Prior to implant placement, a depth gauge 3.5 mm in diameter was used to check the preparation depth, emergence profile, and the expected three-dimensional implant position (Fig 8). The occlusal view shows a site preparation shifted slightly palatally, engaging the palatal wall of the extraction socket (Fig 9).

A Bone Level implant (diameter 4.1 mm, length 14 mm; Institut Straumann AG, Basel, Switzerland) (Fig 10) was placed in the correct three-dimensional position as planned, with the implant shoulder positioned 3 mm away from the planned mucosal margin of the implant-supported restoration (Figs 11 and 12).

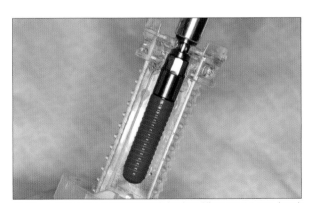

Fig 10 *A Bone Level Regular CrossFit implant (diameter 4.1 mm, length 14 mm).*

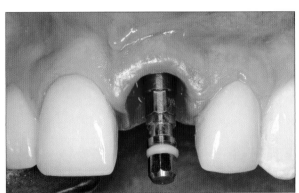

Fig 11 *The Bone Level implant in position.*

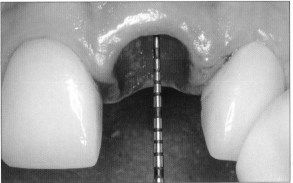

Fig 12 *The periodontal probe is placed at the implant shoulder to demonstrate its position 3 mm apical of the proposed gingival margin.*

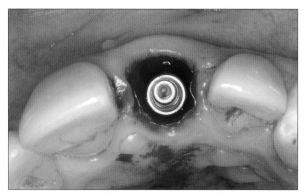

Fig 13   Occlusal view of the Bone level implant placed toward the palatal aspect of the alveolar socket.

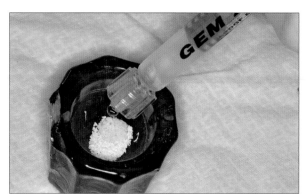

Fig 14   Bovine-derived xenograft being hydrated with recombinant human PDGF.

Removal of the implant mount shows the implant positioned toward the palatal aspect, allowing for an adequate horizontal dimension of the defect for grafting and preservation of the buccal wall (Fig 13).

The horizontal dimension of the defect was grafted using a xenograft derived from bovine hydroxyapatite (Bio-Oss; Geistlich Pharma, Wolhusen, Switzerland) hydrated with recombinant human platelet-derived growth factor (rhPDGF) (Gem21; Osteohealth, Shirley, NY, USA) (Fig 14).

The bone-graft material was positioned along the buccal aspect of the implant (Fig 15), and a connective-tissue graft harvested from the distal aspect of tooth 27 was used as a biological barrier above the bone graft material (Fig 16). The buccal flap was not reflected; the tissue-graft dimensions matched the length, width, and depth of the void above the bone graft and alveolar crest.

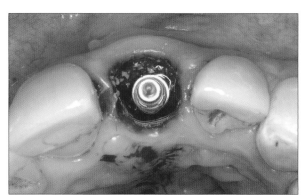

Fig 15   The xenograft in place to bridge the horizontal defect dimension.

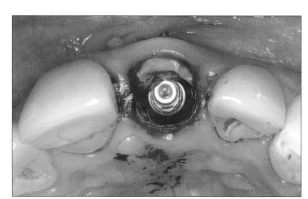

Fig 16   Connective-tissue graft in place acting as a biologic barrier over the xenograft.

A single 5-0 chromic gut horizontal mattress suture (Ethicon; Somerville, NJ, USA) was used to secure the soft-tissue graft (Fig 17). Finally, a customizable Regular CrossFit (RC) polymer healing cap (Institut Straumann AG) was placed for the patient to wear while in transit to her prosthodontist's office for fabrication of the immediate provisional (Fig 18). The postoperative radiograph confirmed the ideal positioning of the dental implant, away from the adjacent roots and any vital structures. (Fig 19).

When the patient had arrived at the prosthodontist's office, provisionalization began by removing the healing cap, placing a RC temporary abutment (RC PEEK abutment), and making marks to guide the reduction of the abutment (Fig 20).

The provisional abutment preparation was then completed (Fig 21). The finish lines were located just below the mucosal margin to facilitate access to the cement line for clean-up.

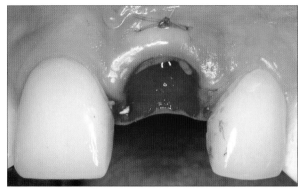

Fig 17   Facial view of the horizontal mattress suture securing the connective-tissue graft to the facial wall of the socket.

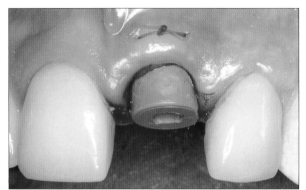

Fig 18   Customized Regular CrossFit polymer healing cap in position.

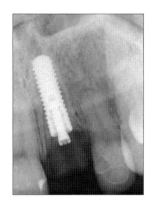

Fig 19   Radiograph taken on completion of the procedure, showing the implant position.

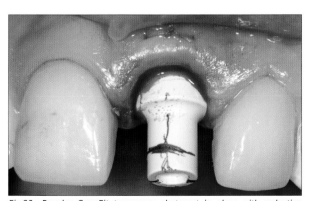

Fig 20   Regular CrossFit temporary abutment in place with reduction marks to guide customization.

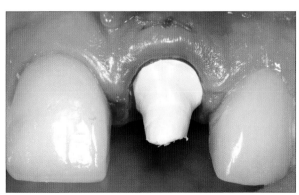

Fig 21   Provisional abutment preparation.

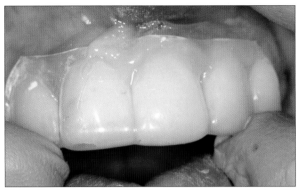

A vacuform matrix filled with cold-curing resin was used to fabricate the provisional crown (Fig 22).

The completed provisional (Fig 23) exhibited ideal contours, allowing for ideal prosthetic volume for the restorative materials and papillae to fill in during healing and maturation. The occlusion was carefully checked to ensure that no contact could occur during excursive or functional movements (Fig 24).

Fig 22   Vacuform template with autopolymerizing resin seated over the provisional abutment.

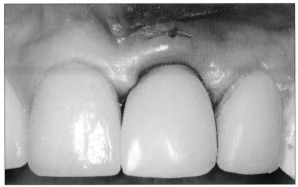

Fig 23   The completed provisional restoration.

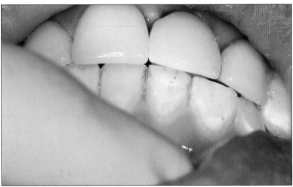

Fig 24   Occlusion check of the provisional restoration.

The two-week follow-up photograph illustrates an uneventful healing response, with tissue rapidly filling the papillary areas (Fig 25).

At two months, the peri-implant tissues were maturing nicely, maintaining the desired mucosal margin position (Fig 26). However, a distinct demarcation between the native tissue and the connective-tissue graft began to emerge.

At five months. although the tissue volume was ideal and the gingival margins were stable, this demarcation was even more prominent. Plans were made to perform dermabrasion to smooth the tissue contours (Fig 27). A follow-up radiograph was taken at this time to verify stable bone levels around the implant (Fig 28).

The fabrication of the custom impression coping began by removing the provisional and the abutment from the patient's mouth and placing it on a RC implant analog. Bite registration material was placed around the analog and provisional to obtain an outline of the crown contours (Fig 29).

With the facial position of the provisional marked in black, the provisional and the abutment were removed and a Bone Level RC impression post placed on the analog, leaving a void that reflected the ideal contours of the proposed restoration. Composite material was slowly added to fill the voids around the impression post and light-cured until set (Fig 30).

The custom impression post was seated in the patient's mouth and provided support for the tissues, as it had the same shape as the provisional. New crowns on teeth 12, 11, and 22 were also planned (Fig 31).

A RC CAD/CAM customized zirconia abutment (CARES) (Institut Straumann AG) was fabricated and delivered prior to cementation of the final crown (Fig 32).

Figure 33 shows the patient's final restorations on the day of delivery. The uneven tissue contact areas were recontoured with a fine diamond bur under copious irrigation.

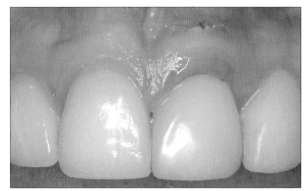

Fig 25   At two weeks. Excellent adaptation of the soft tissue.

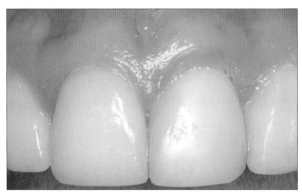

Fig 26   At two months.

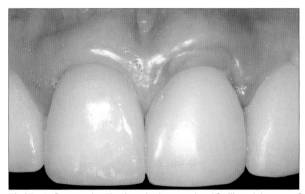

Fig 27   At five months. The tissue had matured and facilitated the start of final restorative process.

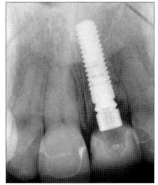

Fig 28   Radiograph of the implant and provisional at the start of the definitive restorative procedures.

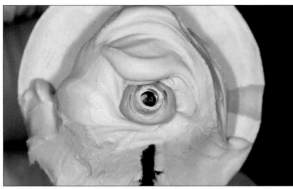

Fig 29   Duplication of the provisional crown contours to create the customized impression coping.

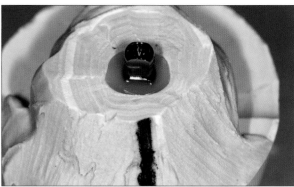

Fig 30   Composite resin placed around the impression post to capture the
provisional contours.

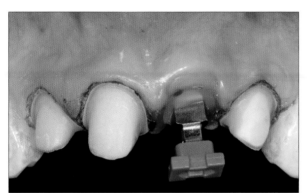

Fig 31   Customized impression post in position prior to taking an impression of the implant and adjacent preparations.

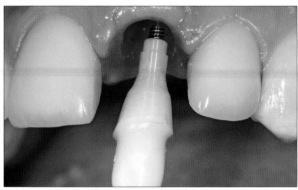

Fig 32   Custom zirconium abutment prior to seating.

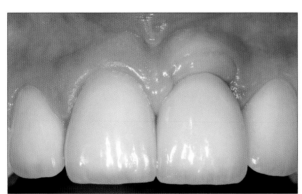

Fig 33   Final restorations in place on the day of delivery.

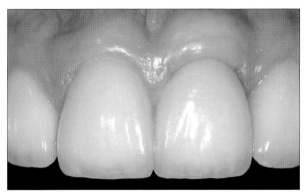

Fig 34 One year after treatment.

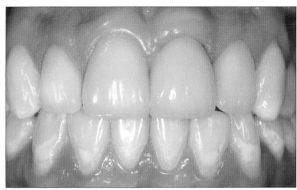

Fig 35 Retracted anterior view at one year.

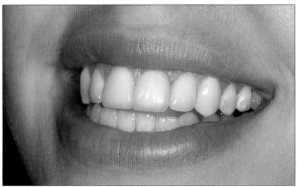

Fig 36 The patient's smile at one year.

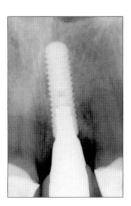

Fig 37 One-year radiograph.

The photograph taken at one year post-treatment demonstrated stable and symmetrical tissue contours (Fig 34).

The anterior retracted view at the same visit again showed excellent results, with harmonious tissue contours that were free of inflammation or other complications (Fig 35).

The one-year photo of the patient's smile illustrated the patient's satisfaction with the final esthetic result (Fig 36).

Stable bone levels were evident around the implant. The emergence profile of the final restoration was in harmony with the bone profile at the implant site (Fig 37).

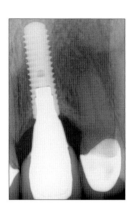

Fig 38   Periapical radiograph taken seven years postoperatively. Long-term stability of the peri-implant alveolar bone.

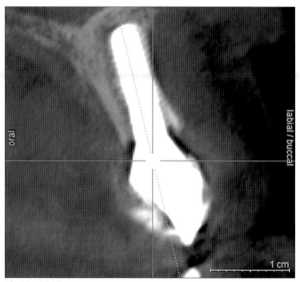

Fig 39   CBCT scan taken at seven years documenting the long-term stability of the buccal plate.

The patient moved to a new city due to work commitments, but her new dentist shared the seven-year periapical radiograph, which shows continued bone-level stability around the entire length of the implant and especially around the implant shoulder (Fig 38).

In consultation with her new dentist, a cone-beam computed tomography (CBCT) scan was taken at the seven-year mark that illustrated the presence of a stable buccal plate around the implant. This validated the long-term result and reassured the patient of the implant's ability to continue functioning well into the future (Fig 39).

Acknowledgments

Laboratory procedures
Nuance Dental Ceramics – Mansfield, TX, USA

Additional radiographic documentation
Dr. Kevin G. Murphy – Baltimore, MD, USA

7.2 Replacement of a Perforated Upper Left Central Incisor: Early Placement of an RC Bone Level Implant

A. Januário, W. Duarte

A 28-year-old patient presented at her general dentist's office and complained about the appearance of her tooth 21 (Fig 1).

The patient had a history of trauma to this tooth. Endodontic treatment had been performed in the past and a crown placed on the tooth. A procedure to replace the old crown was performed by her dentist; however, a perforation on the middle third of the root occurred (Fig 2), and extraction of tooth 21 was suggested. Upon clinical and radiographic examination of the patient, who had been referred to us, replacement of tooth 21 by a dental implant appeared to be indicated.

The patient was in a good general health and her medical history was without significant findings. The teeth and periodontal tissues adjacent to tooth 21 were examined in detail and the result used to assess the esthetic risk for implant therapy (Table 1).

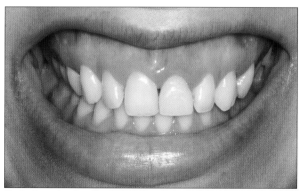

Fig 1 Forced smile with a high lip line. Aspect at initial presentation showing a shortened crown of tooth 21 and a darkened aspect at the gingiva.

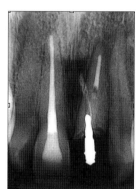

Fig 2 Periapical radiograph. Perforation on the middle third at the mesial aspect of root 21. The post was very short.

Table 1   Esthetic Risk Assessment (ERA)

Esthetic risk factors	Level of risk		
	Low	**Medium**	**High**
Medical status	Healthy, uneventful healing		Compromised healing
Smoking habit	Non-smoker	Light smoker (≤ 10 cigs/day)	Heavy smoker (> 10 cigs/day)
Gingival display at full smile	Low	Medium	High
Width of edentulous span	1 tooth (≥ 7 mm)[1] 1 tooth (≥ 6 mm)[2]	1 tooth (< 7 mm)[1] 1 tooth (< 6 mm)[2]	2 teeth or more
Shape of tooth crowns	Rectangular		Triangular
Restorative status of neighboring teeth	Virgin		Restored
Gingival phenotype	Low-scalloped, thick	Medium-scalloped, medium-thick	High-scalloped, thin
Infection at implant site	None	Chronic	Acute
Soft-tissue anatomy	Soft tissue intact		Soft-tissue defects
Bone level at adjacent teeth	≤ 5 mm to contact point	5.5 to 6.5 mm to contact point	≥ 7 mm to contact point
Facial bone-wall phenotype*	Thick-wall phenotype ≥ 1 mm thickness		Thin-wall phenotype < 1 mm thickness
Bone anatomy of alveolar crest	No bone deficiency	Horizontal bone deficiency	Vertical bone deficiency
Patient's esthetic expectations	Realistic expectations		Unrealistic expectations

* If three-dimensional imaging is available with the tooth in place
[1] Standard-diameter implant, regular connection
[2] Narrow-diameter implant, narrow connection

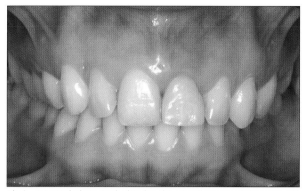

Fig 3   Intraoral photograph showing the overall aspect of the teeth, the condition of the gingival tissue, and the thin gingival phenotype.

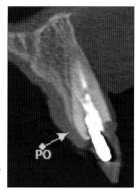

Fig 4   ST-CBCT image showing the apparently absent buccal bone wall, a thin buccal gingiva, and a sufficient amount of bone apically and palatally of tooth 21.

The patient had a thin gingival phenotype (Fig 3). A soft-tissue cone-beam computed tomography (ST-CBCT; Januário and coworkers 2008) confirmed the thin gingival phenotype and showed that the buccal bone wall was either very thin or completely absent (Fig 4). There was sufficient bone apically and palatally of tooth 21 to insert the implant in ideal position.

The probing depths at teeth 21 were 2 mm palatally and buccally and 3 mm interproximally.

Based on the above analysis, it was decided to extract tooth 21 using a minimally invasive approach, first removing the crown and the post (Fig 5) and then performing the extraction. Partial loss of the buccal bone wall was detected (Fig 6), so it was decided to prepare the site for early implant placement (Buser and coworkers 2013).

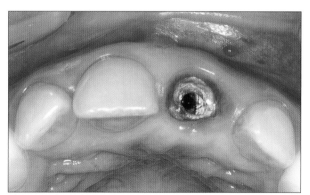

Fig 5   Tooth 21 without the crown and post, prior to extraction.

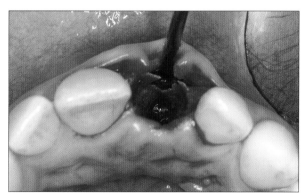

Fig 6   Slight elevation of the buccal gingiva to create a pouch, showing a partial bone loss at the buccal wall.

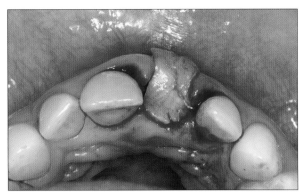

Fig 7   Connective-tissue (CT) graft placed over the socket and buccal gingi-va to show its appropriate mesiodistal and buccopalatal dimensions.

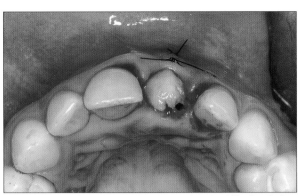

Fig 8   The CT graft was inserted into the pouch and stabilized at the buc-cal gingiva with single sutures.

The buccal gingival tissue was slightly elevated, creating a pouch to accommodate a connective-tissue (CT) graft to cover the socket mesiodistally and to promote a phenotype conversion (Rungcharassaeng and coworkers 2012; Thoma and coworkers 2014) of the buccal gingival tissue. To do that, the CT graft had to be long enough to be inserted into the buccal pouch. It was stabilized to the buccal gingiva with single sutures (Figs 7 and 8).

Sutures were also placed on the mesial and distal papillae. Immediately after the extraction and placement of the CT graft, a provisional bonded crown was inserted to maintain the patient's esthetic and phonetic functions (Fig 9).

Eight weeks later, the soft-tissue healing was completed, and on the incisal view, a slight depression of the buccal aspect was noted, even with the placement of a CT graft (Fig 10). A type II implant placement was scheduled (Hämmerle and coworkers 2004).

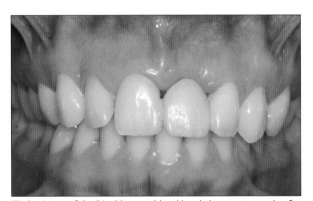

Fig 9   Aspect of site 21 with a provisional bonded crown two weeks after tooth extraction.

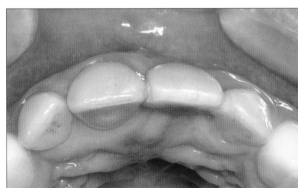

Fig 10   Incisal view after eight weeks of healing with the provisional.

The provisional crown was removed for implant placement. The patient had a high lip line, which increased the esthetic risk and required a highly esthetic result. The frontal and incisal views of the site showed good healing of the soft tissue, and the CT graft was capable of minimizing the buccal tissue collapse and increasing its thickness (Figs 11 to 13).

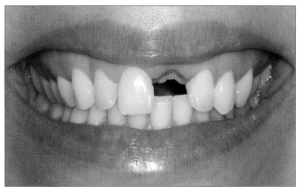

Fig 11   Frontal extraoral view after eight weeks of healing without the provisional.

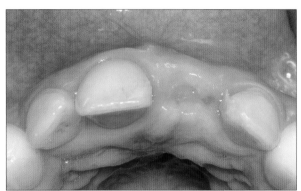

Fig 12   Incisal view after eight weeks of healing without the provisional.

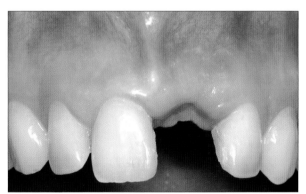

Fig 13   Frontal intraoral view after eight weeks of healing without the provisional.

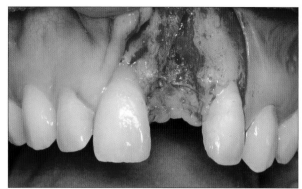

Fig 14   A full-thickness flap was elevated to completely expose the bone defect.

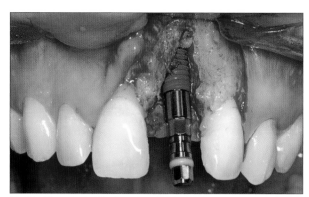

Fig 15   Placement of the Bone Level RC implant.

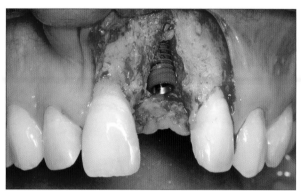

Fig 16   Implant threads exposed.

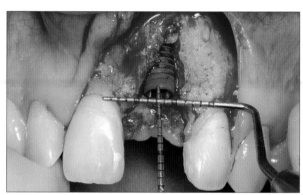

Fig 17   Periodontal probes showing the implant shoulder position 3 mm below the CEJ level of tooth 11.

Since there was a need to correct the defect on the buccal bone wall at the time of implant placement, a full-thickness flap was elevated by placing a vertical releasing incision on the distal aspect of tooth 22. The defect was completely visible and the socket had not yet filled with mature bone (Fig 14).

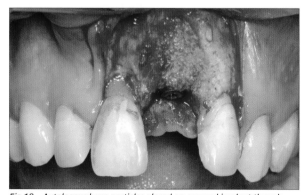

Fig 18   Autologous bone particles placed on exposed implant threads.

A RC Bone Level implant (Bone Level SLActive, diameter 4.1 mm, length 10 mm; Institut Straumann AG, Basel, Switzerland) was placed in its appropriate three-dimensional position. Several implant threads were exposed, requiring a simultaneous GBR procedure (Figs 15 and 16).

The implant shoulder was approximately 3 mm below the level of the cementoenamel junction (CEJ) of the adjacent teeth. This was only possible because of the presence of contralateral central incisor. However, this routine should be avoided in the case of implant placement in different regions of the mouth, since the CEJ level of a non-symmetric tooth will not be an adequate reference for vertical implant placement. In such situations, a vertical guide with the correctly proposed mucosal margin should be considered (Fig 17).

The exposed implant threads were covered with autologous bone particles collected from the bone surrounding the implant site with a small bone chisel (Fig 18).

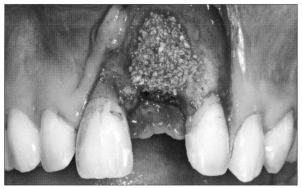

Fig 19   Autologous bone particles covered with demineralized bovine bone matrix.

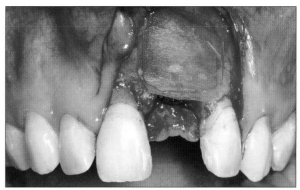

Fig 20   Collagen membrane placed on top of the bone-graft materials.

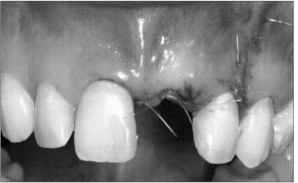

Fig 21   The flap was sutured with single sutures.

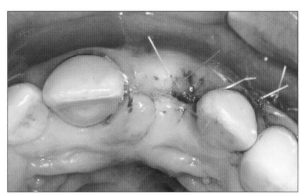

Fig 22   Incisal view of the crestal incision sutured with single sutures.

The bone particles were covered with demineralized bovine bone matrix, and a collagen membrane was placed on top of the bone graft at the buccal aspect to improve the contour. Sufficient bone thickness buccally (approximately 2 mm) is a prerequisite for optimal esthetics results (Figs 19 and 20).

The flap was repositioned and sutured and the bonded provisional restoration was delivered (Figs 21 to 23).

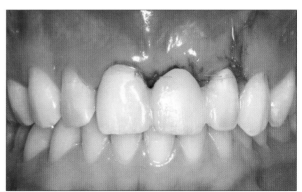

Fig 23   The bonded provisional prosthesis was placed immediately after surgery.

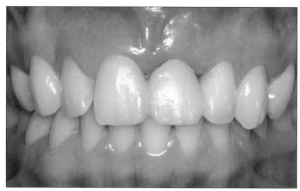

Fig 24   Three months of healing after implant placement and GBR procedure.

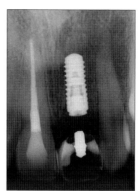

Fig 25   Periapical radiograph at three months after implant placement and GBR procedure.

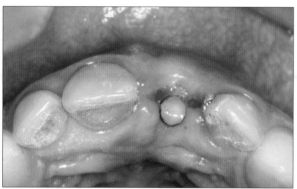

Fig 26   Mucosal punch to expose the healing cap.

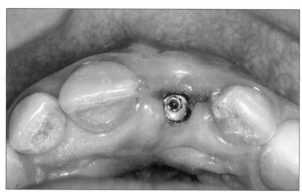

Fig 27   Exposed healing cap.

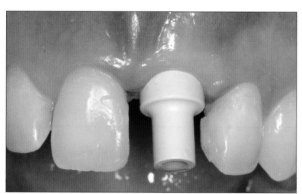

Fig 28   The Bone Level RC temporary abutment in place.

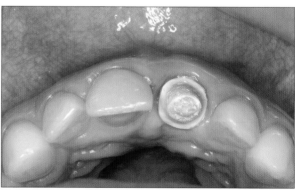

Fig 29   Incisal view of the prepared Bone Level RC temporary abutment.

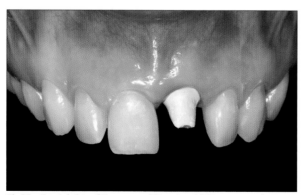

Fig 30   Frontal view of the prepared Bone Level RC temporary abutment.

Three months were allowed for osseointegration (Fig 24). The periapical radiograph shows a correct implant position and the level of the proximal bone (Fig 25).

The second-stage surgery was performed by a mucosal punch on the crest at the position of the implant, which exposed the healing cap (Figs 26 and 27).

A Bone Level RC temporary abutment (PMMA, length 10 mm; Institut Straumann AG) was placed in the implant (Fig 28) and prepared to receive the provisional restoration (Figs 29 and 30).

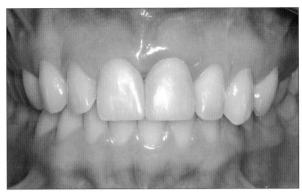

Fig 31 Frontal view of the provisional, showing nice mucosal contours in symmetry with the adjacent gingival margins.

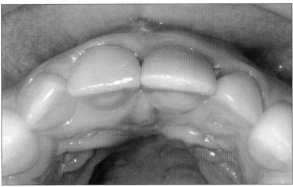

Fig 32 Incisal view of the provisional, showing nice mucosal contours in symmetry with the adjacent gingival margins.

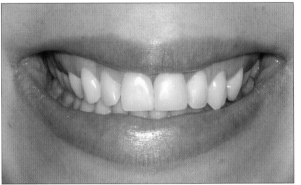

Fig 33 Extraoral frontal view of the patient's smile showing the satisfactory result.

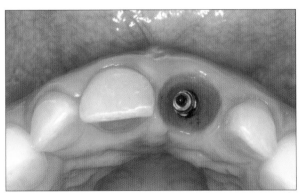

Fig 34 The provisional restoration was removed after two months to take an impression. Excellent facial tissue volume.

The provisional restoration was cemented to the abutment and the mucosal tissue conditioned to its ideal contour. The contour and volume of the peri-implant mucosa were highly satisfactory (Figs 31 to 33).

After two months, the provisional restoration was removed and a final impression taken (Fig 34).

A gold abutment (Gold Abutment, length 8.2 mm; Institut Straumann AG) was used to fabricate a custom abutment (with fired-on ceramics) for the cementation of an all-ceramic crown (Figs 35 and 36).

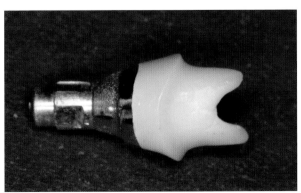

Fig 35 Custom abutment with fired-on ceramics creating ideal emergence contours and cement line position.

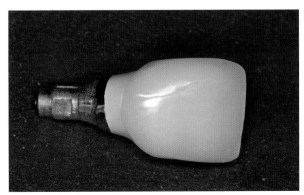

Fig 36 Custom abutment with the all-ceramic crown in place.

After confirming the fit and shade of the custom abutment and crown, the abutment was tightened into the implant (35 N·cm) (Fig 37) and sealed with PTFE and a light-curing temporary restorative material (Fermit; Ivoclar Vivadent, Schaan, Liechtenstein). The ceramic components were treated according to the manufacturer's instructions. The crown was then cemented with a dual-curing resin cement (Variolink II; Ivoclar Vivadent), and light-cured for 40 seconds at each margin. Careful was taken to remove all residual cement. The abutment and the crown integrated ideally with the peri-implant soft tissue (Fig 38).

The periapical radiograph taken at the six-year follow-up showed stable levels of the mesial and distal proximal bone crests (Fig 39). The ST-CBCT showed the presence of a facial bone wall. Furthermore, thick mucosa was present facially, the result of the connective-tissue graft placed at the time of tooth extraction (Fig 40).

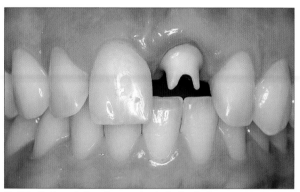

Fig 37   Custom abutment screwed onto the implant.

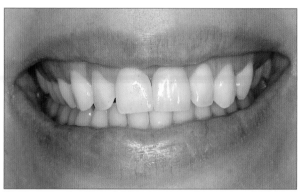

Fig 38   Full smile with the final crown cemented.

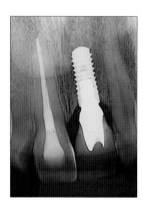

Fig 39   Periapical radiograph six years after implant placement.

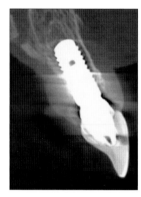

Fig 40   Soft-tissue cone-beam computed tomography six years after implant placement. Observe the buccal bone plate and the width of buccal soft tissue.

A. Januário, W. Duarte

The six-year follow-up photographs show that an excellent esthetic integration and a stable outcome had been reached with a single-tooth replacement therapy (Figs 41 to 43).

Acknowledgment

Prosthetic procedures
Dr. Ney Ferreira do Nascimento – Brasília, Brazil.

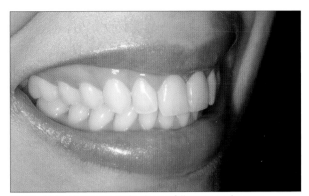

Fig 41   Right lateral view at the six-year follow-up appointment.

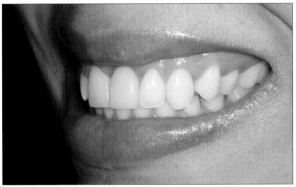

Fig 42   Frontal view at the six-year follow-up appointment.

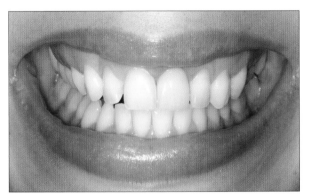

Fig 43   Left lateral view at the six-year follow-up appointment.

7.3   Replacement of an Upper Right Central Incisor with a Root Fracture: Early Placement of an RC Bone Level Implant, Variobase Abutment

C. Kunavisarut

A healthy 28-year-old female patient presented for a consultation on treatment options to restore her upper right central incisor. At the clinical examination, the tooth responded to percussion and palpation. The gingiva was red and slightly swollen, with a mid-facial probing depth of 10 mm. The upper right lateral incisor showed no signs or symptoms, did not respond to exploration and percussion, and the vitality test was positive.

The periapical radiograph (Fig 1) revealed that tooth 11 had been endodontically treated, with no lesion evident at the apex. A small radiopaque calcified structure surrounded by a narrow radiolucent zone (3 × 3 mm) was present at the apex of tooth 12.

Tooth 11 was diagnosed with a vertical root fracture. The lesion at the apex of tooth 12 was diagnosed as a compound odontoma.

The treatment plan was discussed with the patient, who decided to have tooth 11 removed and replace with dental implant. According to the 2013 ITI Consensus (Chen and Buser 2014), a recession of the midfacial mucosa presents a risk when considering immediate implant placement. Early implant placement with an appropriate contour augmentation has been shown to yield a predictable esthetic outcome (Buser and coworkers 2013a). Therefore, an early implant placement protocol was chosen for site 11.

The patient rejected treatment of her odontoma because as she had experienced no symptoms and because tooth 12 could be damaged during surgery. Annual follow-ups including radiograph were therefore planned to check on this lesion.

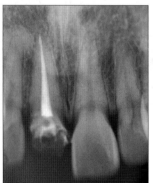

Fig 1   Periapical radiograph of tooth 11. Round radiopaque lesion (3 × 3 mm) at the apex of tooth 12.

Tooth 11 was carefully extracted without elevating a flap. A minimally traumatic technique was used in order to preserve the labial bone. No ridge preservation technique was used. An acrylic removable partial denture was made for patient to use during healing period; it was carefully checked for any excessive soft-tissue contact and compression to help prevent collapse of the soft tissue. Two months after extraction, the soft tissue had completely healed, but a horizontal ridge deficiency was evidently (Figs 2 and 3). The gingival phenotype was thin and highly scalloped, with broad keratinized tissue and slightly tapered teeth.

A CBCT was taken to determine the amount of bone available for proper implant selection and augmentation based upon the contours of the planned restoration (Fig 4). It was determined that the amount of bone available at the site was adequate to achieve primary stability of the implant at placement.

The data obtained from the clinical examination were compiled for the esthetic risk assessment (Table 1).

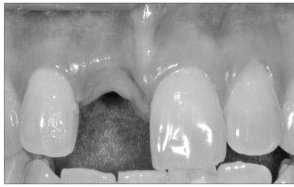

Fig 2   Facial view of teeth 12 to 22 showing high scalloped gingiva with slightly tapered teeth.

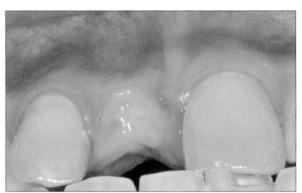

Fig 3   Occlusal view of teeth 12 to 22 showing the horizontal ridge deficiency at site 11.

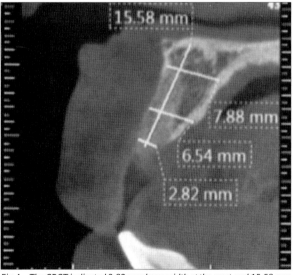

Fig 4   The CBCT indicated 2.82 mm bone width at the crest and 15.58 mm bone height. New bone could be seen forming along the former socket.

Table 1   Esthetic Risk Assessment (ERA)

Esthetic risk factors	Level of risk		
	Low	**Medium**	**High**
Medical status	Healthy, uneventful healing		Compromised healing
Smoking habit	Non-smoker	Light smoker (≤ 10 cigs/day)	Heavy smoker (> 10 cigs/day)
Gingival display at full smile	Low	Medium	High
Width of edentulous span	1 tooth (≥ 7 mm)[1] 1 tooth (≥ 6 mm)[2]	1 tooth (< 7 mm)[1] 1 tooth (< 6 mm)[2]	2 teeth or more
Shape of tooth crowns	Rectangular		Triangular
Restorative status of neighboring teeth	Virgin		Restored
Gingival phenotype	Low-scalloped, thick	Medium-scalloped, medium-thick	High-scalloped, thin
Infection at implant site	None		Acute
Soft-tissue anatomy	Soft tissue intact		Soft-tissue defects
Bone level at adjacent teeth	≤ 5 mm to contact point	5.5 to 6.5 mm to contact point	≥ 7 mm to contact point
Facial bone-wall phenotype*	Thick-wall phenotype ≥ 1 mm thickness		Thin-wall phenotype < 1 mm thickness
Bone anatomy of alveolar crest	No bone deficiency	Horizontal bone deficiency	Vertical bone deficiency
Patient's esthetic expectations	Realistic expectations		Unrealistic expectations

* If three-dimensional imaging is available with the tooth in place
[1] Standard-diameter implant, regular connection
[2] Narrow-diameter implant, narrow connection

After the esthetic risk assessments, the treatment plan was revisited with the patient. Due to the thin and high-scalloped gingiva, a bone-level implant (Bone Level SLActive, diameter 4.1 mm, length 10 mm; Institut Straumann AG, Basel, Switzerland) was selected. Because a dehiscence on the labial aspect was expected, simultaneous guided bone regeneration (GBR) was planned to enhance the contours of the site after implant placement. A screw-retained final restoration was planned to avoid the potential post-insertion complication of residual cement and to make the restoration retrievable.

The following treatment plan was proposed:

- Early placement of a Bone Level SLActive implant (diameter 4.1 mm, length 10 mm) with simultaneous GBR
- Healing period of at least three months
- Screw-retained provisional restoration for at least three months
- Screw-retained zirconia restoration on titanium abutment

Surgical phase

A slightly palatal incision was placed on the crest with a vertical releasing incision at the distolabial line angle of tooth 12. A full-thickness flap was raised. Implant surgery was performed according to the manufacturer's recommended protocol. A three-dimensional implant placement protocol (Buser and coworkers 2004a) was used to ensure an esthetic appearance of the final restoration. The implant was placed 3 mm apical of the midfacial mucosal margin of the planned restoration, at least 1.5 mm away from the adjacent roots and 2 mm behind the ideal point of emergence in the orofacial dimension. A 2-mm gap was found along the entire length of the guide pin after the 3.5-mm drill had been used (Figs 5 to 6). This two-wall defect was favorable for implant placement, since primary stability could be easily achieved, the implant could be positioned inside the alveolar bone, and predictable GBR could be performed thanks to an adequate blood supply from the bony walls.

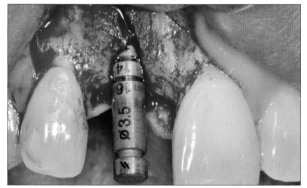

Fig 5 The surgical site was prepared according to the 3D implant placement protocol. A dehiscence of 2 mm was found along the implant length after the last drilling step.

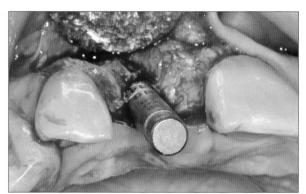

Fig 6 Planning the Implant axis for the screw-retained restoration.

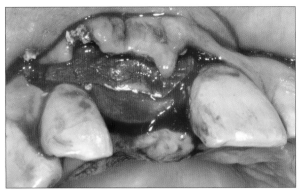

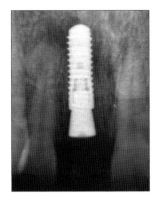

Fig 7 Contour augmentation with a first layer of autologous bone chips, followed by deproteinized bovine bone and a double layer of collagen membrane.

Fig 8 Periapical radiograph taken as a baseline reference.

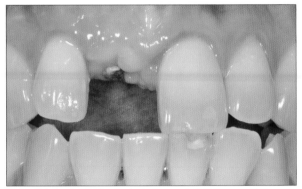

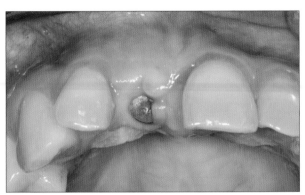

Fig 9 Three months after implant placement. Soft tissue partially covering the healing abutment.

Fig 10 The restored horizontal contour of the edentulous ridge. The implant position was slightly palatal to accommodate a screw-retained restoration.

The implant site was profiled and tapped. A Bone Level implant (Bone Level SLActive, Regular CrossFit, diameter 4.1 mm, length 10 mm; Institut Straumann AG) was placed. Primary stability was achieved. A 4-mm healing abutment was connected finger-tight. A contouring technique (Buser and coworkers 2013a) was used to augment the surgical site. Autologous bone chips were harvested from the close vicinity of the implant site and then placed onto the exposed implant surface. Slowly resorbable grafting material (Bio-Oss; Geistlich Pharma, Wolhusen, Switzerland) was packed over the implant site to provide adequate thickness, which would help maintain the labial contour in the long term. A double-layered

bioabsorbable barrier membrane (Bio-Gide; Geistlich Pharma AG) was applied on the implant site. The periosteum-releasing incision was made at the base of the flap in order to achieve tension-free wound closure. The soft tissue was sutured to achieve semi-submerged healing (Figs 7 and 8).

The patient's acrylic-resin removable partial denture was carefully adjusted to completely relieve any pressure on the surgical site. Three months postoperatively, the soft tissue had partially covered the healing abutment. The horizontal contour of the ridge was restored (Figs 9 and 10).

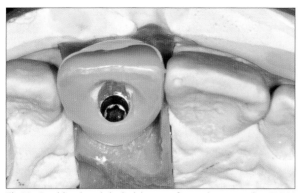

Fig 11 Provisional made in the laboratory from a denture tooth, a PMMA abutment, and acrylic resin. The provisional was screw-retained for easy access and maintenance.

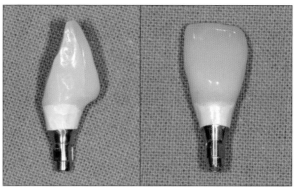

Fig 12 The contour of the provisional restoration was straight or slightly concave on the facial side below the peri-implant mucosal margin. The proximal contour was slightly convex.

In order to change the peri-implant tissue from the circular profile of the healing abutment into triangular profile of a natural tooth, a restoration with a suitable contour was necessary. A provisional restoration was easier to modify and adjust than a permanent restoration and can serve as a tool for communication among the dentist, patient, and technician regarding the desired shape and form of the final restoration. Therefore, it is highly recommended to use a provisional restoration in the esthetic zone.

Both screw-retained and cemented provisional restorations can be used to contour the peri-implant tissue. However, to remove and re-cement a cement-retained provisional restoration several times during this stage could result in tissue trauma and make it impossible to completely remove excess cement, while a screw-retained provisional restoration is much easier to manipulate. Therefore, a screw-retained provisional restoration was made from a denture tooth, a PMMA abutment, and acrylic resin. An impression was taken with polyvinyl siloxane for the fabrication of provisional restoration in the dental laboratory.

The provisional abutment was prepared and several grooves were made for mechanical retention, and a denture tooth was attached to the provisional abutment on the cast with acrylic resin (Fig 11).

The contours of the provisional were shaped such that the zenith of the emergence profile was convex while the contour of the provisional below the soft-tissue margin was straight or slightly concave. The proximal contour was slightly convex to help support the papillae (Fig 12).

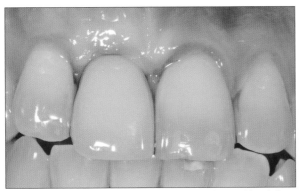

Fig 13 *The tissue blanching seen after inserting the provisional disappeared after 15 minutes.*

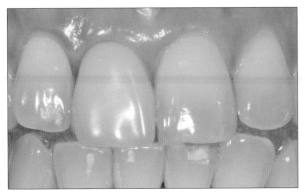

Fig 14 *Three-week follow-up. Tooth 11 was 1 mm shorter than tooth 12. The papillae almost completely filled both embrasures.*

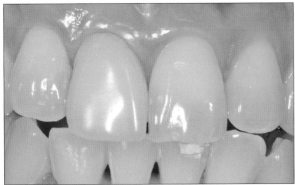

Fig 15 *Six-week follow-up. Same clinical crown length on the provisional and the contralateral tooth.*

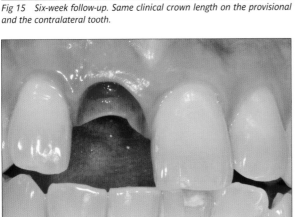

Fig 16 *Facial view of the peri-implant mucosa. Healthy peri-implant tissue.*

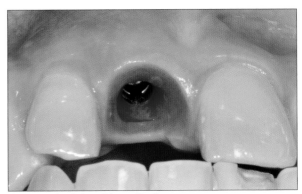

Fig 17 *Occlusal view of the peri-implant mucosa.*

The provisional restoration was tightened to 15 N·cm. Tissue blanching was immediately seen after installation but disappeared after 15 minutes (Fig 13). If the blanching had still persisted after 15 minutes, the contours of the restoration would have had to be adjusted to avoid excessive tissue compression. The patient was instructed to brush and use dental floss around the provisional during the healing phase.

At the three-week follow-up, the clinical crown of the provisional was 1 mm shorter than that of the contralateral tooth. The interdental papillae almost completely filled both embrasures (Fig 14). Acrylic resin was added to the cervical contours of the provisional crown to assist in pushing the peri-implant tissue further apically. It was decided to wait for three more weeks to allow for this tissue movement and maturation.

At the six-week follow-up, the clinical crown on the implant had the same length as that of the contralateral tooth, and the papillae were completely shaped. Since soft-tissue maturation takes place during the first three to six months after surgery, the provisional was left in place for eight more weeks to ensure stability of the peri-implant mucosa (transition zone) before fabricating the final restoration (Fig 15).

Healthy peri-implant mucosa was observed after removing the provisional (Figs 16 and 17). The fabrication of a custom impression coping was necessary to capture the shape of transition zone and transferred it to the cast.

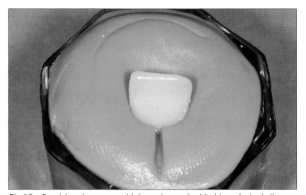

Fig 18   Provisional crown and lab analog embedded in polyvinyl siloxane putty. An indentation was made in the putty to indicate the mid-facial position.

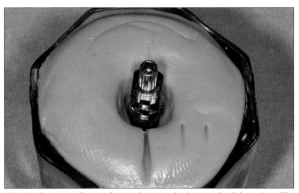

Fig 19   Open-tray impression coping attached on to the lab analog. The gap between the polyvinyl siloxane putty and the impression coping was filled with flowable composite resin.

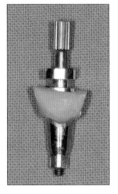

Fig 20   Frontal view of the custom impression coping. The emergence of the transition zone was captured with composite resin.

The provisional was removed and attached to the lab analog. Both the analog and the provisional were inserted in polyvinyl siloxane putty in a small glass container. An indentation in the impression material was made on the mid-facial aspect. After removing the provisional, an open-tray impression coping was attached to the lab analog. Flowable composite resin was used to filled in the gap between the impression coping and the polyvinyl siloxane putty. The composite resin was light-cured for 30 seconds, whereupon the custom impression coping was removed from the lab analog (Figs 18 to 20).

The custom impression coping helped maintain the tissue contours during impression-taking. The final impression was taken with polyvinyl-siloxane. The custom coping allowed the transition zone to be captured (Figs 21 and 22).

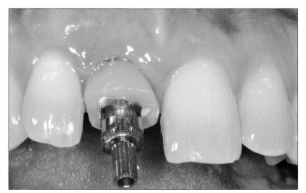

Fig 21   The soft-tissue contours were maintained by using the custom impression coping.

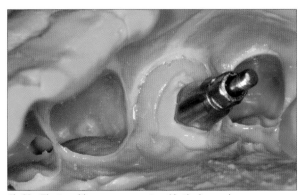

Fig 22   The transition zone was captured in the impression.

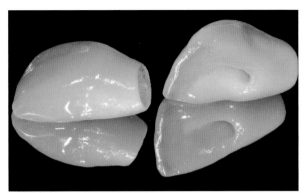

Fig 23   A zirconia coping with a feldspathic veneer. The screw access hole passed through the cingulum.

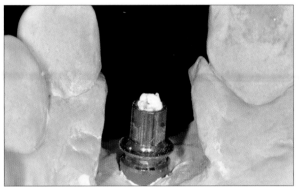

Fig 24   Screw access hole filled with polytetrafluoroethylene before final cementation to protect the screw head.

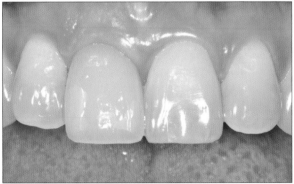

Fig 25   Zirconia restoration on a titanium abutment torqued to 35 N·cm. The gray color of the titanium abutment was completely masked.

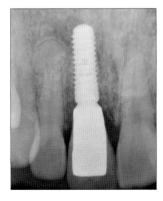

Fig 26   Periapical radiograph. Completely seated restoration.

Several abutments could have been used for the screw-retained permanent restoration, made of gold, zirconia, or titanium. There is only low-level evidence on the effect of wear on these different materials in the implant/abutment contact zone, but to minimize any risk of wear and abutment fracture (Sailer and coworkers 2009b), a titanium abutment (Straumann CARES Variobase; Institut Straumann AG) was selected. A zirconia framework with a feldspathic veneer (Katana Zirconia; Kuraray Noritake Dental, Niigata, Japan) was selected for the final restoration because of the high fracture toughness of the material and to ensure that the grey color of the titanium base was completely masked while still allowing adequate translucency (Fig 23).

A Variobase abutment and the final restoration were tried in the patient's mouth. The shape, color and proximal contacts of the restoration were carefully checked and adjusted accordingly. After polishing the restoration, the screw access hole was filled with polytetrafluoroethylene to protect the screw head before the final cementation. The ceramic restoration was adhesively cemented onto the titanium abutment with a self-curing composite adhesive (Multilink N; Ivoclar Vivadent, Schaan, Liechtenstein); this was done extraorally to ensure complete seating of the restoration and complete removal of any excess cement. The restoration was gently seated on the abutment with slight pressure. The excess cement was remove immediately with a microbrush while pressure was still applied on the restoration.

After complete curing of the adhesive, the restoration was tried in; a slight adjustment was made with a fine diamond bur. The occlusion was adjusted such that a light centric occlusion was established, while protrusive and lateral excursions corresponded to those of the adjacent teeth. A torque of 35 N·cm was applied to the abutment screw. The screw access hole was covered with polytetrafluoroethylene and sealed with composite resin (Fig 25).

Radiographic control was used to ensure proper seating of the restoration. The distance from the contact point to the proximal bone around the adjacent teeth was less than 5 mm, indicating the possibility of completely restored papillae.

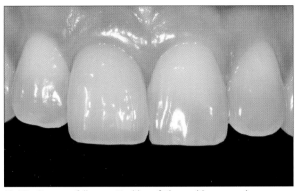

Fig 27 One-year follow up. Healthy soft tissue with no recession.

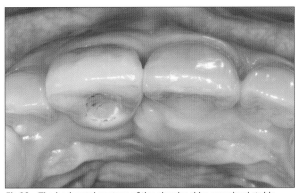

Fig 28 The horizontal contour of the alveolar ridge remained stable.

The patient received oral-hygiene instructions, including brushing and flossing. Regular recall visits were scheduled every three months.

After one year in function, the restoration was well maintained, and the soft tissue was healthy and stable. The patient was satisfied with the result. The radiographic examination showed bone levels similar to those at the time of delivery (Figs 27 to 29).

At the patient's two-year follow-up visit, the esthetic treatment outcome was stable (Figs 30 and 31).

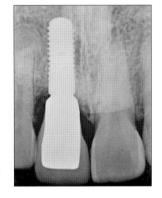

Fig 29 One-year radiological follow-up. The bone level adjacent to the implant was well maintained.

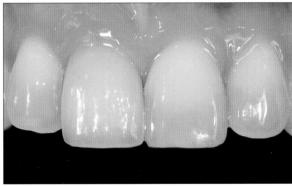

Fig 30 Two-year clinical follow up.

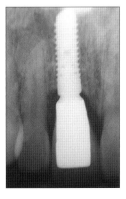

Fig 31 Two-year radiological follow-up.

7.4 Replacement of a Failing Upper Right Central Incisor: Ridge Preservation and Late Placement of a NC Bone Level Implant

W. D. Polido, P. E. Pittas do Canto

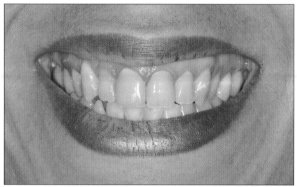

Fig 1   Initial smile.

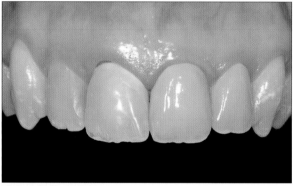

Fig 2   Initial buccal view.

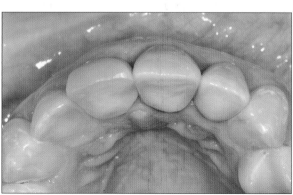

Fig 3   Initial occlusal view.

A 30-year-old patient presented at our clinic with a chief complaint of pain in her endodontically treated right maxillary central incisor (tooth 11) with a post-and-core and a fixed single crown.

She had a very high lip line (Fig 1), a medium to thin soft-tissue phenotype, and a medium scalloped gingival contour. She also had high esthetic expectations because of her young age and beautiful smile. However, her expectations were realistic and she understood the risks of the treatment.

At the initial clinical examination there was a slight mobility of tooth 11; no fistula was observed. The patient also had a single crown on the adjacent tooth 21. Both restorations were old and esthetically deficient (Figs 2 and 3). A digital periapical radiograph showed a very small periapical radiolucency, a thick intraradicular post, and no separation between root fragments. Her dental history included a recent endodontic treatment. A cone-beam computed tomography (CBCT) showed a root perforation, with part of the endodontic obturation paste exiting through the perforation on the buccal side (Figs 4a-d). This was probably the cause of the pain. It was decided to extract tooth 11 and replace it with an implant-supported restoration.

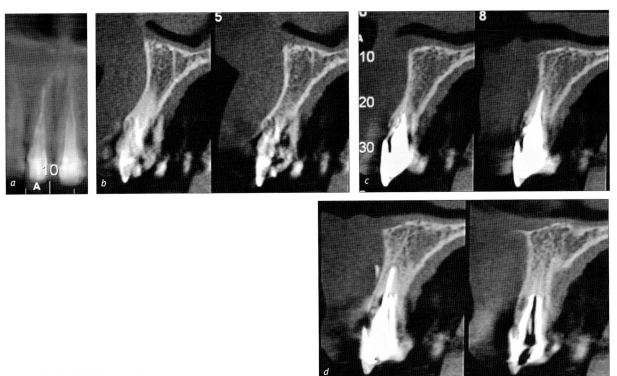

Figs 4a-d   Initial CBCT presentation.

Treatment alternatives for this esthetically demanding case were:

1. Extraction and immediate implant placement (Type 1)
2. Extraction and delayed implant placement (Type 2)
3. Extraction and alveolar socket filling with DBBM and collagen biomaterial for delayed implant placement (ridge preservation)

The CBCT showed a sagittal class I root position according to Kan and coworkers (2011). A very thin facial bone wall, almost imperceptible on the CBCT cross-sections, was believed to be present.

The Esthetic Risk Assessment (ERA; Table 1) was advanced/complex.

We briefly discuss our rationale behind the decision to choose option 3, alveolar bone preservation and delayed implant placement, compared to the other two options.

1. **Extraction and immediate implant placement**
    According to Chen and Buser (2014), recession of the midfacial mucosa is a risk with immediate (type 1) placement. In their systematic review, immediate implant placement was shown to be associated with a greater variability in outcomes and a higher frequency of recession > 1 mm of the midfacial mucosa (eight studies; range 9% to 41% and median 26% of sites, 1 to 3 years after placement) compared to early (type 2 and type 3) implant placement (2 studies; no sites with recession > 1 mm). In two retrospective studies of immediate implant placement with bone grafts, the facial bone wall was not detectable by CBCT in 36% and 57% of sites. These sites had more recession of the midfacial mucosa compared to sites with detectable facial bone. Immediate implant placement also requires the grafting of the gap between the implant and the buccal wall with autologous bone, bone substitute, or soft tissue to achieve a better result (Araújo and coworkers, 2015a). An immediate provisional restoration with an adequate contour is also a key factor—as is a perfect three-dimensional position of the implant—in a flapless approach.

In the present case, a facial bone wall was not detectable on the CBCT, and the alveolar bone was relatively thin, leaving a narrow space for immediate implant placement and a graft, even if a reduced-diameter implant was chosen. The patient had a very high lip line, with a beautiful and wide smile. We felt that even a 1-mm recession would make the difference between a good and an excellent result. Additionally, since the patient had agreed to also replace the crown on the adjacent tooth 21, we had very good support for a provisional restoration during the healing phase. All those

Table 1 Esthetic Risk Assessment (ERA)

Esthetic risk factors	Level of risk		
	Low	**Medium**	**High**
Medical status	Healthy, uneventful healing		Compromised healing
Smoking habit	Non-smoker	Light smoker (≤ 10 cigs/day)	Heavy smoker (> 10 cigs/day)
Gingival display at full smile	Low	Medium	High
Width of edentulous span	1 tooth (≥ 7 mm)[1] 1 tooth (≥ 6 mm)[2]	1 tooth (< 7 mm)[1] 1 tooth (< 6 mm)[2]	2 teeth or more
Shape of tooth crowns	Rectangular		Triangular
Restorative status of neighboring teeth	Virgin		Restored
Gingival phenotype	Low-scalloped, thick	Medium-scalloped, medium-thick	High-scalloped, thin
Infection at implant site	None	Chronic	Acute
Soft-tissue anatomy	Soft tissue intact		Soft-tissue defects
Bone level at adjacent teeth	≤ 5 mm to contact point	5.5 to 6.5 mm to contact point	≥ 7 mm to contact point
Facial bone-wall phenotype*	Thick-wall phenotype ≥ 1 mm thickness		Thin-wall phenotype < 1 mm thickness
Bone anatomy of alveolar crest	No bone deficiency	Horizontal bone deficiency	Vertical bone deficiency
Patient's esthetic expectations	Realistic expectations		Unrealistic expectations

* If three-dimensional imaging is available with the tooth in place
[1] Standard-diameter implant, regular connection
[2] Narrow-diameter implant, narrow connection

factors combined make immediate placement less predictable in this case, even in experienced hands. We use this approach in more favorable situations, with a broader range for recession and thicker alveolar bone and soft tissues.

2. **Extraction with soft-tissue healing and open-flap GBR**

Buser and coworkers (2008) proposed the type 2 placement, which involves tooth extraction, waiting 6 to 8 weeks for complete soft-tissue wound closure, and performing an open-flap procedure. This procedure aims at a perfect 3D implant placement and simultaneous reconstruction of the alveolar volume, especially in the horizontal aspect, by simultaneous contour augmentation using guided bone regeneration with autologous bone chips combined with a low-substitution bone filler plus a resorbable collagen membrane.

This procedure is required in most cases, since thin facial bone-wall phenotypes have shown a progressive vertical bone loss of 7.5 mm on the facial aspect after 8 weeks (Chappuis and coworkers 2013b; Araújo and coworkers 2015).

Although the procedure has proven to have an excellent and stable outcome over time (Buser and coworkers 2013), there are two important aspects that we considered in our presented case. Extraction of the central incisor in this thin bone-wall phenotype will require contour augmentation using GBR to restore the facial bone and the soft-tissue anatomy. In such cases, a vertical releasing incision is necessary, even though it is possible to place the incision further distally, outside the esthetic zone. In the present patient, with a relatively medium/thin soft-tissue phenotype, even a minor soft-tissue scar would have been apparent, compromising the esthetic outcome. The approach is also a more invasive procedure, and in many situations, a third surgery for reopening and abutment connection will be necessary. Secondly, after tooth extraction, a ridge defect may occur, especially where the tissue is thin and the bone loss is more extensive. In patients with a high lip line, this temporary esthetic compromise has to be considered.

3. **Extraction with alveolar ridge preservation and late implant placement**

Alveolar ridge contour preservation is aimed at minimizing horizontal and vertical remodeling after tooth extraction. Recent studies have indicated that with alveolar ridge preservation, horizontal resorption of just over 1 mm will still occur with relative preservation of the vertical bone, whereas the absence of alveolar ridge preservation will generally result in more than 3 mm of horizontal loss and at least 1 mm or more of vertical loss (Horowitz and coworkers 2012).

Having considered options 1 and 2 above, we opted for preservation (option 3) in this case, using a technique similar to that proposed by Elian and coworkers (2007b). Following minimally invasive extraction, we filled the socket with a DBBM and collagen material to preserve the alveolar contour and to able to reduce the need for the future grafting at the time of implant placement. The longer healing time (4 to 5 months) prior to implant placement, plus 2 to 3 months for osseointegration time, was a disadvantage. However, this was of no concern to our patient, since she had a stable cantilevered provisional restoration, cemented on the adjacent tooth.

If preservation of the alveolar volume had not been completely successful, we would still have had the chance for simultaneous GBR at the time of implant placement. The defect morphology would be less favorable 4 to 5 months after socket grafting compared to a type 2 approach, and the site would have had to be grafted twice, increasing treatment time and cost.

In successful procedures with ridge preservation, a connective-tissue graft may still be necessary to optimize the ridge contour.

Figure 5 suggests a timeline for ridge preservation, and Figure 6 compares the three most frequently performed approaches.

The treatment option chosen, given all the above considerations, was option 3, extraction with alveolar preservation and delayed implant placement.

The treatment was initiated by removing the restorations of teeth 11 and 21, preparing tooth 21, taking impressions and fabricating a new cantilevered provisional restoration supported by cementation on 21.

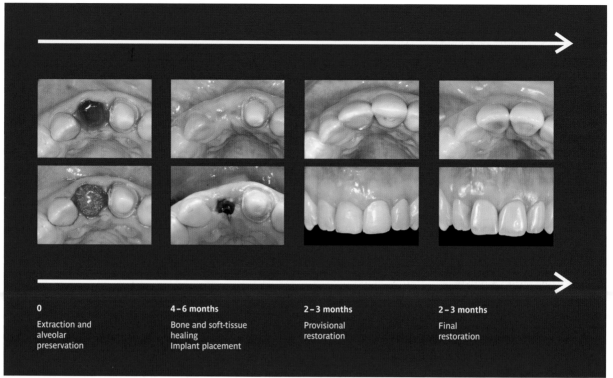

0	4–6 months	2–3 months	2–3 months
Extraction and alveolar preservation	Bone and soft-tissue healing Implant placement	Provisional restoration	Final restoration

Fig 5   Timeline for ridge preservation procedure.

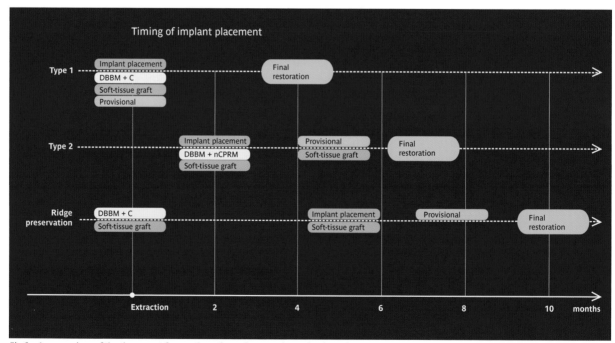

Fig 6   A comparison of the three most frequently performed approaches to implant placement.

The first surgical step involved minimally traumatic extraction of tooth 11, using a fine periotome (Aesculap, Tuttlingen, Germany) to avoid any rotation and rupture of the buccal plate and adjacent soft tissue. Whenever possible, a vertical extraction instrument (Bennex; Meisinger, Neuss, Germany or similar) is indicated so rotation of the root is avoided. After careful removal of tooth 11 (Figs 7 and 8), the buccal plate was probed to detect the presence or absence of buccal alveolar bone. In case of absent or extremely thin buccal bone (also visualized by CBCT), we decided on using a resorbable non-crosslinked porcine-derived collagen membrane (Bio-Gide, Geistlich Biomaterials, Wolhusen, Switzerland) internally in the alveolar socket, with a "socket repair" technique as suggested by Elian and coworkers (2007b) (Figs 9 to 11). A round part was left outside of the socket to close over the resorbable biomaterial placed inside the socket. Then a bone substitute, a demineralized bovine bone mineral with 10% collagen (B Collagen; Geistlich Biomaterials) was placed into the alveolar socket, soaked in blood, to completely fill it. In this case, no soft-tissue graft or soft-tissue substitute was used. According to Horowitz and coworkers (2012), there is no strong evidence that supports the use of a soft-tissue graft or even of primary

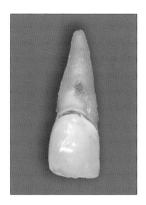

Fig 7   Perforated tooth removed.

closure over the alveolar socket. In our case, the patient exhibited good oral hygiene and compliance, showing up at all follow-ups, so we decided not to use a soft-tissue graft seal.

Medications included an antibiotic (amoxicillin 875 mg every twelve hours for seven days, starting three days before the procedure; ketorolac 10 mg every eight hours in the event of pain; chlorhexidine digluconate 0,12% for oral rinses twice a day, for ten days).

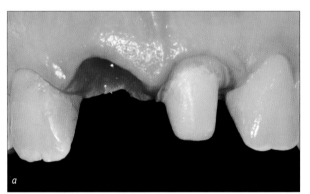
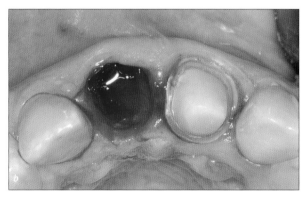

Figs 8a-b   Site 11 after extraction. Frontal and occlusal views.

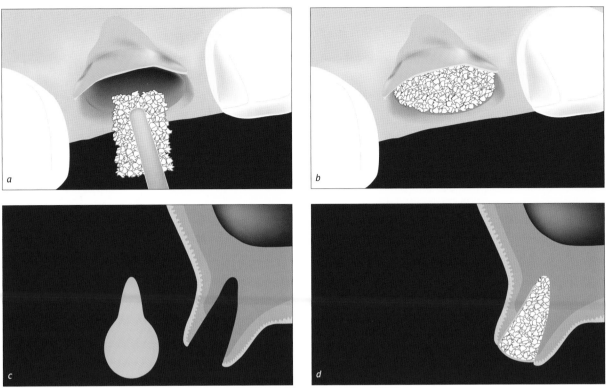

Figs 9a-d   "Socket repair" ridge preservation technique as described by Elian and coworkers (2007b).

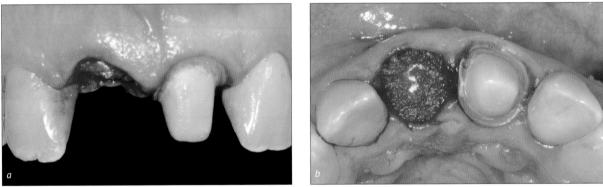

Figs 10a-b   Socket preservation with DBBM and collagen. Frontal and occlusal views.

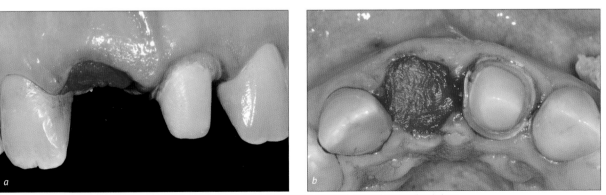

Figs 11a-b   Resorbable membrane on top of the collagenous ridge preservation material. Frontal and occlusal views.

Of importance is the fact that the provisional restoration has to be convex and well-polished, without leaving too much space and without applying pressure to the healing site (Fig 12). Made in this manner, it also helps to protect the area during healing.

After five months of uneventful healing, a new CBCT was taken that showed an alveolar bone slightly remodeled in the horizontal dimension, but still with adequate width and height to place an implant (Figs 13a-c). After measurement (no digital planning software was available at the time for implant placement), we decided to go for a bone-level implant with a reduced diameter and a titanium-zirconium (TiZr) alloy (Bone Level Narrow CrossFit, Roxolid; Institut Straumann AG, Basel, Switzerland). We wanted to preserve as much alveolar bone as possible around the implant, reach good primary stability but without having to use an immediate provisional, and obtain good tissue stability around the cervical area of the implant, provided by the neck design of the BLNC implant according to Cochran and coworkers (2013) and Chappuis and coworkers (2015b). The TiZr alloy was chosen for its increased strength – especially important in this young patient with a long life expectancy and anticipated prolonged use of the implant (Barter and coworkers 2012).

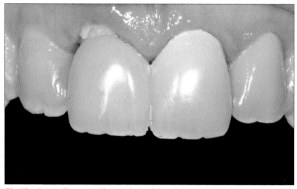

Fig 12   Immediate cantilevered provisional, cemented on tooth 21, after extraction and alveolar ridge preservation.

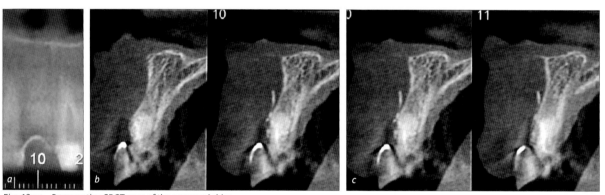

Figs 13a-c   Preoperative CBCT scan of the preserved ridge.

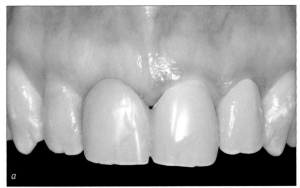
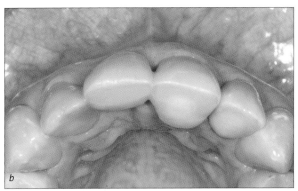

Figs 14a-b   Clinical situation 5 months after ridge preservation and prior to implant placement with provisional in place. Frontal and occlusal views.

The clinical examination showed a very small horizontal recession, but with no concavity evident in the occlusal view (Figs 14a-b). The soft tissues were of medium thickness and without any scars.

The surgical template was manufactured, taking care to stabilize it on the adjacent natural central incisor abutment (as a fixed bridge), and with the ideal cervical height of the future crown. That is of the utmost importance in order to achieve the correct vertical position of the implant.

When the surgical template was put in place, it was noticed that the patient presented with a very nice soft-tissue contour, with keratinized soft tissue of adequate thickness around the planned implant position (Figs 15a-b). These combined factors allowed us to perform implant placement in a flapless manner.

We also wanted to be consistent with a less invasive approach and to avoid an open flap, which would have required a vertical releasing incision with a possible visible scar.

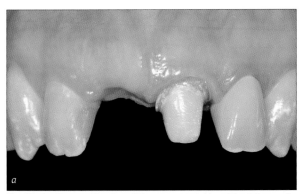
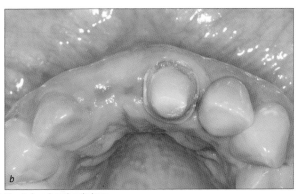

Figs 15a-b   Preoperative view of the augmented ridge without the provisonal. Frontal and occlusal views.

With the surgical guide in place, the correct emergence of the implant was marked with a 15C blade. A round incision was performed (Fig 16), removing the soft tissue. This area was of very good thickness, especially in the connective-tissue component. We saved this tissue; it would be later de-epithelialized and placed as a free graft internally on the buccal aspect, in an envelope fashion, in order to optimize the ridge contour, making it more convex.

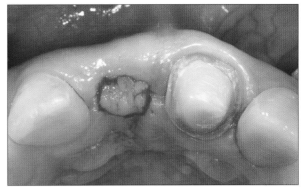

Fig 16   Circular incision for implant placement, in a flapless manner.

After the soft-tissue removal, the surgical guide was put in place again. A mark of the ideal position of the implant was performed with the 1.2-mm round drill. The vertical tissue thickness was measured with a periodontal probe, to find the depth for the implant placement. Ideally, the BL NC implant would have to be positioned vertically at 4 mm from the central area of the future crown. In the case on hand, the distance was only 2 mm. Hence, an additional 2 mm of bone have to be removed in order to position the implant in the appropriate position. We like to accomplish that using the large round bur, also creating a plane platform to initiate the perforations.

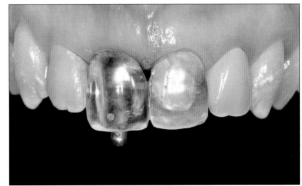

Fig 17   Surgical guide with direction indicator pin in situ.

Through the surgical guide, we did the perforations as per the manufacturer recommendations (Institut Straumann AG, Basel, Switzerland). However, we did not perform the tapping procedure in this case, so as to increase primary stability of the implant. If the palatal wall is thick and dense, the profile drill can be used to adjust the cervical part of the implant in a correct position, but in most of these this will not be necessary. Direction indicators were used to confirm the implant's mesiodistal and buccolingual position and its depth (Fig 17).

In this situation, since we needed 4 mm of depth from the planned mucosal margin of the future restoration, we opted for an implant of 10 mm length. The implant twist drills (2.2 and 2.8 mm in diameter) were used at low speed (600 rpm) with copious irrigation. They were drilled down until the 14-mm mark was flush with the soft-tissue margin, as also confirmed by the direction indicator. Before implant placement, we placed the Bone Level profile drill without any rotation to make sure the preparation of the cervical area was adequate. (If the bone is soft, we avoid drilling and prefer to place the implant at the adequate vertical position. That also helps to optimize primary stability of the implant.)

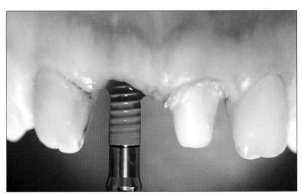

Fig 18   Implant placement (Straumann Bone Level NC implant).

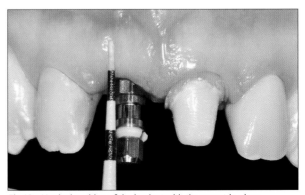

Fig 19   Vertical position of the implant with the mount in place.

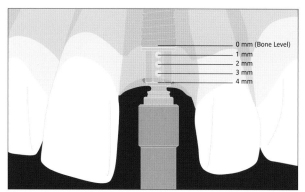

Fig 20   Correct vertical implant positioning using the Loxim implant mount as a tool, using the planned cervical margin of the future restoration as a reference.

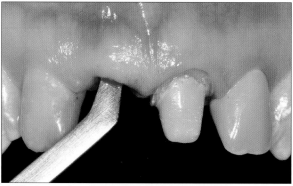

Fig 21   Implant position after placement. Occlusal view.

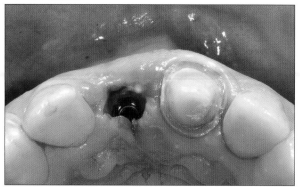

Fig 22   Preparation of an envelope for the soft-tissue graft.

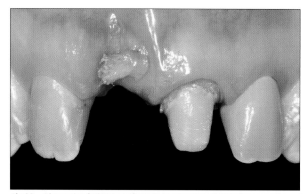

Fig 23   Planned soft-tissue graft position, situation right before insertion of the graft into the envelope.

A bone-level implant (Roxolid, SLActive, Bone Level, Narrow CrossFit, diameter 3.3 mm, length 10 mm; Institut Straumann AG) was placed with the contra-angle handpiece at low speed (25 rpm) (Fig 18). Primary stability was achieved in the correct vertical position with a placement torque of 30 N·cm. The vertical positioning can be finely controlled by observing the Bone Level mount (Fig 19).

In the present case we used the screw implant mount, where the length of the mount had been 3 mm, and the marked color had to be positioned facing the buccal (Fig 19). With the modern (Straumann Loxim) mount, the three round marks represent 3 mm, and the last step to the head of the implant represents an additional 1 mm. The round marks have to be positioned facing buccally (Fig 20).

After removing the mount (with a holding countertorque instrument to avoid excessive torque on the implant) the depth of the implant head was rechecked, and it was found to be in the ideal position (Fig 21).

Then, using a Heidemann composite spatula (Hu-Friedy, Chicago, IL, USA) or similar small and delicate instrument, an envelope dissection was carefully performed on the buccal aspect, creating space for the soft-tissue graft removed from the incision area (Fig 22).

Care was taken to remove the epithelium from the graft, leaving only the connective tissue of adequate thickness (around 4 mm). The soft-tissue graft was placed in a very delicate manner, only with small pressure, without any suture (Fig 23).

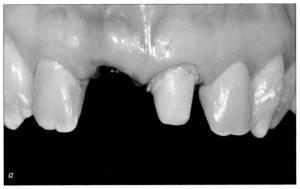 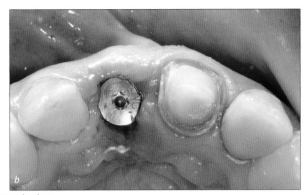

Figs 24a-b   Frontal and occlusal view of the situation with the healing abutment in place.

That was also held in place with the healing abutment (Figs 24a-b) with a diameter of 4.8 mm and a height of 3.5 mm.

The cantilevered provisional restoration was placed as previously, cemented on tooth 21. A healing period of 3 months was defined for osseointegration, even with the use of the TiZr alloy with an SLActive surface, due to the fact that it was a grafted site.

After an uneventful healing period, to start the restorative phase, a periapical radiograph was taken and osseointegration was confirmed by removing the healing cap, retightening it with hand force, and watching for absence of movement. Today we would recommend ISQ measurements (Osstell, Göteborg, Sweden) (Fig 25).

The first step was to design the provisional restoration, to be positioned over the implant 11 and the natural abutment 21. A silicone key made over the diagnostic wax-up was filled with bisacryl resin in order to make a provisional and have an index of the ideal position (Fig 26).

The provisional restoration was positioned over the preparation of the adjacent tooth, with an opening to capture the provisional abutment directly in the mouth (Figs 27a-b).

A NC PEEK provisional abutment (Straumann Bone Level NC) was chosen (Fig 28) and placed in the implant. A small compression was noted with ischemia in the soft tissue, specifically in the mesiofacial area (Figs 29a-b). The abutment was removed and prepared to adjust the emergence contour, reduce the height, and create retention for crown adhesion.

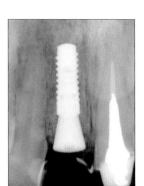

Fig 25   Periapical radiograph twelve weeks after implant placement.

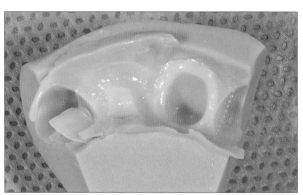

Fig 26   Silicone key impression for fabrication of the provisional restoration.

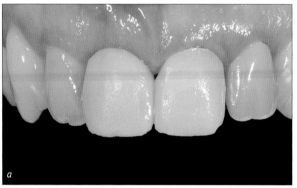

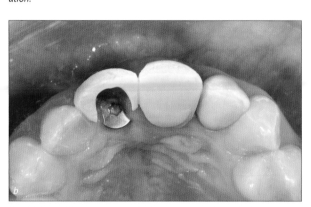

Figs 27a-b   Frontal and occlusal view of the provisional with the implant.

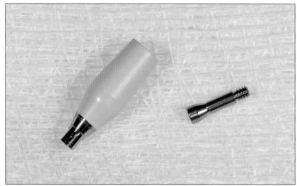

Fig 28   The NC PEEK provisional abutment and screw.

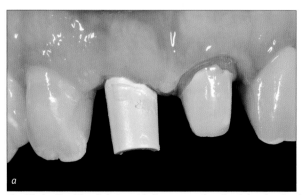

Figs 29a-b   Provisional abutment before preparation. Frontal and occlusal views.

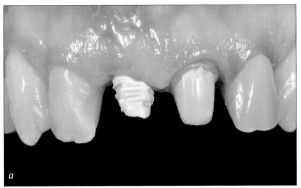
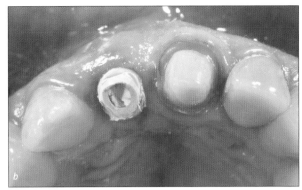

Figs 30a-b   Provisional abutment after preparation. Frontal and occlusal views.

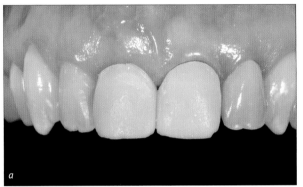
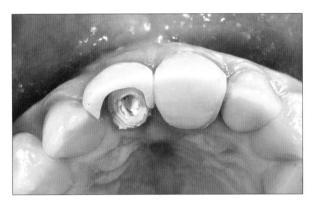

Figs 31a-b   Cantilevered provisional in place. Frontal and occlusal views.

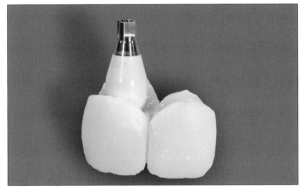

Fig 32   Provisional restoration after intraoral pick-up.

The abutment was replaced (Figs 30a-b) and the pro-visional restoration repositioned (Figs 31a-b). After confirming the contour and the vertical space in occlu-sion, a flowable composite resin (light-curing) was used to attach the provisional restoration to the prepared abutment. It was then carefully removed and separat-ed from the adjacent natural-tooth provisional, and the ideal emergence profile was achieved at chairside, using light-curing flowable composite resin and fine polishing burs (Fig 32). After finishing, the provisional was screwed in place to 15 N·cm, and the access hole was closed with PTFE material and an interim light-curing resin adhesive

(Flow Resin; 3M, St. Paul, MN, USA) (Figs 33a-b). A con-trol periapical radiograph was taken to confirm full seat-ing of the provisional restoration (Fig 34).

Usually it takes two to three months for the soft-tissue contour to stabilize. Ideally one should manipulate the provisional as little as possible, making only strictly nec-essary contour adjustments. Once the ideal contour is achieved, with selective application of composite to com-press the relevant areas, the impression for the final res-toration was taken.

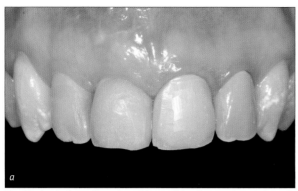

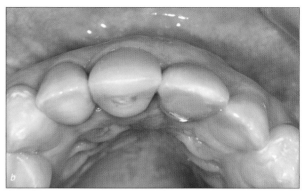

Figs 33a-b   An immediate view of the provisional restoration 45 days after implant placement. Frontal and occlusal view.

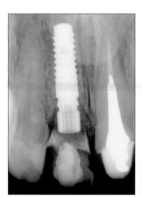

Fig 34   Periapical radiograph 45 days after implant placement, with the immediate provisional restoration in place.

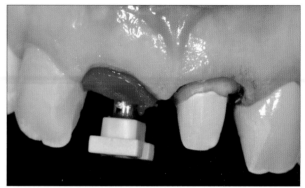

Fig 35   The impression was taken on the tooth and the implant simultaneously.

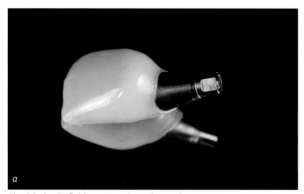

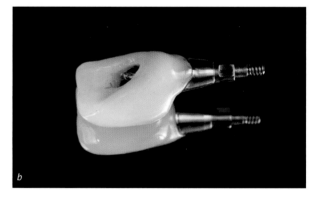

Figs 36a-b   Definitive restoration prior to placement.

In this case, an opaque composite was placed over the post of tooth 21, and a retraction cord was positioned to obtain an optimized impression of the final margin. On implant 11, the impression was customized using an impression coping with Duralay resin to capture the transition zone from the implant to the mucosal margin. An impression was taken of both the tooth and implant at the same time (Fig 35).

An anatomic abutment (Straumann BL NC) was indicated in this situation. It was decided to customize it using a Lava zirconica coping (3M, São Paulo, Brazil) on which a ceramic crown had been cemented extraorally, resulting in a screw-retained definitive restoration (Figs 36a-b).

In today's clinical practice, this same treatment would be achieved with a CAD/CAM abutment, something that was not available at the time of this treatment.

The access hole was filled with a PTFE cord and sealed with a light-curing composite resin.

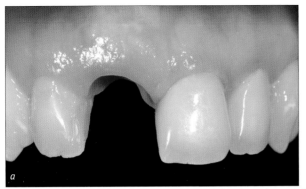

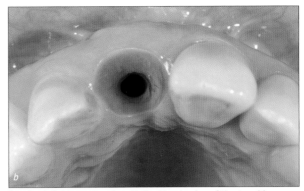

Figs 37a-b Facial and occlusal view of the clinical situation prior to delivering the definitive restoration. Notice the shaping of the transition zone, achieved by the use of the screw-retained provisional restoration.

The definitive restoration was placed six months after the implant. The occlusal and buccal views of the soft-tissue contour after placement of the definitive restoration show excellent tissue stability obtained with a combination of ridge preservation, a small soft-tissue augmentation at implant placement, and a long period in situ of a provisional restoration with adequate contours (Figs 37a-b).

The situation was stable at the one-year follow-up (Figs 38 to 42), three-year follow-up (Figs 43 to 45) and five-year follow-up (Figs 46 to 50).

Since the restoration was screw-retained, it was retrievable.

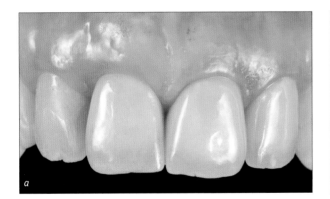

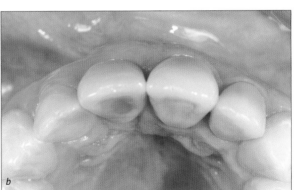

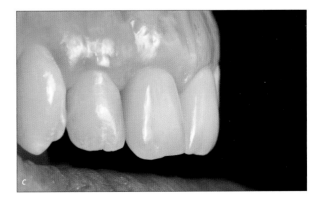

Figs 38a-c The intraoral situation at the one-year follow-up.

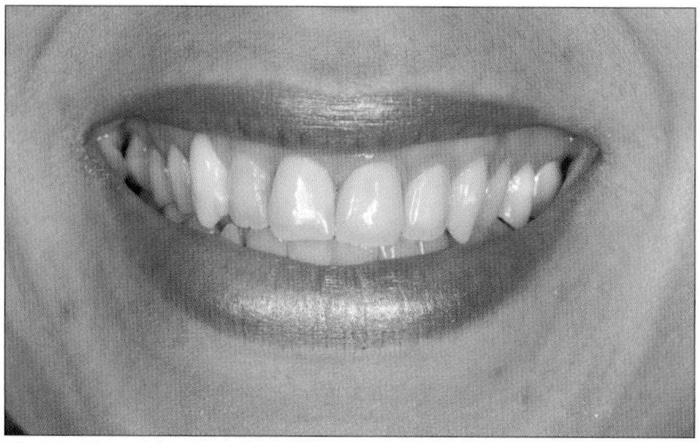

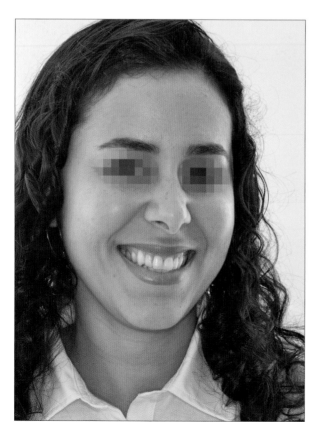

Fig 39   The patient's smile at the one-year follow-up.

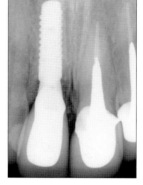

Fig 40   One-year follow-up periapical radiograph.

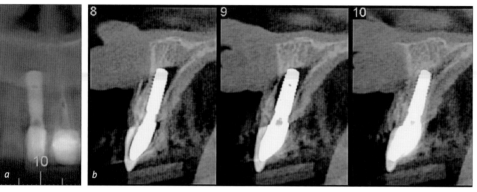

Figs 41a-b   One-year follow-up CBCT.

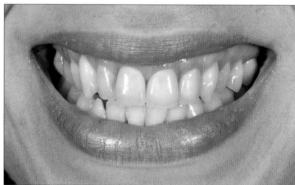

Fig 43   The patient's smile at the three-year follow-up.

Fig 42   The patient's face at the one-year follow-up visit.

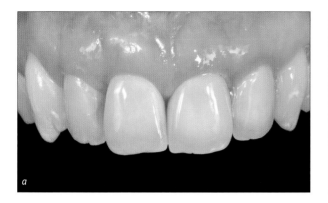

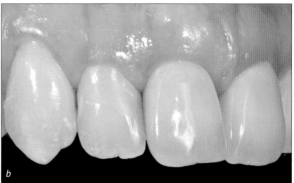

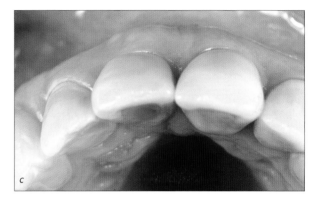

Figs 44a-c   The intraoral situation at the three-year follow-up.

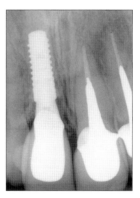

Fig 45   Three-year follow-up periapical radiograph.

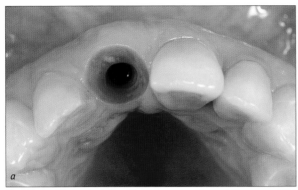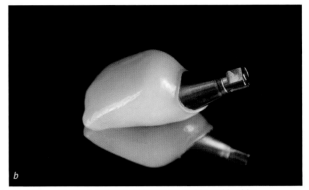

Figs 46a-b   The implant site without the restoration and the crown at the five-year follow-up. The peri-implant tissues are stable and healthy.

At the five-year follow-up appointment, we were able to remove the restoration for lab polishing and noticed an excellent soft-tissue contour.

The mucosal margin (soft-tissue vertical position) as well as the soft-tissue horizontal position (occlusal view) remained with the same characteristics as when the case was finished. Pleasing pink and white esthetic scores were obtained after five years (Belser and coworkers 2009).

The TiZr implant was performing as expected, as supported by a recent paper by Altuna and coworkers (2016).

Radiographically, the bone remained stable, with minimal remodeling around the implant, both in a periapical radiograph and in a CBCT (horizontal view), confirming the correct decision to be as conservative as possible, with the ridge preservation approach and a minor soft-tissue graft at implant placement with a Roxolid Bone Level Narrow CrossFit implant for a central incisor, preserving the bone and soft tissue while at the same time maintaining tissue stability.

The choice of a reduced-diameter implant (Bone Level Narrow CrossFit) intended to preserve the augmented

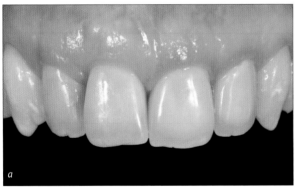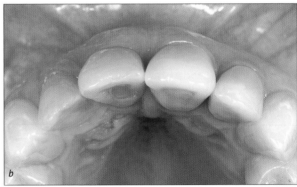

Figs 47a-b   The intraoral situation with the crown in situ at the five-year follow-up. Occlusal and labial views.

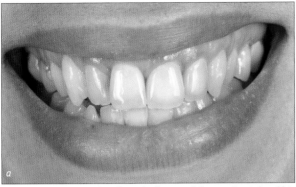
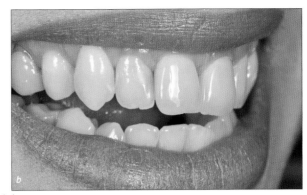

Figs 48a-b   The patient's smile at the five-year follow-up. Frontal and lateral views.

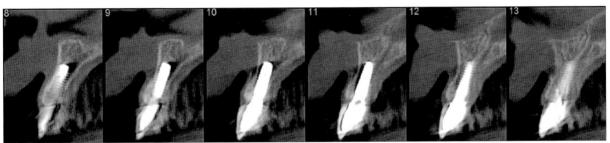

Fig 49   Five-year follow-up CBCT. Note retraction of the upper lip, allowing better observation of the buccal soft tissues and buccal-plate thickness, and graft stability (Januário and coworkers 2008).

bone and the esthetic longevity of the restoration. This patient had a medium to thin alveolar bone even after successful ridge preservation. If a regular-diameter implant had been used, the remaining facial plate would be thinner. If any horizontal resorption occurs with time (in a 30-year-old patient, longevity means at least a 40-year perspective), the thicker the facial tissue, the better the chance of maintaining a good esthetic outcome. The reduced area for osseointegration in a reduced-diameter implant was compensated by using a TiZr implant with a SLActive surface with an appropriate length of at least 10 mm to maximize the bone-to-implant contact in a smaller implant.

When a reduced-diameter implant is chosen for a larger tooth restoration (like on this case, a central incisor), we recommend placing the implant 4 mm deep below the planned mucosal margin of the restoration, in order to obtain vertical space in the transition zone for the correct emergence profile of the restoration. If a regular-diameter implant is placed, 3 mm of depth would be used from the planned mucosal margin to the top of the BL implant. Today this is our preferred approach for similar situations.

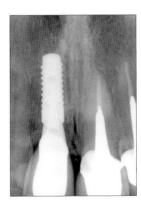

Fig 50   Five-year follow-up periapical radiograph.

7.5 Replacement of an Upper Right Central Incisor with Root Resorption: Ridge Preservation, Delayed Placement of an NC Bone Level Roxolid Implant

P. Casentini

A 32-year-old female Caucasian patient with a compromised maxillary right central incisor was referred to us by a general dentist. Her chief complaints were discomfort and mobility of tooth 11 with unsatisfactory esthetics due to discoloration. The patient reported a previous trauma, some years earlier, as the origin of pathology on the afflicted tooth. Anamnesis was negative for any other dental or periodontal pathology in the remaining dentition. The patient did not take any medication and reported to be a light smoker (5–10 cigs/day). She had high esthetic expectations of her treatment.

The extraoral examination revealed a high smile line with full exposure of her maxillary teeth and surrounding soft tissue in the area between the second premolars (Fig 1).

Intraoral examination confirmed the presence of a discolored tooth 11. The tooth had been restored with composite, exhibited increased mobility (class II). A fistula was detected at the mucogingival line (Figs 2 and 3).

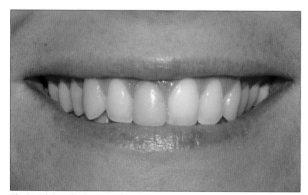

Fig 1   High smile line with full exposure of the maxillary anteriors.

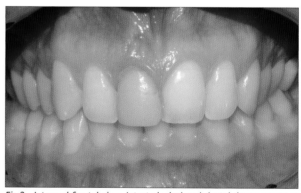

Fig 2   Intraoral frontal view. Intact gingival and dental tissues except at site 11.

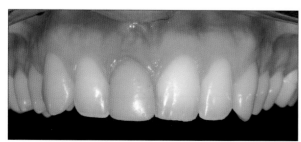

Fig 3   Frontal view of the maxillary anteriors. Tooth 11 was discolored and presented a fistula at the mucogingival line.

The soft-tissue phenotype was classified as thin and high-scalloped. Buccal displacement of the affected tooth contributed to reducing the thickness of the soft tissue, which was less than 1 mm on the buccal side. (Fig 4).

Referring to average esthetic parameters (Magne and Belser 2002), the two central incisors presented different axes and shapes. The incisal edges of the four incisors were aligned along a straight line (Fig 5).

An intraoral radiograph revealed external resorption of the root, which was surrounded by a radiolucent area (Fig 6).

The Esthetic Risk Assessment (ERA; Table 1) revealed a medium risk profile: the main risk factors were the high lip line and the thin and high-scalloped soft-tissue phenotype. The presence of a chronic infection, the interrupted buccal cortical plate, and the smoking habit were also considered as secondary risk factors. Finally, the patient's esthetic expectations were considered realistic (in view of the clinical situation) but nevertheless high.

Based on the clinical and radiological situation, the following treatment plan was proposed:

- Extraction of tooth 11 and ridge preservation using a bone substitute, followed by temporary restoration with a RRFDP
- Delayed placement of an implant after 6 months of healing
- Temporary prosthetic restoration followed by final ceramic crown; a composite restoration of the adjacent left central incisor was also considered, in order to optimize the esthetic result

The choice of treatment modality was related to local conditions, particularly the thin and highly scalloped soft tissue and the absence of an intact bone wall of the socket. The inclination and position of the root was asymmetric, which was not considered favorable for immediate implant placement. The patient's high esthetic expectations were also taken into account.

For all these reasons, immediate placement was not considered an option. A staged approach was preferred, as it facilitated further improvements and corrections at every step.

The patient agreed to the proposed treatment plan and gave her written informed consent. Moreover, the patient was recommended to avoid smoking after the surgical procedures.

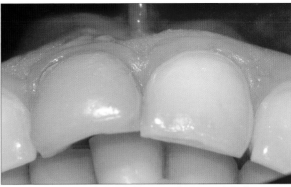

Fig 4 Occlusal view of the maxillary anteriors. Buccal displacement of tooth 11 and extremely thin buccal soft tissue.

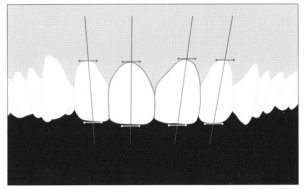

Fig 5 The esthetic analysis showed asymmetric shapes and axes of the central incisors and the absence of a "convex smile" at the incisal edges.

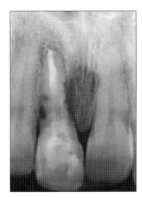

Fig 6 Periapical radiograph. External resorption of root 11 and periradicular radiolucency.

Table 1   Esthetic Risk Assessment (ERA)

Esthetic risk factors	Level of risk		
	Low	**Medium**	**High**
Medical status	Healthy, uneventful healing		Compromised healing
Smoking habit	Non-smoker	Light smoker (≤ 10 cigs/day)	Heavy smoker (> 10 cigs/day)
Gingival display at full smile	Low	Medium	High
Width of edentulous span	1 tooth (≥ 7 mm)[1] 1 tooth (≥ 6 mm)[2]	1 tooth (< 7 mm)[1] 1 tooth (< 6 mm)[2]	2 teeth or more
Shape of tooth crowns	Rectangular		Triangular
Restorative status of neighboring teeth	Virgin		Restored
Gingival phenotype	Low-scalloped, thick	Medium-scalloped, medium-thick	High-scalloped, thin
Infection at implant site	None	Chronic	Acute
Soft-tissue anatomy	Soft tissue intact		Soft-tissue defects
Bone level at adjacent teeth	≤ 5 mm to contact point	5.5 to 6.5 mm to contact point	≥ 7 mm to contact point
Facial bone-wall phenotype*	Thick-wall phenotype ≥ 1 mm thickness		Thin-wall phenotype < 1 mm thickness
Bone anatomy of alveolar crest	No bone deficiency	Horizontal bone deficiency	Vertical bone deficiency
Patient's esthetic expectations	Realistic expectations		Unrealistic expectations

* If three-dimensional imaging is available with the tooth in place
[1] Standard-diameter implant, regular connection
[2] Narrow-diameter implant, narrow connection

After the preliminary impressions, an interim resin-retained fixed dental prosthesis (RRFDP) made of composite resin with metal wings was produced by the dental laboratory (Fig 7).

Minimally traumatic extraction was performed under local anesthesia. The site was carefully debrided (Fig 8).

Following the extraction, partial damage to the thin buccal wall was confirmed. The extraction socket was filled with a bovine xenograft (Bio-Oss Collagen; Geistlich Pharma, Wolhusen, Switzerland) and sealed with a punch graft of connective tissue harvested from the palate (Figs 9 and 10).

The compromised socket wall and the delicate soft-tissue anatomy were the main reasons for choosing a ridge-preservation approach over delayed post-extraction implant placement. The risk of socket collapse was considered too high in this case, while ridge preservation allowed an almost complete restoration of the crest and adjacent papillae. The connective-tissue punch created thick and stable peri-implant soft-tissue contours.

The soft-tissue punch was completely immobilized by means of 6.0 resorbable polyglycolic-acid sutures (Vicryl; Ethicon, New Brunswick, NJ, USA). The donor site was protected with a collagen sponge stabilized with the same kind of suture. Once the ridge preservation procedure

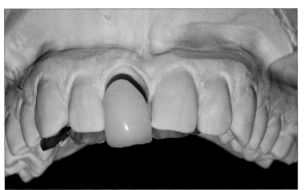

Fig 7 Interim resin-retained fixed dental prosthesis (RRFDP) in metal and composite resin was shaped with a moderate ovate pontic in the extraction area.

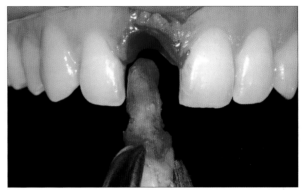

Fig 8 Minimally traumatic extraction of the compromised tooth. The extraction socket was carefully debrided.

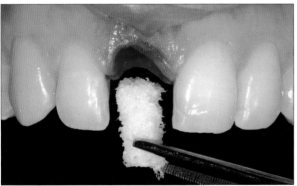

Fig 9 The extraction socket was filled with a bovine xenograft.

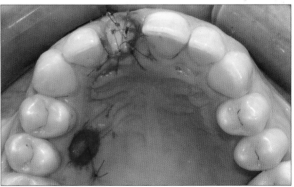

Fig 10 A soft-tissue punch graft harvested from the palate was used to seal the socket.

was completed, the RRFDP was immediately bonded to the adjacent teeth (Fig 11) with a dual-curing composite cement (RelyX Unicem; 3M, St. Paul, MN, USA).

Antibiotic medication began on the day before surgery and was continued for six days postoperatively. Chlorhexidine mouth rinses were also prescribed for three weeks, together with a non-steroidal antiinflammatory medication in case of pain.

The patient was advised to reduce her smoking and to avoid brushing in the treated area.

At suture removal after 15 days, healing was uneventful (Fig 12). The patient reported no significant symptoms.

After six months of uncomplicated healing, the preservation of the ridge volume was confirmed both in the vertical and horizontal dimensions (Figs 13 and 14). A control radiograph documented adequate integration of the xenograft (Fig 15).

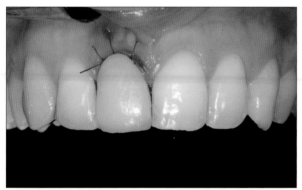

Fig 11   Frontal view of the anterior maxillary teeth after delivery of the RRFDP.

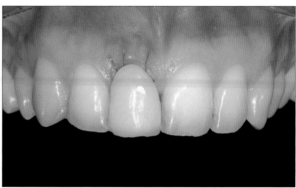

Fig 12   Frontal view of the maxillary anteriors at two weeks. Tissue healing was uneventful.

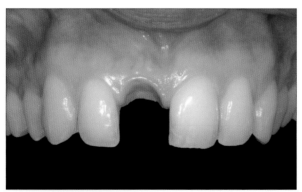

Fig 13   Frontal view of the anterior maxillary teeth after six months of healing. The volume of the ridge was nicely maintained.

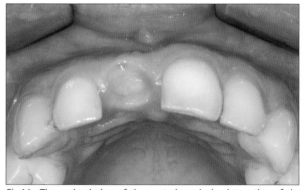

Fig 14   The occlusal view of the crest showed nice integration of the soft-tissue punch graft and reduced ridge contraction in the horizontal dimension.

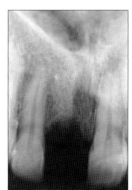

Fig 15   Periapical radiograph six months after ridge preservation.

At implant placement, the choice of a reduced-diameter implant combined with a perfect prosthetically-driven position was considered adequate to avoid a wider dehiscence of the implant surface, simplifying the regenerative procedure and increasing its predictability. The use of a titanium-zirconium alloy implant with an active surface (Straumann Roxolid SLActive; Institut Straumann AG, Basel, Switzerland) was preferred for its higher fracture resistance and faster osseointegration. On the other hand, reports or a fracture of an anterior implant in the correct prosthetic position are very rare. In general, reduced-diameter implants in the esthetic zone can often help avoid "danger zones" and reduce the risk of esthetic complications.

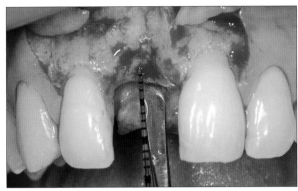

Fig 16   Frontal view of the surgical site after flap elevation.

Implant surgery was performed under local anesthesia. After flap elevation, the xenograft appeared well integrated and presented a favorable shape (Figs 16 and 17). The implant bed was prepared following the usual protocol, and drilling was prosthetically guided using a surgical template (Fig 18).

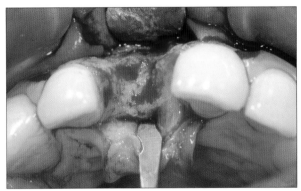

Fig 17   Occlusal view of the surgical site after flap elevation.

One Straumann Bone Level Narrow CrossFit Roxolid implant (diameter 3.3 mm, length 10 mm) with a SLActive surface (Institut Straumann AG) was inserted (Fig 19) and achieved adequate primary stability.

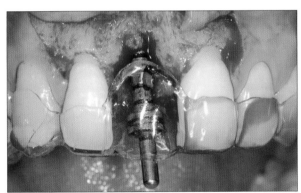

Fig 18   A surgical guide assisted the prosthetically driven implant placement.

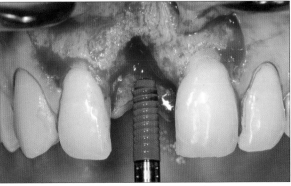

Fig 19   Insertion of the implant with a SLActive surface.

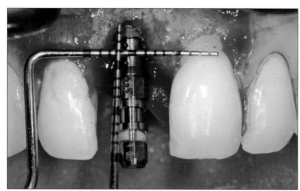

Fig 20   *The correct apicocoronal position of the implant was confirmed with a periodontal probe.*

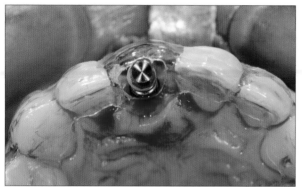

Fig 21   *Occlusal view after implant placement, with the surgical guide still in place, confirmed the correct three-dimensional position of the implant.*

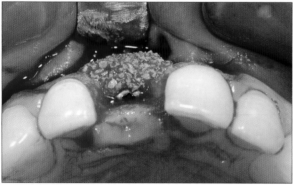

Fig 22   *Autologous bone chips and DBBM granules were used as a filling material during the GBR procedure.*

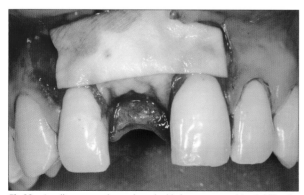

Fig 23   *A collagen membrane in a double layer was used to stabilize the graft.*

The implant shoulder was placed 2 mm apically of the cementoenamel junction (CEJ) of the adjacent teeth, and a buccopalatal axis compatible with a screw-retained restoration was selected (Figs 20 and 21).

Since a small buccal dehiscence of the implant surface (1.5 mm) was present, it was decided to treat it and further improve the shape of the ridge by means of a guided bone regeneration (GBR) procedure.

After small perforations in the surrounding cortical bone were performed, to improve revascularization of the graft, a first layer of autologous bone chips harvested from the nasal spine area was placed over the dehiscence. A second layer of deproteinized bovine bone mineral (DBBM) protected by a double-layer collagen membrane (Bio-Oss and Bio-Gide; Geistlich Pharma) completed the regenerative technique (Figs 22 and 23).

The flap was closed by primary intention without tension by means of mattress and single sutures after interrupting the periosteal layer and releasing the flap; 6.0 resorbable sutures (Vicryl; Ethicon) were utilized (Fig 24).

The temporary RRFDP was adapted to avoid excessive pressure, and rebonded immediately after surgery.

Postoperative instructions and medications were the same as after the first surgery.

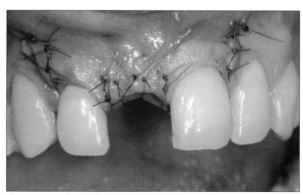

Fig 24   *Frontal view after suture.*

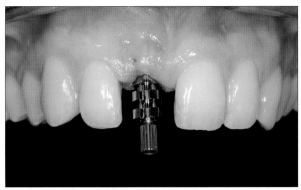

Fig 25   First impression for the provisional.

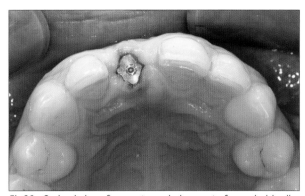

Fig 26   Occlusal view after reentry and placement of a conical healing screw.

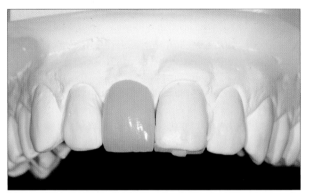

Fig 27   The temporary provisional restoration and additional composite veneer on the stone cast before delivery. Frontal view.

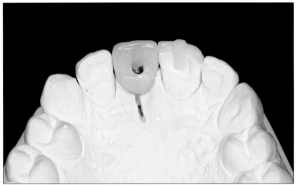

Fig 28   The temporary provisional restoration and additional composite veneer on the stone cast before delivery. Palatal view.

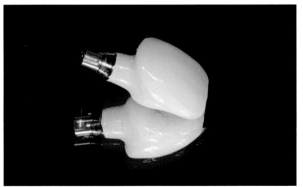

Fig 29   The temporary crown.

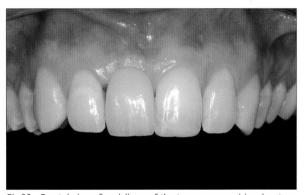

Fig 30   Frontal view after delivery of the temporary provisional restoration.

After four months of healing, reentry was performed using small midcrestal mesiodistal incision under local anesthesia. The adjacent papillae were not involved in the incision. A polyether open-tray impression was taken at the same appointment (Fig 25). A conical healing screw was inserted before replacing the RRFDP (Fig 26).

A screw-retained provisional crown was fabricated by the dental laboratory using a titanium temporary abutment. To improve the esthetic outcome, an indirect composite restoration was also produced to reconstruct the incisal edge of the adjacent central incisor (Figs 27 and 28).

To avoid excessive pressure on the peri-implant soft tissues, a concave profile of the temporary crown was initially provided (Fig 29).

During the following appointment, the temporary crown was delivered, and the additional composite veneer was bonded to the adjacent central incisor with pre-heated composite resin (Fig 30).

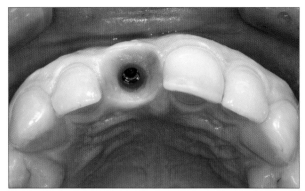

Fig 31   Occlusal view of the peri-implant soft tissue after conditioning.

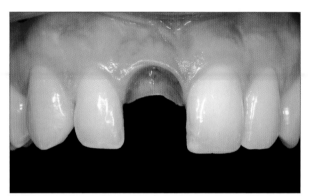

Fig 32   Frontal view of the peri-implant soft tissue after conditioning.

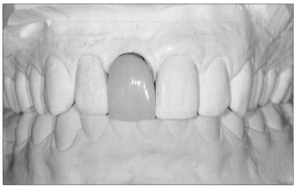

Fig 33   Frontal view of the final crown on the stone cast before delivery.

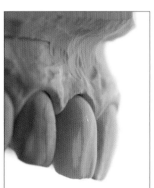

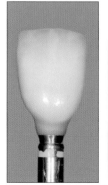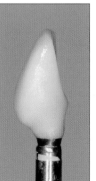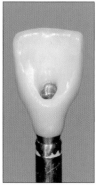

Fig 34   Surface texture of the final crown.

Fig 35   Emergence profile of the final crown. Frontal, mesiodistal, and palatal views.

Soft-tissue conditioning involved filling the overlap of the temporary crown with flowable composite. Two appointments after four and eight weeks were necessary to achieve an adequate emergence profile of the implant-supported restoration (Figs 31 and 32).

The final impression for the definitive restoration was taken after twelve weeks of soft-tissue conditioning by the provisional crown.

A screw-retained crown was realized by the dental laboratory using a zirconia framework veneered with ceramics and bonded to a titanium abutment. The connection between the crown and the implant was assured by an original Straumann titanium abutment. Since the Straumann Variobase abutment had not yet been available at the time of this treatment, an abutment for cemented prostheses was used (Figs 33 and 34).

Despite the reduced diameter (3.3 mm) of the implant/prosthetic platform, the appropriate three-dimensional position of the implant guaranteed the correct emergence profile of the crown and adequate support for the peri-implant soft tissue (Figs 35a-c).

One factor that could limit the use of reduced-diameter implants is a history of bruxism: in this case, the patient's anamnesis was negative for bruxism, and no signs of this condition were present.

Before delivery of the crown, the internal cavity of the implant was disinfected with chlorhexidine gel. The crown was screwed in place at a torque of 35 N·cm, and the access cavity to the screw was sealed with PTFE paper and some flowable composite.

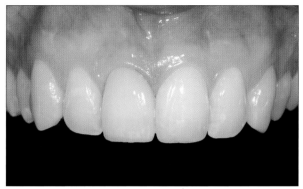

Fig 36   Frontal view after delivery of the definitive crown.

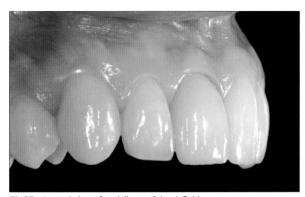

Fig 37   Lateral view after delivery of the definitive crown.

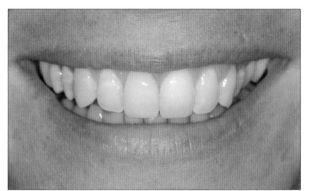

Fig 38   Extraoral view of the smile after treatment.

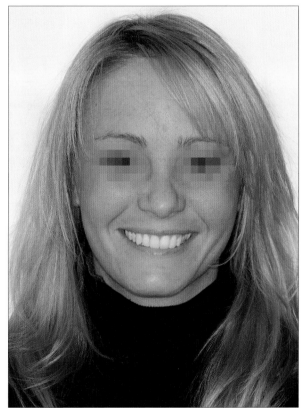

Fig 39   The patient's smile.

The final crown integrated well with the surrounding natural dentition in terms of tooth size, shape, color, and surface texture. The patient expressed her full satisfaction with the final treatment outcome (Figs 36 to 39).

From a radiological point of view, the peri-implant bone appeared stable and well mineralized (Fig 40).

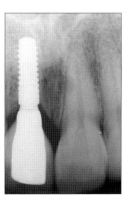

Fig 40   Final control radiograph.

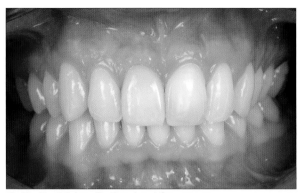

Fig 41   *Frontal view of both arches at five years.*

At the five-year clinical and radiological follow-up, the soft tissue and bone contours were perfectly stable. The implant-supported restoration was well integrated with the surrounding tissues and the patient's smile demonstrates full satisfaction of her expectations (Figs 41 to 46).

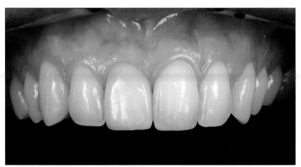

Fig 42   *Frontal view of the anterior maxillary teeth at five years.*

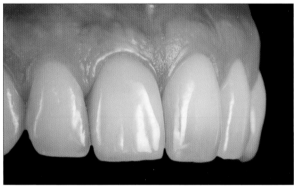

Fig 43   *Lateral view of the anterior maxillary teeth at five years.*

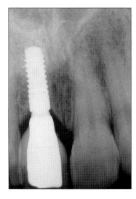

Fig 44   *Control radiograph at five years.*

The five-year follow-up gave rise to a positive mid-term prognosis and seemed to support the clinician's treatment choices.

The use of a reduced-diameter implant to support a crown for a maxillary central incisor cannot yet be considered standard. In selected cases, however, it could help simplify the treatment.

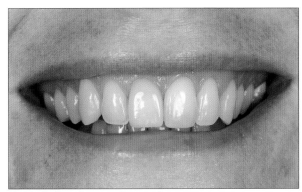

Fig 45   Smile at five years. Close-up view.

Acknowledgments

Laboratory procedures
MDT Alwin Schönenberger, Vision Dental – Chiasso, Switzerland

Vision-Dental Academy Training Center – Busto Arsizio, Italy

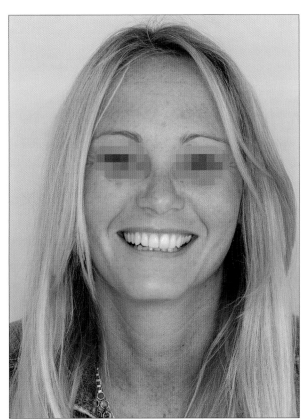

Fig 46   Smile at five years. Full-face view.

7.6   Replacement of an Upper Right Central Incisor with Root Resorption: Ridge Preservation, Early Placement of an RC Bone Level Implant

S. Chen

A 49-year-old female patient was referred for implant therapy to replace the upper right central incisor (tooth 11). The tooth had been assessed by an endodontist who diagnosed a vertical fracture of the root (Fig 1). The tooth had a hopeless prognosis and needed to be extracted.

The patient was healthy and was not taking any medications. She was allergic to penicillin. The patient had high esthetic demands but her expectations were realistic.

The extraoral examination revealed no facial asymmetries. The right temporomandibular joint demonstrated an opening click but was otherwise asymptomatic. The lip line was high with a significant gingival display (Figs 2a-b).

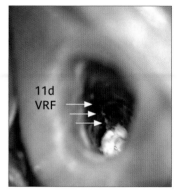

Fig 1   Microscopic view of the root canal of tooth 11 demonstrating a vertical root fracture on the distal wall

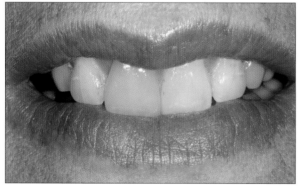

Fig 2a   Lip line at rest.

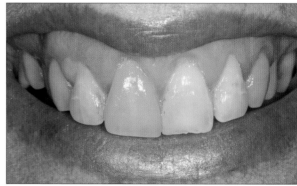

Fig 2b   Full display of the gingiva at full smile.

The intraoral examination revealed that the oral mucosa was healthy. The occlusion was class 2 division 1, with an overjet 5 mm and an overbite of 5 mm (Fig 3). Periodontally, the probing pockets were within normal limits. There was mild generalized gingivitis and minor bleeding on probing. The patient's oral hygiene was generally inadequate. An assessment of the maxillary anterior teeth showed that the teeth had long clinical crowns and were triangular in outline. The interdental papillae were long. The tissue phenotype was medium thick.

A deep pocket was present on the midfacial aspect of tooth 11, indicative of a vertical root fracture. A periapical radiograph confirmed that the tooth had been endodontically treated. There was blunting of the interdental septum between the two central incisors. Furthermore, the distance between the bone crest both mesially and distally was 5 to 6 mm to the contact points (Fig 4a). CBCT scans revealed a thick facial bone plate and a prominent concavity of the ridge immediately apical to the root (Fig 4b).

The problem list was as follows:

- High esthetic expectations
- Damaged facial bone wall of the socket
- Maxillary central incisors that are triangular in outline
- Class 2 division 2 occlusion with retroclined maxillary anterior teeth

The Esthetic Risk Assessment (ERA) was complex (Table 1).

Following discussions with the patient, she understood the complexity of the proposed treatment and accepted the esthetic risk. Under these conditions, an early placement protocol (type 2) was recommended in accordance with the ITI recommendations to minimize the esthetic risk (Morton and coworkers 2014).

The treatment plan was follows:

- Periodontal therapy to improve oral hygiene and gingival health.
- Decoronation of tooth 11 and delivery of a removable acrylic partial denture to serve as an interim prosthesis.
- Extraction of tooth 11
- Eight weeks later, placement of an implant at site 11 with simultaneous grafting and contour augmentation with DBBM according to the principles of guided bone regeneration (GBR)
- Following integration of the implant, construction of the implant-supported prosthesis

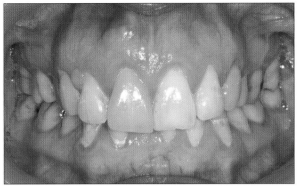

Fig 3   Facial view of the dentition and initial presentation. Class 2 division 2 occlusion and deep bite.

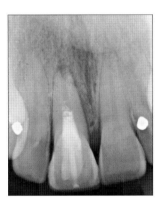

Fig 4a   Periapical radiograph of tooth 11.

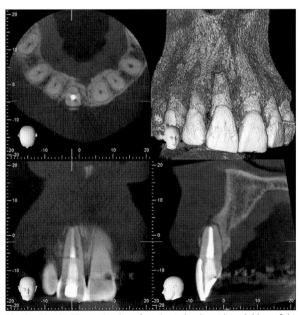

Fig 4b   The CBCT examination of tooth 11 site showed partial loss of the facial bone plate, extended bone defects on the mesial and distal aspects of the root, and an apical fenestration. There was a ridge concavity immediately apical to the root due to the marked axial discrepancy between the tooth and the alveolar process.

Table 1   Esthetic Risk Assessment (ERA)

Esthetic risk factors	Level of risk		
	Low	**Medium**	**High**
Medical status	Healthy, uneventful healing		Compromised healing
Smoking habit	Non-smoker	Light smoker (≤ 10 cigs/day)	Heavy smoker (> 10 cigs/day)
Gingival display at full smile	Low	Medium	High
Width of edentulous span	1 tooth (≥ 7 mm)[1] 1 tooth (≥ 6 mm)[2]	1 tooth (< 7 mm)[1] 1 tooth (< 6 mm)[2]	2 teeth or more
Shape of tooth crowns	Rectangular		Triangular
Restorative status of neighboring teeth	Virgin		Restored
Gingival phenotype	Low-scalloped, thick	Medium-scalloped, medium-thick	High-scalloped, thin
Infection at implant site	None	Chronic	Acute
Soft-tissue anatomy	Soft tissue intact		Soft-tissue defects
Bone level at adjacent teeth	≤ 5 mm to contact point	5.5 to 6.5 mm to contact point	≥ 7 mm to contact point
Facial bone-wall phenotype*	Thick-wall phenotype ≥ 1 mm thickness		Thin-wall phenotype < 1 mm thickness
Bone anatomy of alveolar crest	No bone deficiency	Horizontal bone deficiency	Vertical bone deficiency
Patient's esthetic expectations	Realistic expectations	Moderate expectations	Unrealistic expectations

* If three-dimensional imaging is available with the tooth in place
[1] Standard-diameter implant, regular connection
[2] Narrow-diameter implant, narrow connection

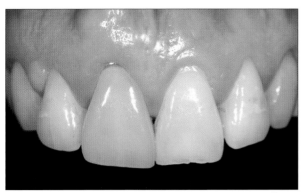

Fig 5a   The crown of tooth 11 was removed and a removable acrylic partial denture provided to serve as an interim prosthesis.

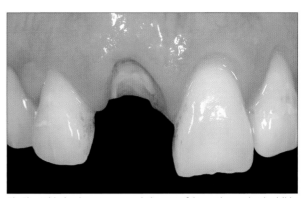

Fig 5b   With the denture removed, the root of the tooth was clearly visible.

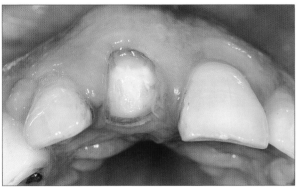

Fig 5c   Occlusal view of root 11.

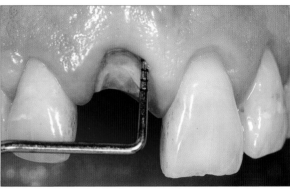

Fig 5d   A periodontal probe demonstrated the presence of a deep pocket on the facial aspect of the root in the region of the vertical root fracture.

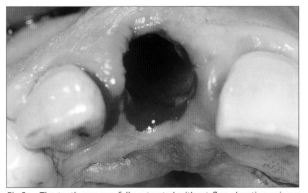

Fig 5e   The tooth was carefully extracted without flap elevation using a combination of fine luxators and root forceps.

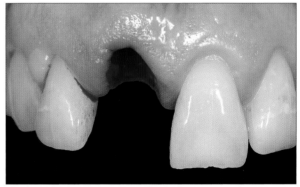

Fig 5f   Facial view of site 11 immediately after root extraction.

On completion of the periodontal therapy, the patient returned to the prosthodontist for removal of the tooth crown and delivery of an interim removable prosthesis. She later returned for extraction of the root. The high soft-tissue scallop and damage to the facial bone wall of the socket were confirmed (Figs 5a-d). Using a combination of periotomes and forceps, the tooth was extracted without elevating a surgical flap (Figs 5e-f). Care was taken to remove all granulation tissue within the socket.

The patient returned eight weeks later for implant placement. At this time, the soft tissue had healed with almost complete closure over the socket (Fig 6a). A full-thickness two-sided mucoperiosteal flap was raised that extended from tooth 21 to tooth 12 (Figs 6b-c). The vertical releasing incision was placed on the mesial aspect of tooth 12. The healing socket was carefully debrided to remove all soft tissue. About 5 mm of vertical resorption of the facial bone crest was noted. Additionally, two

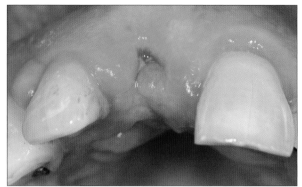

Fig 6a Ten weeks after extraction, the extraction site had healed with almost complete closure over the entrance of the socket.

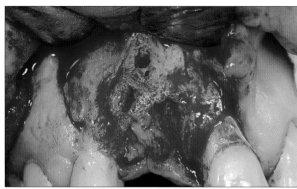

Fig 6b A two-sided full-thickness mucoperiosteal flap was raised to completely expose the healing socket and root eminences of adjacent teeth. Damage to the facial bone wall with two fenestration defects and crestal bone loss of approximately 5 mm. Concavity in the ridge apical to the healing socket.

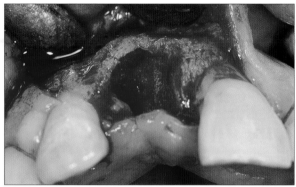

Fig 6c Occlusal view of tooth 11 following removal of granulation tissue from the healing socket.

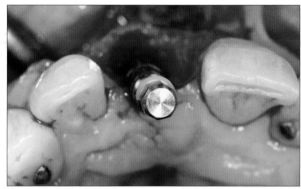

Fig 6d Occlusal view of the implant in position with implant mount attached, showing the orofacial and mesiodistal orientation of the implant.

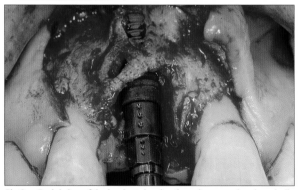

Fig 6e Facial view of the implant showing the apicocoronal and mesiodistal position of the implant in relation to the adjacent teeth. The implant was placed in the correct three-dimensional prosthodontic position. Note the residual peri-implant defects and the presence of fenestration of the facial bone in the apical area.

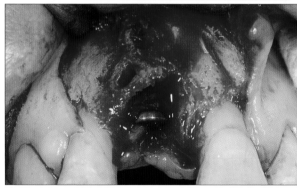

Fig 6f A 2-mm RC healing abutment was attached to the implant, and autologous bone chips were harvested from the vicinity using bone scrapers. The bone chips were applied to the exposed implant surface.

fenestration defects in the facial bone were identified. The deep concavity apical to the base of the socket as also noted. The facial bone had a thickness of about 1 mm at the crest. The osteotomy was prepared according to a surgical template and the implant was placed in a favorable three-dimensional position (Straumann Bone Level RC SLActive, diameter 4.1 mm, length 10 mm; Institut Straumann AG, Basel, Switzerland). Due to the

underlying class 2 division 2 occlusion in which the central incisors are retroclined, care was taken to ensure that the implant correctly emerged through the anticipated cingulum of the final restoration (Figs 6d-h). The implant was therefore retroclined even more so than the adjacent central incisor, which was necessary due to the underlying occlusion.

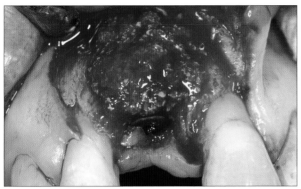

Fig 6g *Particles of DBBM soaked in venous blood were applied to the facial aspect of the implant to augment the contour of the ridge. The graft extended to the level of the top of the healing abutment.*

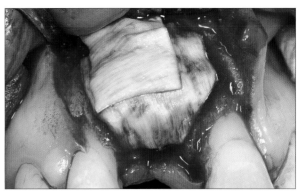

Fig 6h *Two layers of a resorbable collagen membrane were placed over the bone graft to act as a barrier and to stabilize the bone graft.*

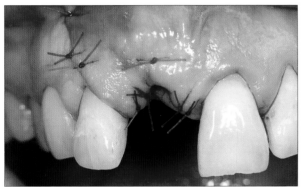

Fig 6i *The periosteum of the flap was released at the base and the flap advanced coronally by 3 to 4 mm to facilitate complete closure over the implant and biomaterials.*

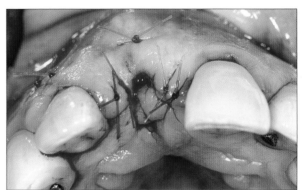

Fig 6j *Occlusal view of the surgical site following flap closure.*

Given the defects in the facial bone wall, a significant portion of the implant surface was exposed. A 2-mm healing abutment (RC healing abutment; Institut Straumann AG) was connected to the implant. Autologous bone chips were locally harvested using a bone scraper and chisels. The bone chips were placed over the exposed surface of the implant, and a thick layer of particulate deproteinized bovine bone mineral (DBBM) (Bio-Oss; Geistlich Pharma, Wolhusen, Switzerland) was used to fill residual defects in the socket and to cover the facial surface of the ridge. The contour was "overbuilt" to augment the ridge contour. Two layers of a resorbable collagen membrane (Bio-Gide; Geistlich Pharma) were used to cover and protect the graft. The flap was then advanced coronally to achieve primary closure (Figs 6i-j). Due to the early placement, sufficient soft-tissue healing and an increase in soft-tissue volume had occurred and allowed primary closure with minimal coronal repositioning of the flap.

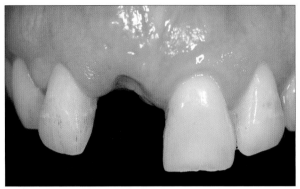

Fig 7a   Facial view of site 11 ten weeks after implant placement.

A healing period of ten weeks was scheduled. The mucosa healed with full coverage of the site. After administration of local anesthesia, a small opening was made in the mucosa at the crest to connect a longer transmucosal healing abutment (Figs 7a-d). Radiographic examination confirmed continuous contact of bone against the walls of the implant and ideal crestal bone conditions (Fig 7e).

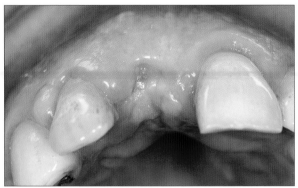

Fig 7b   Ten weeks after implant placement after uneventful healing. Occlusal view confirming complete soft-tissue closure over the implant.

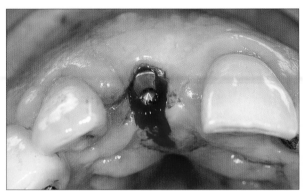

Fig 7c   A circular incision over the top of the implant was made to expose the implant, and a longer healing abutment (RC 4 mm) was attached.

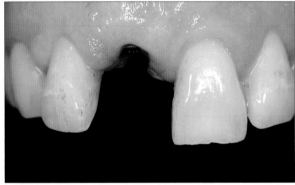

Fig 7d   Facial view of the implant site after connecting a longer healing abutment.

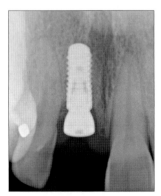

Fig 7e   Radiographic control at ten weeks.

The patient returned to the prosthodontist for the restorative procedures (Figs 8a-g). An impression was taken with addition silicone material and a standardized implant impression post in place. A CAD/CAM design for a direct screw-retained all-ceramic implant-supported single crown was prepared using proprietary software (3Shape, Copenhagen, Denmark). The definitive crown was fabricated using Straumann CARES (Institut Straumann AG) with a zirconia substructure and a ceramic build-up.

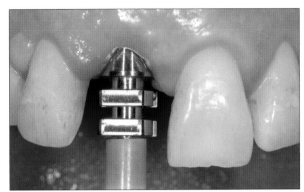
Fig 8a   Standardized implant impression post in place.

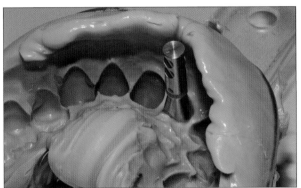
Fig 8b   Addition condensation silicone impression with BLI laboratory analog in place.

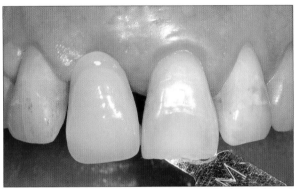
Fig 8c   Shade calibration for an enhanced direct analog "map" of the adjacent tooth for the definitive ceramic build-up.

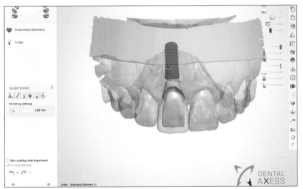
Fig 8d   CAD/CAM design for a direct screw-retained all-ceramic implant-supported single crown using 3Shape software (3Shape, Copenhagen, Denmark).

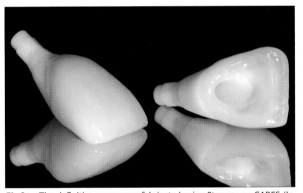
Fig 8e   The definitive crown was fabricated using Straumann CARES (Institut Straumann AG) with a zirconia substructure with layered ceramic.

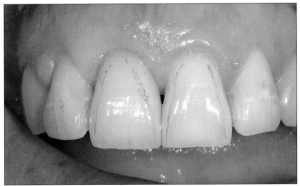
Fig 8f   Trial seating and contour evaluation prior to adjustment.

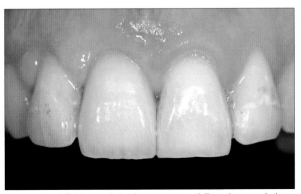
Fig 8g   The definitive single implant crown was delivered two weeks later.

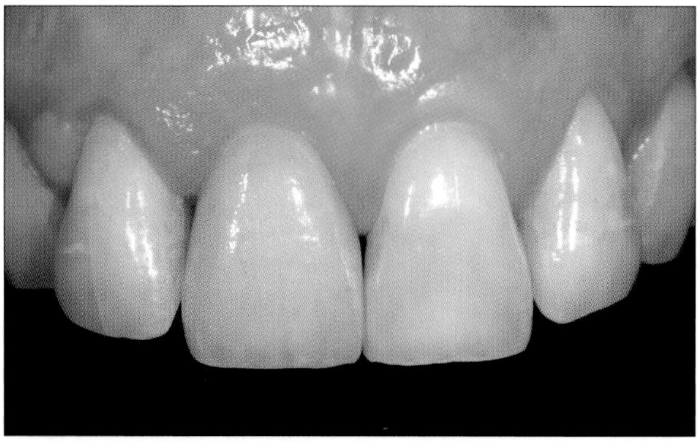

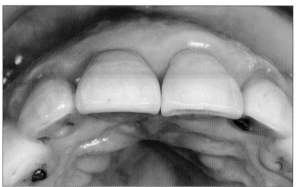

Fig 9a   Facial view one year after implant placement.

The clinical and radiographic examination one year after implant placement confirmed the presence of healthy peri-implant tissues and stable crestal bone as well as a satisfactory esthetic outcome (Figs 9a-c).

The early implant placement protocol (type 2) provided the opportunity to reconstruct the facial contour of the ridge to enhance the esthetic outcome. An occlusal view of the implant-supported restoration confirmed the ideal ridge contour on the facial aspect. At the two-year recall, maintenance of peri-implant soft-tissue health and contours and radiographic bone levels were noted (Figs 10 a-e). A CBCT examination at that time showed the presence of a thick facial bone wall that had been reconstructed by GBR, and crestal bone coronal to the implant/abutment junction.

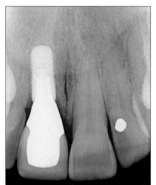

Fig 9b   Occlusal view of the implant one year after implant placement. Ideal facial ridge contour as a consequence of grafting for contour augmentation at the time of implant placement.

Fig 9c   Radiographic control one year after implant placement.

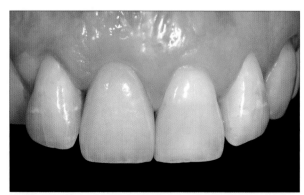

Fig 10a   Healthy and stable peri-implant tissues at the two-year recall.

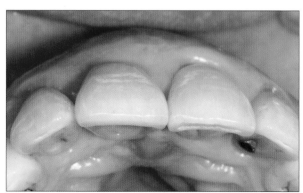

Fig 10b   Occlusal view of implant 11. The contour augmentation on the facial aspect was stable.

The successful functional and esthetic outcome of treatment was due to a number of factors considered critical.

- Early implant placement after extraction (type 2) was selected to allow soft-tissue healing so that the soft-tissue volume was maximized at the time of implant placement.
- The implant was placed in an ideal prosthodontic position in 3 dimensions – coronoapically, mesiodistally, and orofacially.
- The selected implant had an osteoconductive surface and a design that permits bone regeneration coronal to the implant/abutment junction. The implant has an internal tapered connection and a stable implant/abutment junction under functional load. This minimized the required dimensions of the implant/abutment microgap and allowed the use of GBR to recreate a bone crest coronal to the implant/abutment junction.
- In addition to an autologous bone graft to the exposed implant surface, a bone substitute with a low substitution rate was selected to reconstruct the facial contour of the ridge. This is important in achieving a good esthetic outcome. Finally, the prosthodontic and laboratories ceramic procedures were precise and allowed ideal tooth esthetics to be achieved.

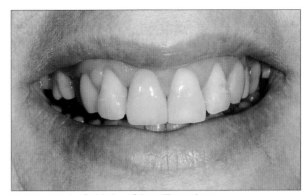

Fig 10c   Anterior facial view of the smiling patient.

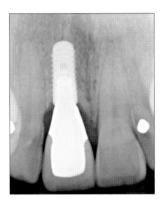

Fig 10d   Two-year radiographic control. Stable crestal bone at the neck of the implant.

Acknowledgment

Prosthetic procedures
Dr. Anthony Dickinson – Melbourne, Australia

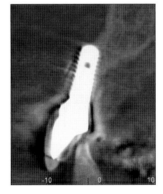

Fig 10e   A CBCT scan obtained two years after implant placement. A thick bone wall was present on the facial aspect of the implant.

7.7 Replacement of an Ankylosed Central Incisor with a Gingival Recession: Tooth Extraction with Socket Grafting and Late Implant Placement with Simultaneous Contour Augmentation

D. Buser, U. Belser

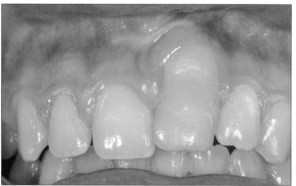

In 2008, a healthy 15-year-old female, non-smoking patient presented at our clinic with a major esthetic problem of tooth 21. Her dental history revealed that the tooth had been avulsed by trauma years before. As a result, the replanted and temporarily splinted tooth had ankylosed and was in severe apical malposition (Fig 1). The ankylosed tooth exhibited a significant gingival recession that disturbed the patient greatly.

Due to the patient's low age and with her skeletal growth not completed, periodic follow-up visits were scheduled to monitor the situation until the patient was old enough for implant therapy.

Figures 2 and 3 show the clinical situation two years later, at age 17. The patient's skeletal growth combined with the ankylosis of tooth 21 had further exacerbated the vertical discrepancy of the incisal edge positions of teeth 11 and 21 and the gingival recession at the ankylosed tooth 21.

The adjacent teeth 11 and 22 were periodontally healthy. Their bone-crest levels adjacent to tooth 21 were well maintained, so that they would provide favorable papillary support at the future implant site.

As routinely performed in daily practice, an esthetic risk assessment (Martin and coworkers 2006) was performed (Table 1).

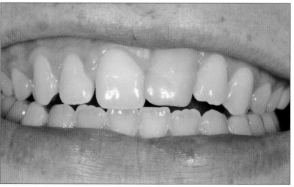

Fig 1   Initial clinical situation in 2008, at age 15. Severe gingival disharmony and apical malposition of tooth 21.

Fig 2   Close-up of the infrapositioned and ankylosed tooth 21 at age 17.

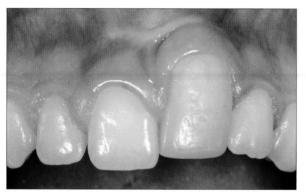

Fig 3   Medium to high smile line.

Table 1   Esthetic Risk Assessment (ERA)

Esthetic risk factors	Level of risk		
	Low	**Medium**	**High**
Medical status	Healthy, uneventful healing		Compromised healing
Smoking habit	Non-smoker	Light smoker (≤ 10 cigs/day)	Heavy smoker (> 10 cigs/day)
Gingival display at full smile	Low	Medium	High
Width of edentulous span	1 tooth (≥ 7 mm)[1] 1 tooth (≥ 6 mm)[2]	1 tooth (< 7 mm)[1] 1 tooth (< 6 mm)[2]	2 teeth or more
Shape of tooth crowns	Rectangular		Triangular
Restorative status of neighboring teeth	Virgin		Restored
Gingival phenotype	Low-scalloped, thick	Medium-scalloped, medium-thick	High-scalloped, thin
Infection at implant site	None	Chronic	Acute
Soft-tissue anatomy	Soft tissue intact		Soft-tissue defects
Bone level at adjacent teeth	≤ 5 mm to contact point	5.5 to 6.5 mm to contact point	≥ 7 mm to contact point
Facial bone-wall phenotype*	Thick-wall phenotype ≥ 1 mm thickness		Thin-wall phenotype < 1 mm thickness
Bone anatomy of alveolar crest	No bone deficiency	Horizontal bone deficiency	Vertical bone deficiency
Patient's esthetic expectations	Realistic expectations		Unrealistic expectations

* If three-dimensional imaging is available with the tooth in place
[1] Standard-diameter implant, regular connection
[2] Narrow-diameter implant, narrow connection

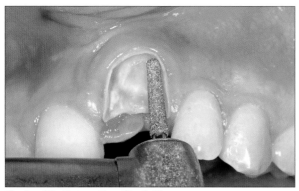
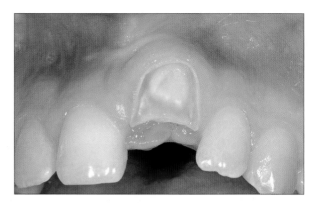

Figs 4 and 5   Decoronation of tooth 21.

Based on the findings comprising several high risk factors, the situation was rated Complex (C) according to the SAC Classification (Dawson and Chen 2009).

As a first treatment step, tooth 21 was decoronated in October 2012 to provide space for increasing the amount of keratinized mucosa (KM) at the future implant site (Figs 4 and 5). This technique has been used in implant patients for more than 20 years (Langer 1994). At that time, the patient was 19 years old.

Eight weeks after decoronation and uneventful wound healing with a considerable gain in KM (Fig 6), the root was further shortened a second time. The mucosal wound was left to heal by secondary intention (Fig 7).

Another eight weeks later, the patient returned to our clinic for removal of the root. Site 21 presented clinically healthy, with a significant gain in KM around the shortened root (Fig 8).

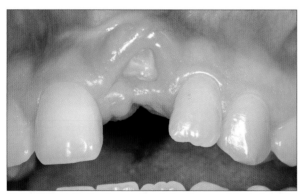

Fig 6   Eight weeks after decoronation, before the second shortening of the root.

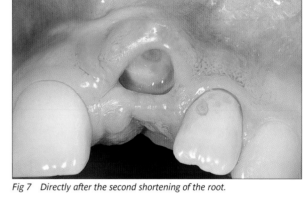

Fig 7   Directly after the second shortening of the root.

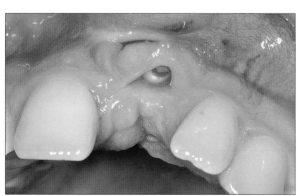

Fig 8   Clinical situation before root removal. A significant gain in KM in the future implant site could be achieved.

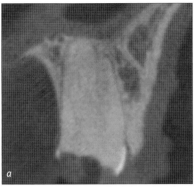
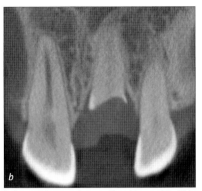
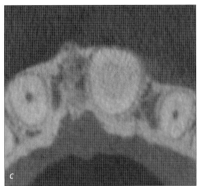

Figs 9a-c   CBCT scans: sagittal, frontal, and coronal views of the anterior maxilla with root 21 still in place. Most striking: the lack of bone volume apical to the root.

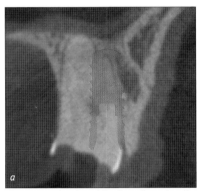
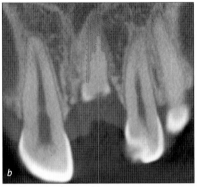
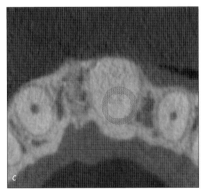

Figs 10a-c   Planning of the three-dimensionally correct future implant position.

At this stage, a cone-beam computer tomography (CBCT, Accuitomo 170; Morita, Kyoto, Japan) of the anterior maxilla was taken. The CBCT scans showed that there was no bone available apical to the ankylosed root (Fig 9a). In addition, there was no facial bone wall in the crestal area, while the bone height in the proximal area of the adjacent teeth was favorable (Fig 9b). In addition, the crest was more than 6 mm wide both mesially and distally of the root (Fig 9c).

The correct 3D position of the future implant was then determined with a view to optimal placement (Figs 10a-c).

Clinical considerations for treatment planning

Based on the local bone anatomy, the treatment plan was discussed with the patient. The clinical and radiographic examination demonstrated that we had a rare indication for late implant placement (Type 4). Based on the ITI treatment guidelines from the last ITI Consensus Conference in Bern (Morton and coworkers 2014) and the current guidelines used at the University of Bern (Buser and coworkers 2017) this treatment approach can be necessary for patient- and site-specific reasons,

which were both present, since at an age of 15 years, the patient was clearly too young for implant therapy, and she had no bone volume apical to the ankylosed root, which would have been necessary to achieve good primary stability of an inserted implant. Therefore, late implant placement was the treatment of choice, letting the patient grow up.

The following treatment plan was agreed upon:

- Removal of root 21 combined with a simultaneous socket grafting for ridge preservation using a low-substitution bone filler
- Six months later, late implant placement (Type IV) in area 21 with a simultaneous contour augmentation using GBR
- At least eight weeks of healing, followed by reentry using a punch technique
- Delivery of a screw-retained, implant-supported temporary acrylic crown for at least two years, given the patient's young age
- Delivery of the final all-ceramic implant-supported crown

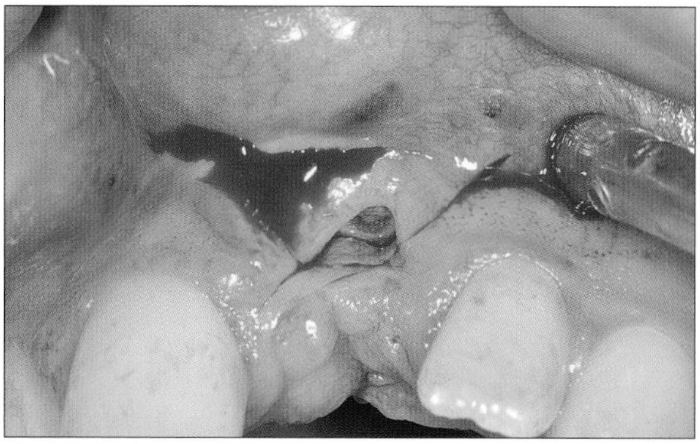

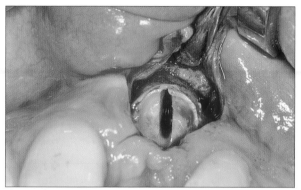

Fig 11   The site was opened with a small trapezoidal flap.

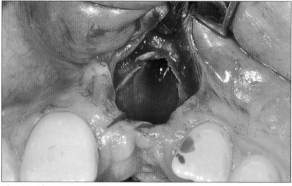

Fig 12   The root was separated along its longitudinal axis.

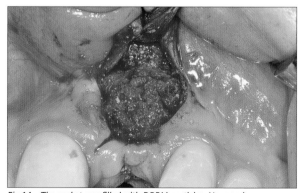

Fig 13   After root removal

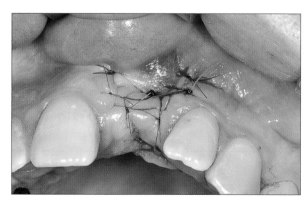

Root removal and socket grafting for ridge preservation

In March 2013, root 21 was carefully removed using a low-trauma technique, raising a small trapezoidal muco-periosteal flap with a papilla-sparing incision (Fig 11). To minimize the pressure on the very delicate and thin facial bone wall in the apical area during tooth extraction, the root was separated along its longitudinal axis in an orofacial direction (Fig 12). The hemisected root fragments were very carefully removed. Due to the ankylosis of the root, some ankylosed root remnants had to be removed with a diamond bur, causing a bleeding bone surface.

Subsequently, the socket (Fig 13) was filled with low-substitution bone-filler particles (Bio-Oss deproteinized bovine bone mineral/DBBM, Geistlich Pharma, Wolhusen, Switzerland) (Fig 14), and the surgery was completed with a tension-free primary wound closure (Fig 15).

Fig 14   The socket was filled with DBBM particles. No membrane was applied to keep the flap opening as small as possible.

Fig 15   After tension-free primary wound closure with interrupted single sutures.

This socket grafting for ridge preservation is strongly recommended by the ITI in cases with late implant placement (Morton and coworkers 2014), since it helps to reduce the amount of ridge atrophy. Socket grafting is a well-documented surgical technique (Darby and coworkers 2009), but it cannot stop bundle-bone resorption since the ridge volume is still reduced in the crestal area (Araújo and Lindhe 2009a; Araújo and coworkers 2015a). In this situation, the main advantage of socket grafting is that the reduction of any potential ridge atrophy helps avoid ridge augmentation with a block graft using a staged approach.

Wound healing progressed without any complications. After six months, the site presented nicely healed. A favorable amount of KM was present at the future implant site. The volume of the alveolar ridge seemed to be maintained sufficiently (Figs 16 and 17a), although the facial aspect of the ridge was slightly flattened (Fig 16).

A periapical radiograph confirmed a normal bone structure at the grafted site. As usual, the radiopaque low-substitution DBBM filler was still visible in the area of the former socket (Fig 17b).

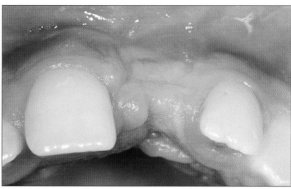

Fig 16   Contour of the alveolar ridge six months after root removal and socket grafting with DBBM.

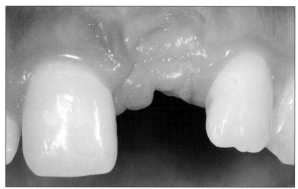

Fig 17a   Facial view of the future implant site six months after root removal and socket grafting.

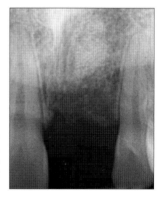

Fig 17b Periapical radiograph six months following socket grafting confirms the favorable bone height at adjacent teeth and a normal bone structure at site 21.

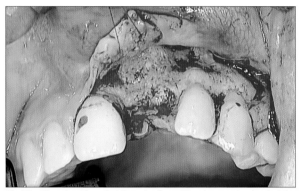

Fig 18   After elevation of a triangular flap with only one releasing incision on the distal aspect of tooth 23.

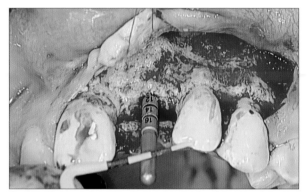

Fig 19   Alignment pin and periodontal probe visualizing correct implant axis and preparation depth.

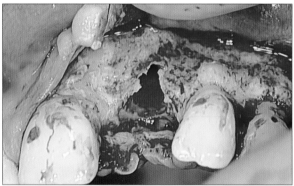

Fig 20   Following implant bed preparation.

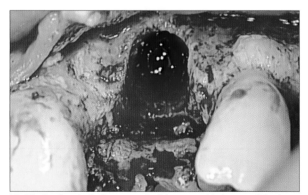

Fig 21   Implant bed after removal of the paper-thin bone wall in the crestal area.

Implant placement with simultaneous contour augmentation using GBR

Implant surgery was performed under local anesthesia with a sedative premedication. The implant site was exposed using a triangular mucoperiosteal flap with a distal releasing incision at the left canine (Fig 18).

This flap design has been favored for roughly 10 years for single-tooth replacement in the esthetic zone, since it provides a flap with good vascularity, good visual access to the implant site, and a low risk for scarring lines in the esthetic zone. Elevation of the flap revealed a well-healed edentulous ridge with a minor facial flattening of the crest. This allowed for implant placement in a correct 3D position with good primary stability (Fig 19), followed by simultaneous contour augmentation using GBR.

After implant-bed preparation (Fig 20), the paper-thin facial bone wall in the crestal area of the implant bed was carefully removed with a round diamond bur to create a facial bone defect with bleeding bony walls (Fig 21).

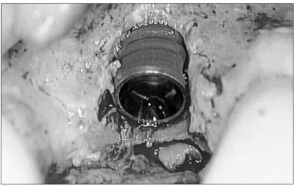

Fig 22   The implant shoulder was positioned around 3 mm apically to the facial mucosal margin of the planned implant crown. The implant shoulder is located subcrestally on the mesial, palatal and distal aspect of the implant. On the facial aspect, a crater-like dehiscence defect is present, as expected.

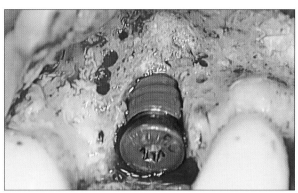

Fig 23   The 2-mm healing cap was inserted into the implant.

A 10-mm Bone Level implant with a diameter of 4.1 mm (Institute Straumann AG, Basel, Switzerland) was inserted. Thanks to successful socket grafting, the implant could be placed in a correct 3D position, with the implant platform within the comfort zones in the mesiodistal, coronoapical and orofacial directions (Buser and coworkers 2004a) (Fig 22). The implant shoulder was located approximately 3 mm apically to the future mucosal margin of the planned implant crown. A 2 mm healing cap was inserted to allow bone augmentation to the rim of the healing cap (Fig 23). As expected, the facial flattening required a simultaneous contour augmentation using GBR, which is a well-documented surgical technique for horizontal ridge augmentation (Buser and coworkers 2008a).

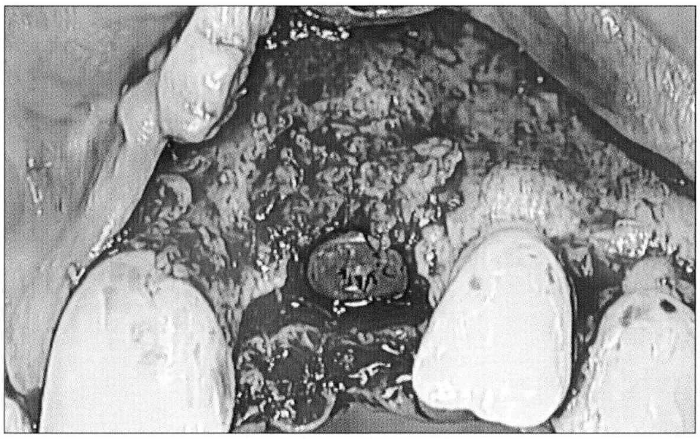

The peri-implant cortical bone surface was perforated with multiple bur holes to open the marrow cavity. The dehiscence defect on the facial aspect of the implant was augmented with two bone fillers to regenerate and overcontour the facial bone wall. A layer of autologous bone chips was applied to fill the bone defect to the rim of the healing cap (Fig. 24).

Fig 24   Locally harvested autologous bone chips were used to cover the exposed implant surface and to fill the facial bone defect up to the rim of the healing cap.

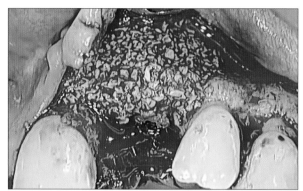

Fig 25   Facial view of the overcontoured alveolar ridge after application of the DBBM particles on top of the first layer of bone chips.

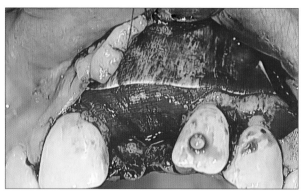

Fig 26   The augmentation material was covered with a collagen membrane using a double-layer technique to prolong its barrier function and to improve its stability during initial healing.

These bone chips had been locally harvested within the same flap area with a bone scraper (Hu-Friedy, Chicago, IL, USA). This first layer was covered by a second layer of DBBM particles (Bio-Oss; Geistlich Pharma) characterized by a low substitution rate (Fig 25). The DBBM particles were covered with a bioresorbable, non-crosslinked collagen membrane (Bio-Gide; Geistlich Pharma) using the double-layer technique to improve membrane stability (Fig 26).

In sites with a favorable two-wall defect morphology, bioabsorbable non-crosslinked collagen membranes have been preferred by our group since the late 1990s, since they are easy to handle during surgery and they do not require open-flap reentry. In addition, they have a low risk of complications in case of a soft-tissue dehiscence following GBR procedures (von Arx and Buser 2006). However, these collagen membranes have only a short barrier function of four to eight weeks (von Arx and coworkers 2005). So these resorbable membranes need to be combined with appropriate bone fillers to compensate for the short barrier function.

In the late 1990s we started using a combination of two bone fillers, autologous bone chips and bovine DBBM particles (Buser and coworkers 2004a; Buser and coworkers 2008b). This combination offers synergistic properties for optimized regenerative outcomes with the GBR technique. Autologous bone grafts are used to accelerate new bone formation not only at the implant surface to accelerate osseointegration, but also in the superficial layer of bone substitutes to obtain DBBM particles embedded in bone. The superiority of autologous bone

chips has been confirmed in several histomorphometric experimental studies (Buser and coworkers 1998b; Jensen and coworkers 2006; Jensen and coworkers 2007; Jensen and coworkers 2009).

As a second bone filler, DBBM particles are routinely used to cover the applied layer of autograft chips. These DBBM particles improve the contour of the alveolar crest around dental implants. This technique for contour augmentation is intended to optimize the esthetic outcomes around dental implants (Buser and coworkers 2008b). DBBM particles are characterized by a low substitution rate, as demonstrated in several preclinical studies (Buser and coworkers 1998a; Jensen and coworkers 1996; Jensen and coworkers 2006; Jensen and coworkers 2007, Jensen and coworkers 2009).

The synergistic play between both fillers has been confirmed by stable and favorable esthetic outcomes in two case series studies examining single-tooth replacement with early implant placement and simultaneous contour augmentation using GBR (Buser and coworkers 2008a; Buser and coworkers 2009). Both groups of patients were prospectively analyzed again using CBCT to examine the status of the facial bone wall (Buser and coworkers 2013a; Buser and coworkers 2013b). Both studies demonstrated a fully intact facial bone wall in 95% of patients. In addition, a recent histomorphometric study with 12 human biopsies in 10 patients confirmed the low substitution rate of DBBM particles, since the mean percentage of DBBM was 32% at 14 to 80 months after augmentation (Jensen and coworkers 2014).

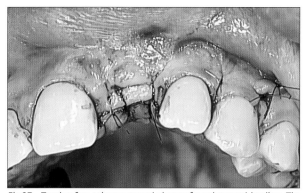

Fig 27 *Tension-free primary wound closure for submerged healing. The wound was closed with a mattress suture and multiple interrupted single sutures.*

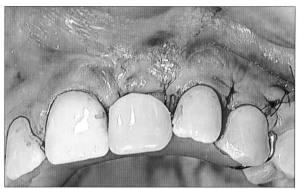

Fig 28 *The cut-back interim removable dental prosthesis in place after surgery. Care was taken that no pressure was applied to the augmented site during the first four weeks of healing.*

Following the release of the periosteum, the surgery was completed with a tension-free primary wound closure using a horizontal mattress suture (4-0) and multiple interrupted single sutures (5-0) to facilitate submerged healing (Fig 27). The interim removable dental prosthesis was reduced in the gap area to avoid pressure on the augmented site (Fig 28). The postsurgical radiograph confirmed the correct 3D implant position (Fig 29).

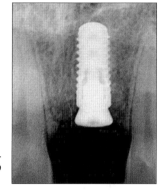

Fig 29 *The postsurgical radiograph confirms the correct 3D position of the implant.*

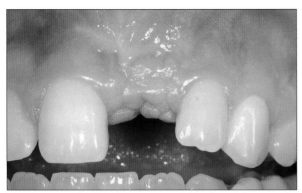

Fig 30 Implant site following an uneventful healing of three months. Some minor scars are visible in the area of the former root.

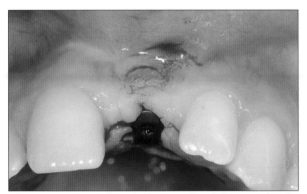

Fig 31 Reentry was performed using a punch technique. Insertion of a 3.5 mm healing cap. The mucosal surface was freshened with a large diamond bur.

Reentry and prosthetic treatment

After a complication-free healing period of three months, the implant site had healed nicely but showed some minor scars in the area of the former root (Fig 30). The site was reentered using a punch technique. The mucosal surface was freshened with a large diamond bur to minimize the scars. In addition, the short 2-mm healing cap was replaced by a longer 3.5-mm healing cap (Fig 31).

In 2014, an open-tray impression was taken and a provisional directly screw-retained implant crown fabricated in the dental laboratory and subsequently inserted to initiate peri-implant soft-tissue conditioning. At this stage, the patient was 21 years old. As it was planned to leave the temporary implant crown in the patient's mouth for a prolonged period, it was based on a titanium coping and veneered with high-quality acrylic using a traditional layering technique (Figs 32 and 33).

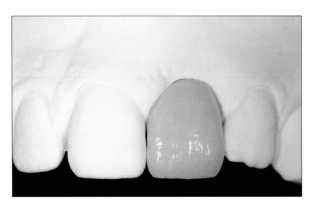

Fig 32 Facial close-up view of the provisional implant crown composed of a prefabricated titanium coping and layered acrylic veneering.

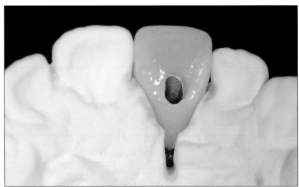

Fig 33 The palatal aspect of the directly screw-retained implant provisional documents an ideally located screw access channel in the center of the cingulum area as a result of an optimal 3D implant position.

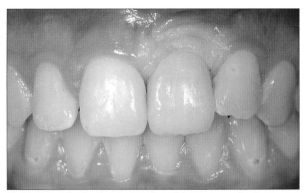

Fig 34   Immediately after the insertion of the temporary implant crown. Marked blanching of the marginal peri-implant soft tissue due to an increased emergence profile compared to that of the healing cap.

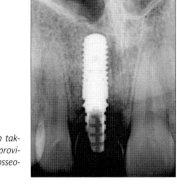

Fig 35   Periapical radiograph taken after the insertion of the provisional implant crown. Stable osseointegration.

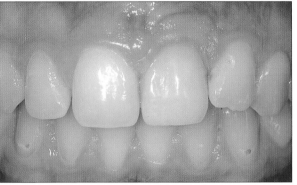

Fig 36   Three-year follow-up of the provisional implant crown. Stable and harmonious peri-implant soft-tissue contours.

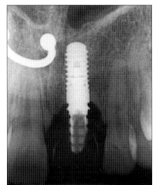

Fig 37   Periapical radiograph taken three years after the insertion of the temporary implant crown, documents the completed bone remodeling. Optimal bone density was established at the level of the implant shoulder.

The provisional was inserted under local anesthesia and caused the usual transient blanching of the peri-implant mucosa (Fig 34). The periapical radiograph taken in the spring of 2014 shows the well-integrated Bone Level implant restored with the titanium-based temporary crown (Fig 35).

Finally, the provisional crown was left in place for more than two years to await the completion of any additional skeletal growth. After this period, no more significant additional growth was noticed (Fig 36). The corresponding periapical radiograph revealed completed bone remodeling, including a particularly dense bone structure adjacent to the implant shoulder (Fig 37). Consequently, final impressions were taken (Fig 38) for the fabrication of an all-ceramic definitive implant crown.

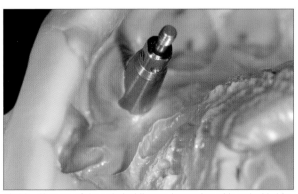

Fig 38   Close-up of the polyvinylsiloxane impression with embedded impression post using the open-tray technique.

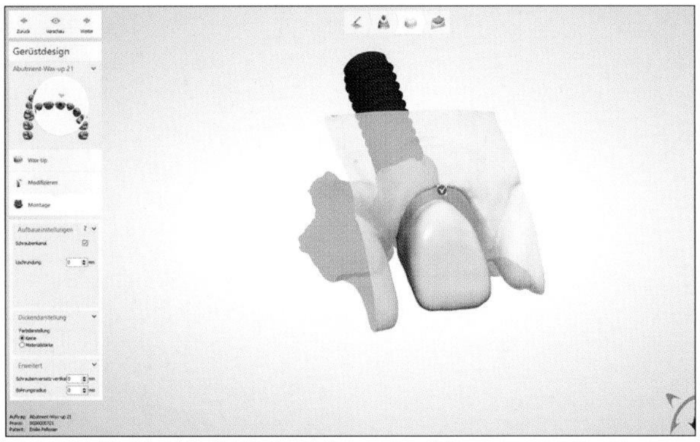

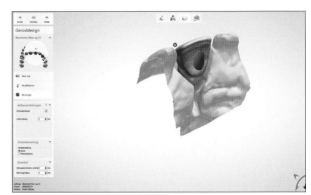

Fig 39a   Facial view of the planned zirconia substructure. Minimal and uniform space reserved for the subsequent veneering with cosmetic ceramics.

Fig 39b   Palatal view.

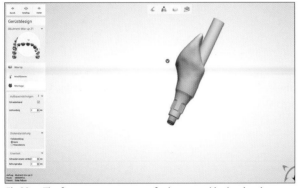

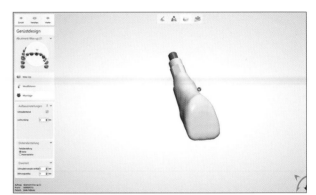

Fig 39c   The future screw access, perfectly centered in the cingulum area and providing adequate distance to the incisal edge.

Fig 39d   The cervical aspect of the CAD/CAM zirconia substructure was characterized by a flat emergence profile. This was a direct consequence of an optimal 3D implant position.

It was decided to use a directly screw-retained design, based on a custom-made CAD/CAM zirconia abutment and subsequent manual veneering to provide mechanical strength and optimum esthetics. The corresponding scanning and designing process is documented by Figures 39a-d, and the final esthetic veneering by Figures 40a-b.

In this context, particular emphasis was placed on the completed all-ceramic implant crown to have adequate incisal translucency and overall luminosity, as well as form and volume that nicely integrated with the natural adjacent anterior maxillary dentition (Figs 41a-b).

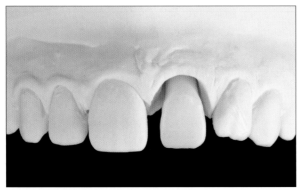

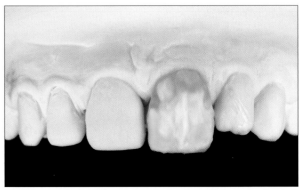

Fig 40a   The CAD/CAM-generated zirconia abutment, repositioned on the master cast, visualizes the uniform and adequately dimensioned space for the subsequent layer of cosmetic ceramics.

Fig 40b   In order to achieve the required optical effects, a complex stratification involving various pigments in different colors and opacities were applied.

D. Buser, U. Belser

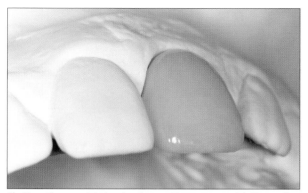

Fig 41a   The completed restoration on the master model. Harmonious integration of form, volume, and surface texture.

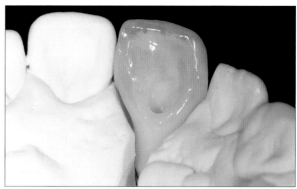

Fig 41b   Palatal view. Note the subtle translucency of the incisal third.

In conclusion, the clinical and radiographic follow-up three years after implant surgery (Figs 42a-d), displaying both harmonious peri-implant soft-tissue contours and stable osseointegration conditions, underlines the efficacy of the chosen treatment approach.

Acknowledgment

The authors wish to express their gratitude to Pascal Müller, CDT and Master Ceramist (Glattbrugg, Switzerland), for his expert work during the fabrication of the implant-supported FDPs featured in this clinical case.

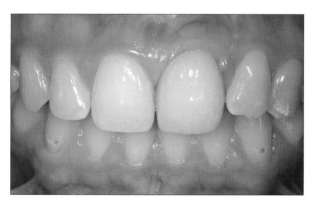

Fig 42a   Final view of the directly screw-retained all-ceramic implant crown 21. Symmetrical levels of the midfacial mucosal margins of the two central incisors. Convex profile of the peri-implant mucosa as a result of successful contour augmentation performed during implant placement.

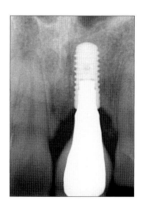

Fig 42b   Periapical radiograph taken three years after implant surgery. Stable bony conditions and coronal bone-to-implant contacts at the level of the implant shoulder.

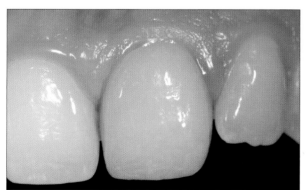

Fig 42c   Facial close-up view of the anterior maxillary region. The implant restoration integrates harmoniously with the adjacent natural dentition.

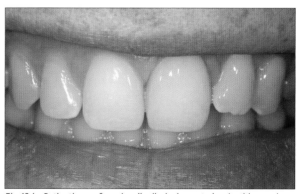

Fig 42d   Patient's non-forced smile displaying anterior dentition and surrounding gingival tissues. An esthetically pleasing overall result.

7.8 Replacement of a Compromised Upper Right Central Incisor: Hard- and Soft-tissue Augmentation, Late Placement of an RC Bone Level Implant

P. Casentini

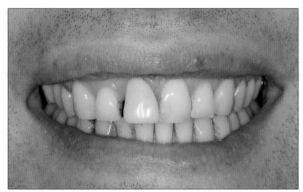

Fig 1   The patient's smile. Pronounced exposure of the anterior maxillary teeth and the surrounding soft tissues.

A 36-year-old male patient with a compromised maxillary central incisor was referred by his general dentist for consultation.

The patient's chief complaints were the gradual debonding of a temporary crown on the right central incisor and unsatisfactory esthetics due to an increasing diastema between the right central and lateral incisors. The patient reported a traumatic event some years previously, when a crown had been placed after root-canal treatment. The referring dentist wanted to provide a new crown restoration, but was concerned about the condition of the residual root. Anamnesis was negative for any other dental or periodontal pathology in the remaining dentition. The patient reported taking no medications: He was a smoker (10 to 15 cigs/day) and had realistic esthetic expectations.

The extraoral examination revealed a high smile line with full exposure of the maxillary teeth and surrounding soft tissues in the area between the second premolars (Fig 1).

The intraoral examination showed a temporary crown on the right central maxillary incisor and a diastema. An asymmetry in soft-tissue levels at the central incisors was also found, with the margin located 1 mm further apically on the restored tooth. This asymmetry, in addition to differences in mesiodistal spaces, also resulted in different perceived shapes of the two central incisors, where tooth 11 seemed more triangular than tooth 21.

The soft-tissue phenotype was classified as medium in terms of thickness and scalloping, and the teeth exhibited a square shape. After removal of the temporary crown, the root proved to be partially fractured, with thin residual walls (Figs 2 and 3).

An intraoral radiograph taken after removal of the temporary crown confirmed the presence of a root with a minimum amount of residual tooth structure. No periapical pathology was present (Fig 4).

The Esthetic Risk Assessment (ERA; Table 1) revealed a medium risk profile: main factors of risk identified were the high lip line, the presence of a soft-tissue defect and a diastema, and the need to manage the mesiodistal space, as well as the smoking habit.

Based on the clinical and radiological situation, the following treatment plan was proposed:

- Extraction of the central incisor and ridge preservation using a bone substitute, followed by temporary restoration with a removable partial denture. An immediate implant was not considered a safe procedure because a soft-tissue recession was already present on the tooth to be extracted.
- Delayed placement of an implant after 6 months of healing, eventually combined with hard- and soft-tissue augmentation.
- Temporary prosthetic restoration followed by final ceramic crown. It was also decided to place an additional ceramic veneer on the adjacent left central incisor to close the diastema.

The patient agreed with the proposed treatment plan and gave his written informed consent. Moreover, the patient was recommended to avoid smoking after the surgical procedures.

The first part of the treatment was performed by the referring dentist; clinical documentation of this phase is missing.

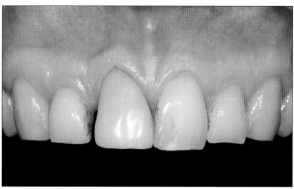

Fig 2   Frontal view of the maxillary teeth highlighting the asymmetrical shape of the two central incisors and the presence of a diastema.

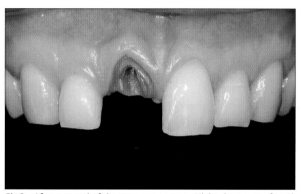

Fig 3   After removal of the temporary crown. Minimal amount of tooth structure left.

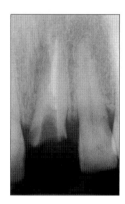

Fig 4   Initial periapical radiograph.

Table 1 Esthetic Risk Assessment (ERA)

Esthetic risk factors	Level of risk		
	Low	**Medium**	**High**
Medical status	Healthy, uneventful healing		Compromised healing
Smoking habit	Non-smoker	Light smoker (≤ 10 cigs/day)	Heavy smoker (> 10 cigs/day)
Gingival display at full smile	Low	Medium	High
Width of edentulous span	1 tooth (≥ 7 mm)[1] 1 tooth (≥ 6 mm)[2]	1 tooth (< 7 mm)[1] 1 tooth (< 6 mm)[2]	2 teeth or more
Shape of tooth crowns	Rectangular		Triangular
Restorative status of neighboring teeth	Virgin		Restored
Gingival phenotype	Low-scalloped, thick	Medium-scalloped, medium-thick	High-scalloped, thin
Infection at implant site	None	Chronic	Acute
Soft-tissue anatomy	Soft tissue intact		Soft-tissue defects
Bone level at adjacent teeth	≤ 5 mm to contact point	5.5 to 6.5 mm to contact point	≥ 7 mm to contact point
Facial bone-wall phenotype*	Thick-wall phenotype ≥ 1 mm thickness		Thin-wall phenotype < 1 mm thickness
Bone anatomy of alveolar crest	No bone deficiency	Horizontal bone deficiency	Vertical bone deficiency
Patient's esthetic expectations	Realistic expectations		Unrealistic expectations

* If three-dimensional imaging is available with the tooth in place
[1] Standard-diameter implant, regular connection
[2] Narrow-diameter implant, narrow connection

Following the extraction, the buccal bone wall was partially damaged. The extraction socket was filled with a bovine xenograft (Bio-Oss Collagen; Geistlich Pharma, Wolhusen, Switzerland) and sealed with a collagen sponge. A removable interim prosthesis was immediately delivered after extraction. Antibiotic medication began on the day before surgery and was continued for six days postoperatively. Chlorhexidine mouth rinses were also prescribed for three weeks. The patient was recommended to reduce smoking and avoid brushing in the surgical area.

After six months of uneventful healing, the site was re-evaluated for implant placement. The soft tissues now presented a more favorable shape as compared to the initial situation. While the ridge volume had been maintained almost completely, there was some horizontal ridge resorption. A control radiograph showed adequate integration of the xenograft, with the typical radiopaque appearance (Figs 5 to 7).

Implant surgery was performed under local anesthesia. After flap elevation, the xenograft appeared well integrated and presented a favorable volume and shape (Figs 8 and 9).

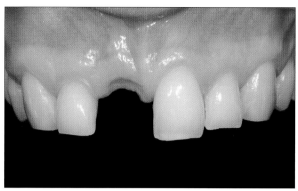

Fig 5 Frontal view before implant placement. Improved soft-tissue volume.

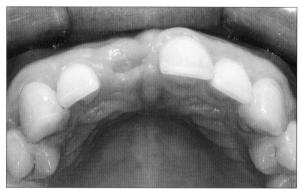

Fig 6 Occlusal view before implant placement. Slight horizontal ridge resorption.

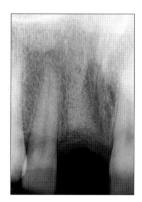

Fig 7 Periapical radiograph six months after ridge preservation. Good integration of the xenograft.

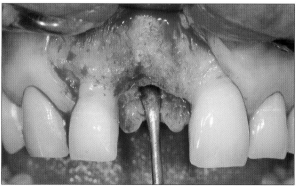

Fig 8 Frontal view after flap elevation. Favorable ridge preservation.

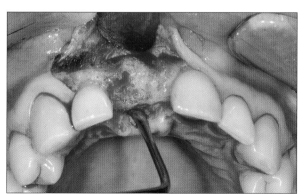

Fig 9 Occlusal view after flap elevation.

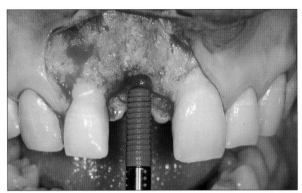

Fig 10 *Prosthetically driven implant placement in the correct mesiodistal position.*

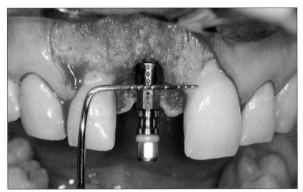

Fig 11 *Prosthetically driven implant placement in the correct orofacial position.*

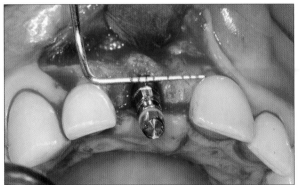

Fig 12 *Prosthetically driven implant placement in the correct apicocoronal position.*

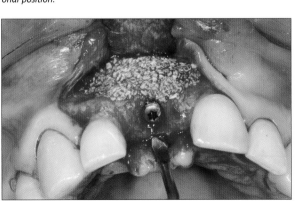

Fig 14 *Placement of the grafting material.*

After the implant bed was prepared following the usual protocol, a Straumann Bone Level Regular CrossFit implant (diameter 4.1 mm, length 12 mm) with a SLActive surface (Institut Straumann AG, Basel, Switzerland) was inserted and achieved adequate primary stability.

The placement of the implant was prosthetically driven. The implant shoulder was placed 1 mm palatal to the emergence of the adjacent teeth and 2.5 mm apical to the cementoenamel junction of the adjacent teeth. The buccopalatal implant axis was also controlled in order to realize a screw-retained restoration (Figs 10 to 12).

The mesiodistal position of the implant was determined, keeping in mind the final restorative space after mesially veneering the adjacent central incisor (Fig 13).

Although the bone volume was adequate after ridge preservation, it was decided to further improve the ridge profile by means of a guided bone regeneration (GBR) procedure, in order to create a thicker buccal peri-implant bone wall. Deproteinized bovine bone mineral (DBBM) was placed and stabilized with a double-layer collagen membrane (Bio-Oss and Bio-Gide; Geistlich Pharma) (Figs 14 and 15).

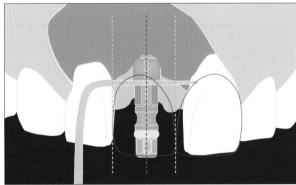

Fig 13 *The mesiodistal implant position took into consideration the planned restoration of the adjacent central incisor.*

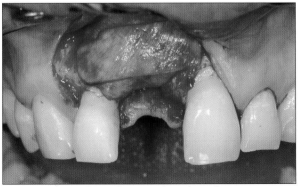

Fig 15 *Placement of the collagen membrane in two layers.*

A connective-tissue graft harvested from the palatal mucosa was used to increase the thickness of the soft tissue. The soft-tissue graft was attached to the internal layer of the buccal flap with 6-0 resorbable sutures (Figs 16 and 17).

The flap was closed by primary intention without tension by means of mattress and single sutures after interrupting the periosteal layer and releasing the flap; 6:0 resorbable sutures (Vicryl Ethicon, New Brunswick, NJ, USA) were utilized (Fig 18).

The temporary removable prosthesis was adapted to avoid excessive pressure and re-delivered to the patient immediately after surgery.

Postoperative instructions and medications were the same as after the first surgery.

After four months of healing, reentry was performed using a small midcrestal mesiodistal incision under local anesthesia. The adjacent papillae were not involved in the incision. A conical healing screw was connected to the implant (Figs 19 and 20).

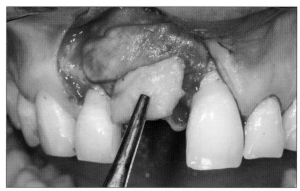
Fig 16   Placement of a connective-tissue graft.

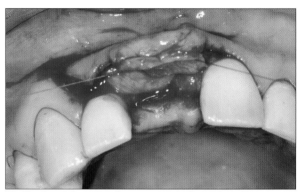
Fig 17   Connective graft being secured to the buccal flap with sutures.

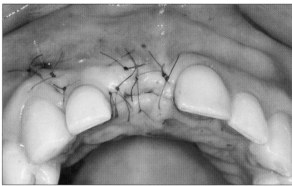
Fig 18   Occlusal view after repositioning and suturing the flap.

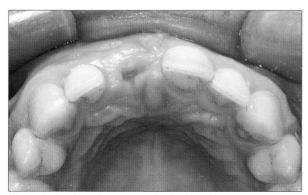
Fig 19   Occlusal view four months after implant placement.

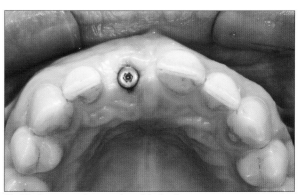
Fig 20   Reentry and connection of the healing screw.

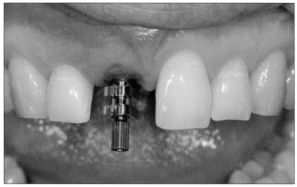

Fig 21 *Connection of the pick-up (open-tray) impression post.*

One week after reentry, a polyether open-tray impression was taken (Figs 21 and 22).

A bite registration was also performed in conjunction with a plastic index being placed parallel to the interpupillary line. The registration allowed the dental laboratory to place the models in the articulator correctly. This is considered important in particular in case of restorations involving the midline, as in this case. Finally, the shade was selected, and pictures with similar color samples were taken (Figs 23 to 25).

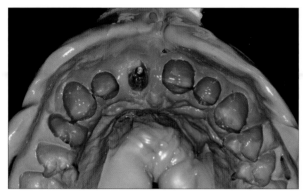

Fig 22 *Impression with polyether material.*

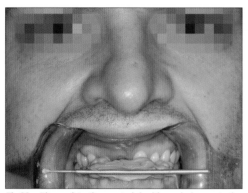

Fig 23 *Bite registration material with an index capturing the interpupillary line.*

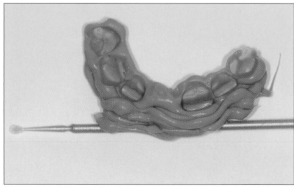

Fig 24 *Bite index.*

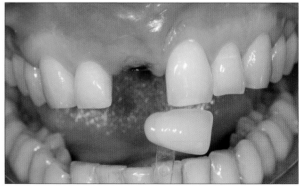

Fig 25 *Shade selection.*

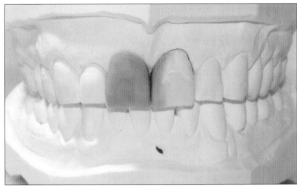

Fig 26   Wax-up of the planned restorations.

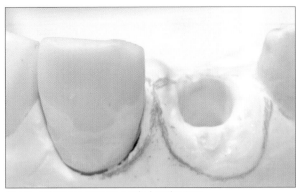

Fig 27   Emergence contours marked on the stone.

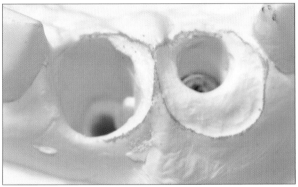

Fig 28   Reduction of the coronal aspect.

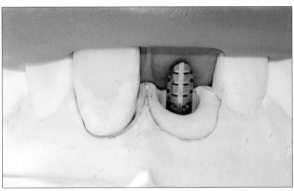

Fig 29   Temporary titanium abutment shaped to adapt to the prevailing local conditions.

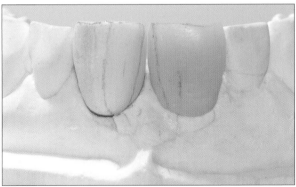

Fig 30   Veneering of the resin material.

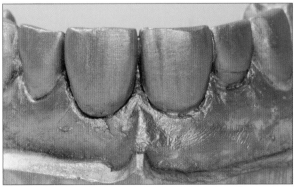

Fig 31   Gold spray was used to check the shape and the surface texture of the temporary crown and ceramic veneer.

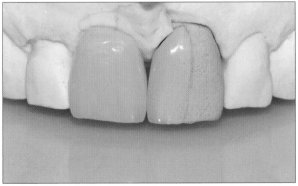

Fig 32   Temporary crown and ceramic veneer on the cast after finishing.

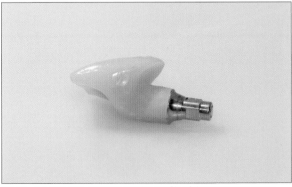

Fig 33   Lateral view. Concave overlap profile of the temporary crown.

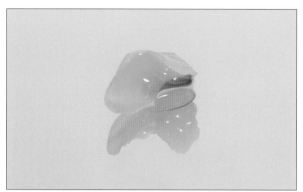

Fig 34   Etching of the ceramic veneer with 9% hydrofluoric acid.

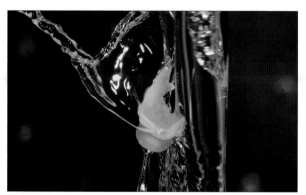

Fig 35   Rinsing with water.

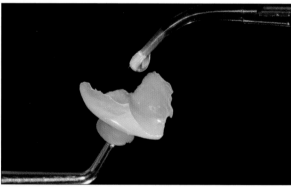

Fig 36   Application of the silane.

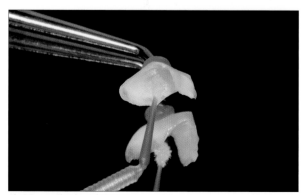

Fig 37   Application of the bonding agent.

After pouring the casts, the dental laboratory performed a wax-up for the temporary screw-retained crown and the adjacent ceramic veneer. Once the emergence profile had been marked with a red pencil, the wax was removed and the stone reproducing the soft tissues was superficially shaped with a bur. The screw-retained provisional crown was fabricated using a titanium temporary abutment. To avoid excessive pressure on the peri-implant soft tissues, the temporary crown featured a concave overlap design, and the emergence profile was cylindrical on the first few millimeters. The left central incisor was duplicated in refractory material for the feldspathic ceramic veneer (Figs 26 to 33).

During the following appointment, the ceramic veneer was bonded to the adjacent tooth and the screw-retained temporary crown was delivered. The ceramic veneer was etched with hydrofluoric acid for 90 seconds, then washed, placed in an ultrasonic cleaner with pure ethanol for 4 minutes, silanized and bonded (Figs 34 to 37).

The mesial sulcus of the central incisor was opened with a retraction cord, and the field was isolated with rubber dam. The ceramic veneer was bonded with flowable composite resin (Figs 38 to 41).

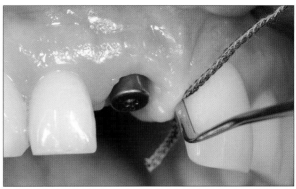

Fig 38   Placement of a retraction cord into the gingival sulcus of the contralateral central incisor.

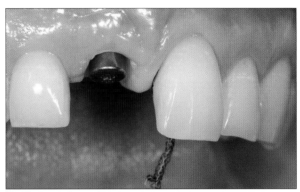

Fig 39   Retraction cord in place.

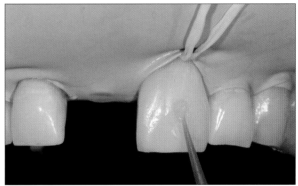

Fig 40   Bonding of the ceramic veneer.

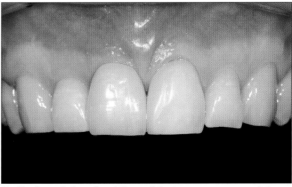

Fig 41   Frontal view after delivery of the temporary crown and the ceramic veneer.

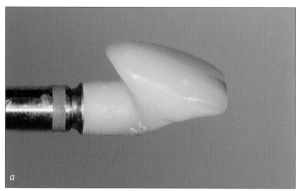 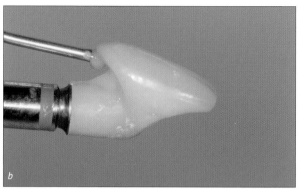

Figs 42a-b   Emergence profile of the provisional restoration, modified at chairside by adding flowable composite resin.

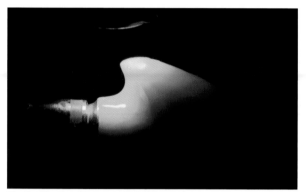

Fig 43   The flowable composite is light-cured.

After four and eight weeks, soft-tissue conditioning was obtained, gradually filling the overlap of the provisional restoration with flowable composite until an adequate emergence profile of the implant-supported restoration was achieved (Figs 42 to 46).

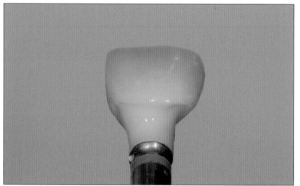 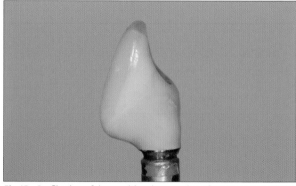

Fig 44   Adding some more flowable composite resin at chairside.

Fig 45   Profile view of the provisional restoration after the second relining procedure.

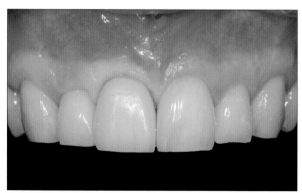

Fig 46   Screw-retained provisional crown inserted using slight pressure on the surrounding mucosa.

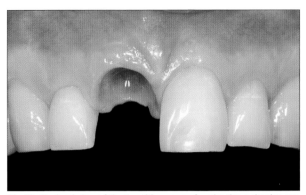

Fig 47 *Occlusal view of the transition zone after the tissue-shaping procedure was complete.*

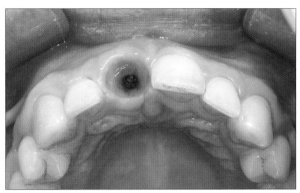

Fig 48 *Peri-implant soft tissue after conditioning in an occlusal view.*

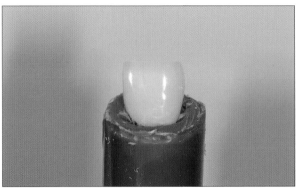

Fig 49 *Provisional restoration connected with an implant analog and inserted into impression material.*

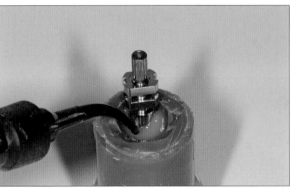

Fig 50 *Impression cap, individualized and adapted to the specific emergence profile by adding some flowable composite resin.*

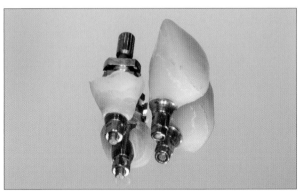

Fig 51 *Provisional restoration and customized impression post, now exhibiting the same profile.*

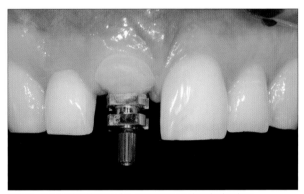

Fig 52 *Customized impression post connected to the implant.*

After twelve weeks of conditioning, the soft-tissue contours in the transition zone were considered adequate and the final impression was taken (Figs 47 and 48).

An extraoral impression of the provisional restoration allowed for fabrication of a customized impression post that copied the submucosal emergence profile (transition zone). An open-tray impression in polyether was taken (Figs 49 to 53).

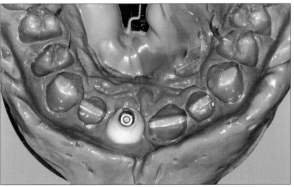

Fig 53 *Final open-tray impression.*

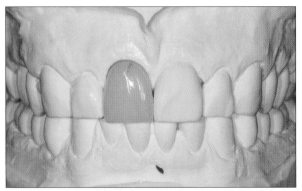

Fig 54   Frontal view of the final crown on the stone cast before delivery.

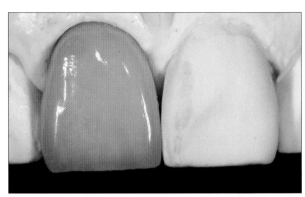

Fig 55   Close-up of the crown on the stone cast before delivery.

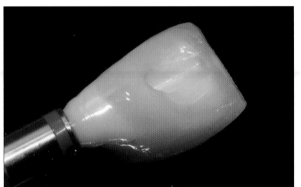

Fig 56   Palatal view of the final zirconia crown.

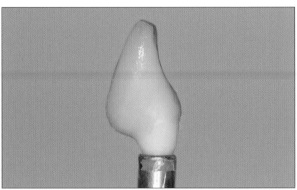

Fig 57   Profile view of the final zirconia crown.

A screw-retained crown was realized by the dental laboratory a CAD/CAM zirconia framework (CARES, Institut Straumann AG) veneered with ceramics (Figs 54 to 57).

Before delivery, the internal cavity of the implant and the crown were disinfected with chlorhexidine gel. The crown was screwed in place at a torque of 35 N·cm, and the access cavity to the screw was sealed with PTFE taper and some flowable composite resin.

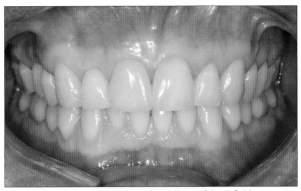

Fig 58   Frontal view, both arches, after delivery of the definitive crown.

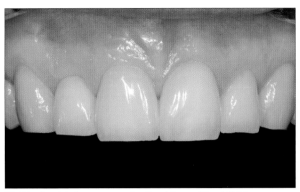

Fig 59   Frontal view, upper arch, after delivery of the definitive crown.

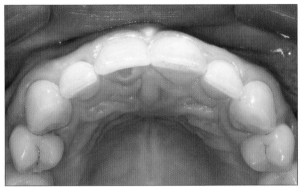

Fig 60   Occlusal view after delivery of the definitive crown.

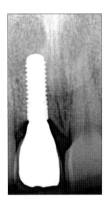

Fig 61   Periapical radiograph after delivery of the definitive crown.

The final crown integrated well with the surrounding natural dentition in terms of tooth size, shape, color, and surface texture. The patient expressed her full satisfaction with the final treatment outcome (Figs 58 to 60).

From a radiological point of view, the peri-implant bone appeared mineralized, and no signs of peri-implant bone resorption were present (Fig 61).

At the five-year follow-up, a minimal migration of the left central incisor caused the appearance of a diastema between the two central incisors. The migration of the contralateral central incisor was probably related to bruxism. The patient reported increasing stress in his daily life and a recent habit of grinding his teeth during the day. The occlusion was checked again; some occlusal adjustments were performed and the patient was recommended to avoid excessive pressure between the two arches. The patient was not interested in having the small interincisal diastema corrected and declared himself fully satisfied with the esthetic outcome of the rehabilitation.

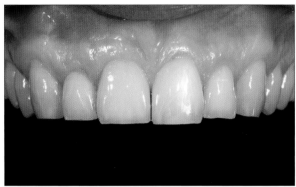

Fig 62   *Follow-up at five years. Frontal view of the maxillary anteriors.*

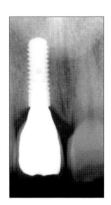

Fig 63   *Radiographic follow-up at five years.*

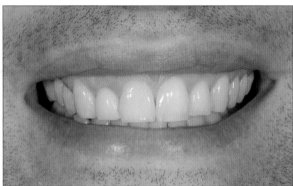

Fig 64   *Smile at five years. Close-up view.*

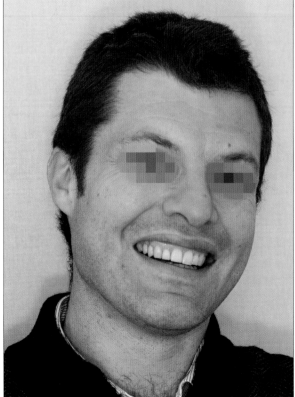

Fig 65   *Smile at five years. Full-face view.*

On the other hand, peri-implant soft-tissue positions and bone levels were stable, and the small diastema was not visible in the extraoral view (Figs 62 to 65).

Acknowledgments

Extraction and ridge preservation procedure
Dr. Fabio Quarta – Milano, Italy

Laboratory procedures
MDT Alwin Schönenberger Vision-Dental – Chiasso, Switzerland
Vision-Dental Academy Training Center – Busto Arsizio, Italy
Giuseppe Voce, MDT – University of Zürich, Switzerland

7.9 Replacement of a Failing Restored Upper Right Central Incisor: Ridge Preservation and Early Placement of an RC Bone Level Implant

D. Thoma

A 23-year-old female, healthy and non-smoking patient had had tooth 11 temporarily restored following a trauma in adolescence. As the patient's growth had since come to an end and the crown had fractured (Fig 1), she requested an implant-supported restoration of tooth 11. Moreover, the contralateral tooth 21 presented an old composite restoration at the mesial incisal edge (Fig 2). The periodontal tissues were healthy with periodontal probing depth values below 3 mm, but some inflammation was observed around the semi-submerged root of tooth 11 (Fig 3).

The patient exhibited a medium to high lip line exposing a high-scalloped gingiva and a thin gingival phenotype. The level of the gingiva at site 11 was further apical than at the contralateral tooth 21. It was therefore foreseeable that a major bone augmentation procedure with a rigid membrane and soft-tissue grafting would be necessary to ensure a long-term esthetic outcome in the anterior region (Fig 4).

The Esthetic Risk Assessment (ERA; Table 1) was complex.

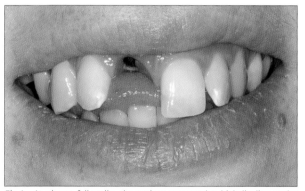

Fig 1 *At almost full smile, the patient presented a high lip line and a vertical soft-tissue deficit at site 11 compared to the contralateral natural tooth 21.*

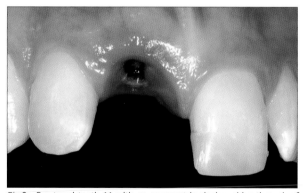

Fig 2 *Fractured tooth 11 with an asymmetric gingiva, shine-through of the root, thin phenotype with high-scalloped gingiva.*

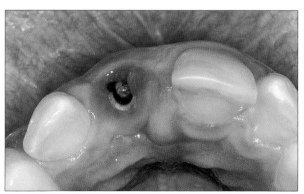

Fig 3 *Inflamed tissues around the residual root 11.*

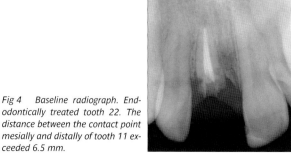

Fig 4 *Baseline radiograph. Endodontically treated tooth 22. The distance between the contact point mesially and distally of tooth 11 exceeded 6.5 mm.*

Table 1   Esthetic Risk Assessment (ERA)

Esthetic risk factors	Level of risk		
	Low	**Medium**	**High**
Medical status	Healthy, uneventful healing		Compromised healing
Smoking habit	Non-smoker	Light smoker (≤ 10 cigs/day)	Heavy smoker (> 10 cigs/day)
Gingival display at full smile	Low	Medium	High
Width of edentulous span	1 tooth (≥ 7 mm)[1] 1 tooth (≥ 6 mm)[2]	1 tooth (< 7 mm)[1] 1 tooth (< 6 mm)[2]	2 teeth or more
Shape of tooth crowns	Rectangular		Triangular
Restorative status of neighboring teeth	Virgin	Old restoration on tooth 21 at incisal edge	Restored
Gingival phenotype	Low-scalloped, thick	Medium-scalloped, medium-thick	High-scalloped, thin
Infection at implant site	None	Chronic	Acute
Soft-tissue anatomy	Soft tissue intact		Soft-tissue defects
Bone level at adjacent teeth	≤ 5 mm to contact point	5.5 to 6.5 mm to contact point	≥ 7 mm to contact point
Facial bone-wall phenotype*	Thick-wall phenotype ≥ 1 mm thickness		Thin-wall phenotype < 1 mm thickness
Bone anatomy of alveolar crest	No bone deficiency	Horizontal bone deficiency	Vertical bone deficiency
Patient's esthetic expectations	Realistic expectations		Unrealistic expectations

* If three-dimensional imaging is available with the tooth in place
[1] Standard-diameter implant, regular connection
[2] Narrow-diameter implant, narrow connection

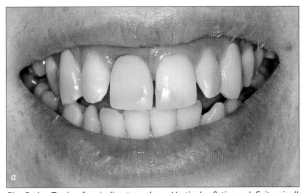 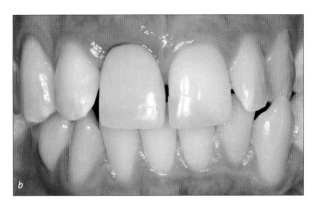

Figs 5a-b   Try-in of an indirect mock-up. Vertical soft-tissue deficit apically.

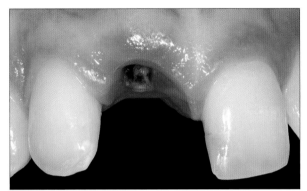

Fig 6   Buccal view prior to tooth extraction.

As a first step, an alginate impression was taken. The dental technician fabricated an indirect mock-up to assess the treatment goal and to discuss the treatment procedures with the patient. The mock-up try-in demonstrated a vertical soft-tissue deficit at site 11 compared to the contralateral tooth 21 (Figs 5a-b).

The present clinical case involved a number of clinical challenges. This included a high lip line, a thin tissue phenotype, high-scalloped gingiva, a vertical soft-tissue deficit, a narrow ridge, and a large distance between the interproximal bone and the prospective contact point.

Following discussions with the patient and the dental technician presenting several treatment options, a staged approach was chosen.

From an esthetic point of view, the zenith of the tooth 12 was slightly more apical than the zenith of tooth 22, indicating that tooth 11 could be slightly extended in an apical direction. To compensate for missing soft tissue and to optimize the soft-tissue quality and quantity prior to implant placement, ridge preservation (socket seal technique) was planned on the day of extraction. This approach is well-documented in the literature, even bearing in mind that the collagen matrix used for the socket seal has evidence for six months only (Jung and coworkers 2013b) (Fig 6).

Following careful tooth extraction, a slight collapse of the ridge profile was observed, indicating a deficit of the buccal bone plate (Figs 7a-b). The mucosal margin of the extraction socket were deepithelialized using a diamond drill to prevent the formation of scar tissue and initiated angiogenesis (Fig 8). Subsequently, a stable deproteinized bovine bone material (DBBM) with 10% collagen was placed in the extraction socket (Fig 9), extending to the level of the lingual bone and interdental crest (Fig 10).

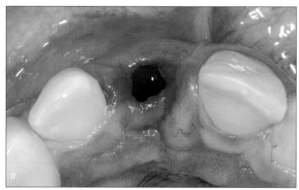
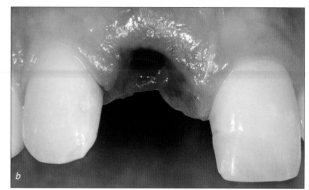

Figs 7a-b   Occlusal and buccal view after tooth extraction. Slight collapse of the buccal contour.

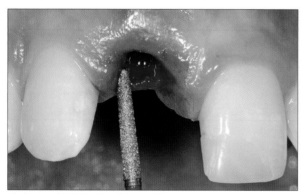
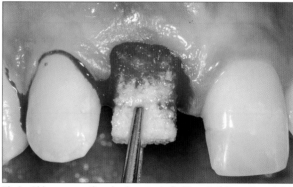

Fig 8   Deepithelialization of the marginal gingiva using a diamond drill.

Fig 9   Ridge preservation via placement of a biomaterial to reduce shrinkage following tooth extraction.

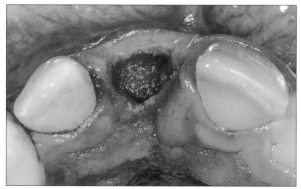

Fig 10   The biomaterial was placed flush with the interdental and palatal bone crest. Due to a partial loss of the buccal bone crest, the biomaterial was in contact with the buccal soft tissue.

Traditionally, free gingival grafts or connective-tissue grafts from the palate are used to seal the extraction socket over the bone substitute (Jung and coworkers 2004a). Disadvantages, however, include higher morbidity and possible complications, the often imperfect adaptation of the graft to the color and texture of the surrounding tissue, and the somewhat difficult handling of the graft. Therefore, a bilayered collagen matrix (Fig 11) was sutured on top of the bone substitute to seal the socket (Figs 12a-b). This collagen matrix has been demonstrated to enhance early healing and to be a suitable replacement for autologous free gingival grafts for the same indication (Thoma and coworkers 2012). Even though no or only minimal hard-tissue regeneration can be expected within the two months following ridge preservation, the soft-tissue seal technique optimize wound closure and maintain the ridge contour during the first six to eight weeks.

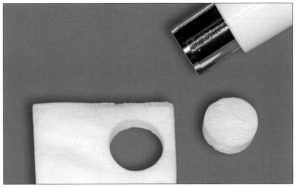

Fig 11   Collagen matrix shaped to match the size of the extraction socket.

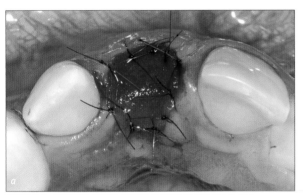
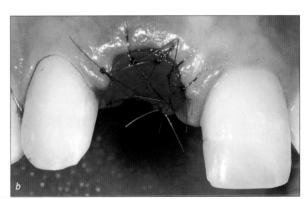

Figs 12a-b   Collagen matrix sutured in place to seal the socket.

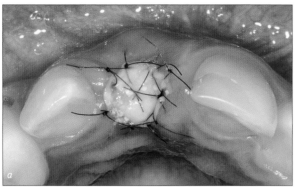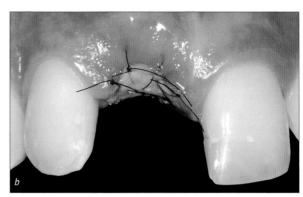

Figs 13a-b   One week after ridge preservation. Collagen matrix still in place.

At suture removal (Figs 13a-b), healthy tissues were observed and the collagen matrix was still in place. Because of the relatively narrow ridge with a partially missing buccal bone plate and thin soft tissue, guided surgery was planned to ensure an optimal implant position. For that purpose, a cone-beam computed tomography (CBCT) was taken (Fig 14).

The dental technician then fabricated a wax-up, optimized based on the mock-up try-in. This wax-up was scanned and superimposed on the CBCT for digital implant planning. Cross-sections of the CBCT demonstrated a narrow ridge and a partially missing buccal bone

plate, such that primary implant stability could be obtained only in the apical region. Moreover, the implant had to be placed slightly further buccally to guarantee 1 mm of native bone on the palatal aspect of the implant and to accommodate the nerve. According to the digital planning, the entire buccal surface of the implant would be exposed, and a major guided bone regeneration procedure with a stable membrane would be needed (Fig 15).

Six weeks after ridge preservation, the clinical examination showed healthy tissues and fully keratinized tissue at site 11 (Figs 16a-b).

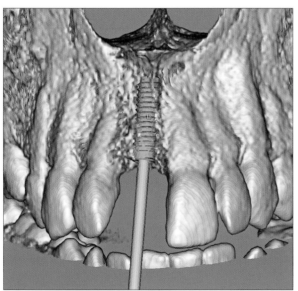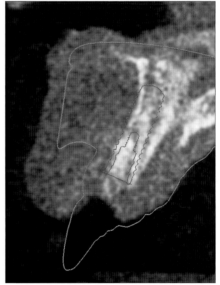

Fig 14   Implant planning for guided surgery. The planned implant position will lead to a large buccal dehiscence.

Fig 15   Cross-section indicating the planned implant position (slightly buccal, 1 mm of native bone on the palatal aspect). The outline of the wax-up is indicated in purple.

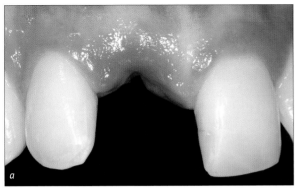

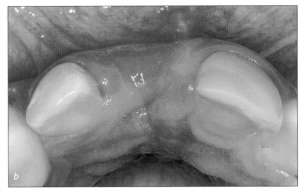

Figs 16a-b   Clinically healthy soft tissue with full keratinization, six weeks after ridge preservation.

A full-thickness flap was elevated and the surgical guide, fabricated by means of a 3D printer, was positioned (Figs 17 and 18). Guided implant-bed preparation (SMOP; Swissmeda, Zürich, Switzerland) and guided implant placement were performed (Fig 19).

Our use of the most recent techniques of taking a CBCT without a scanning template and of superimposing the digital file of the wax-up allowed planning and placing the implant in an optimal position.

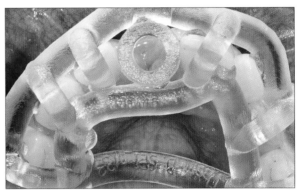

Fig 17   Digitally designed and 3D-printed surgical guide in position.

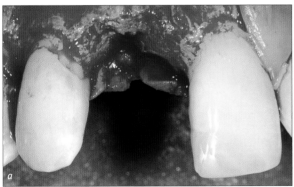

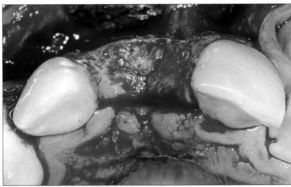

Figs 18a-b   After flap elevation, the contour of the ridge was maintained. Biomaterial particles were embedded in a healing extraction socket.

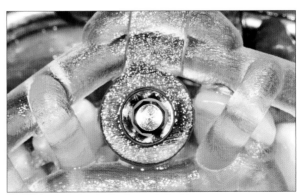

Fig 19   Implant placed using the surgical guide.

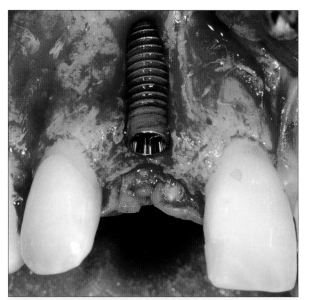

As anticipated by digital planning, a large dehiscence was present on the buccal side of the implant (Fig 20).

The occlusal view showed a slightly buccal position of the implant, leaving 1 mm of native bone on the palatal side. Guided bone regeneration was performed using a stable non-resorbable membrane and DBBM (Figs 21a-b).

Non-resorbable membranes offer benefits in cases without supporting neighboring bone walls. This results in an enhanced stability of the augmented site and allows the regeneration of bone outside the ridge curvature in two-wall defects. Primary wound closure was obtained in the present case (Figs 22a-b).

Fig 20   Large dehiscence defect on buccal side of the implant, similar to the planned implant position.

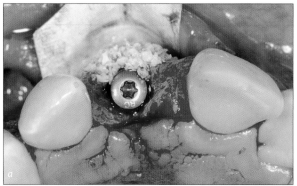
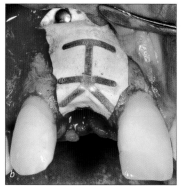

Figs 21a-b   Guided bone regeneration using a stable non-resorbable membrane and DBBM.

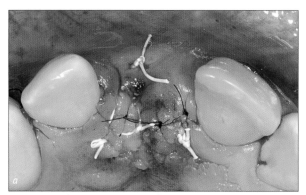
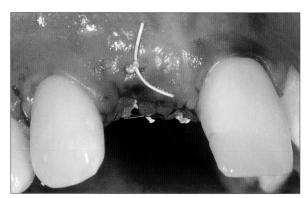

Figs 22a-b   Primary wound closure after implant surgery.

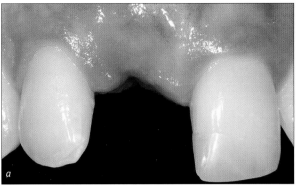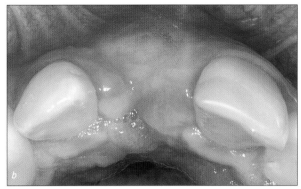

Figs 23a-b Six months after implant placement. The non-resorbable membrane was visible through the mucosa. Slight volume deficit on the buccal side.

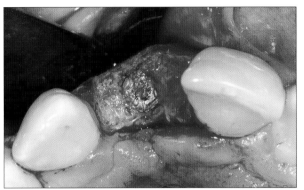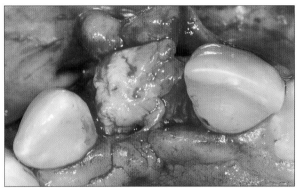

Fig 24 Removal of the non-resorbable membrane. Buccal bone regeneration was evident.

Fig 25 A connective-tissue graft was placed to compensate for the remaining volume deficit.

Six months later, the clinical examination showed a slight loss in buccal volume and a shine-through of the non-resorbable membrane (Figs 23a-b).

To compensate for the missing volume, soft-tissue grafting was applied (Thoma and coworkers 2016b). According to the literature, the use of a subepithelial connective-tissue graft (SCTG) is considered the gold standard (Thoma and coworkers 2014a). Following the removal of the non-resorbable membrane (Fig 24), the SCTG was harvested from the patient's own palate and placed on the occlusal and buccal aspect of the implant (Fig 25). The combination of hard- and soft-tissue grafting procedures is essential in cases with a thin tissue phenotype in the esthetic zone, with soft-tissue grafting contributing to 40% of the final volume (Schneider and coworkers 2011).

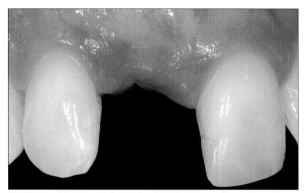

Fig 26   Healthy tissue eight weeks after soft-tissue grafting.

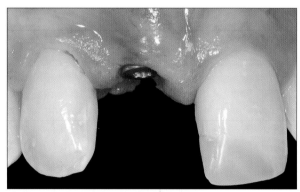

Fig 27   Minimally invasive abutment connection using a sharp elevator.

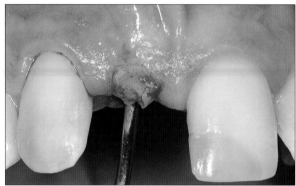

Fig 28   Following abutment connection, a buccal prominence was visible due to the roll flap.

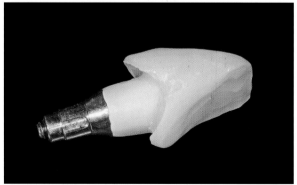

Fig 29   Provisional restoration with narrow submucosal emergence profile and a fully contoured buccal shell.

Eight weeks later (Fig 26), minimally invasive abutment connection was performed, preparing a roll flap and optimizing the buccal tissue architecture (Fig 27).

At the same time, an impression was taken on the implant level and a healing abutment placed (Fig 28).

The dental technician made a screw-retained provisional restoration based on the initial wax-up (Fig 29).

Typically, the provisional restoration has two aims: to create the emergence profile and to compensate for the changes in tissue architecture that occur, predominantly during the early phase (3 months) (Grunder 2000). The submucosal part of the provisional restoration was slowly changed by adding flowable composite to mimic the emergence profile of the contralateral tooth (Figs 30 to 33).

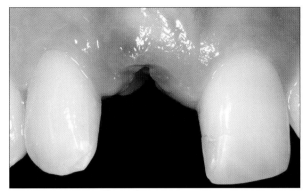

Fig 30   Emergence profile creation.

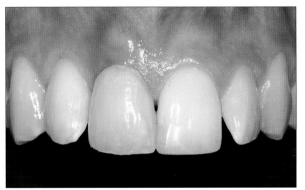

Fig 31   Provisional restoration in situ.

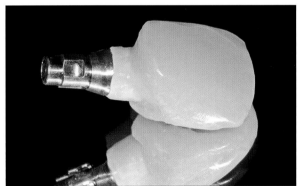

Fig 32   Fully customized provisional restoration with emergence profile.

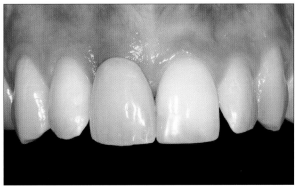

Fig 33   Clinical situation at the end of the provisional phase.

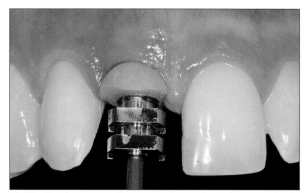

Fig 34   Final impression using a custom impression coping to transfer the emergence profile to the master cast.

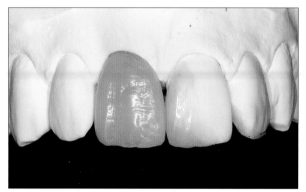

Fig 35   Wax-up for the implant-supported crown 11 and the tooth-supported crown 21.

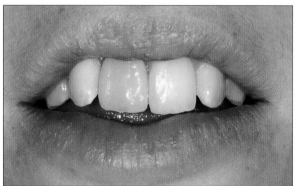

Fig 36   Try-in of wax-up. Relatively flat shape of tooth 11.

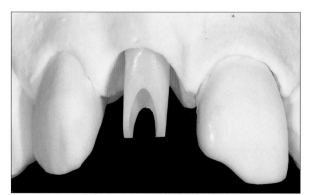

Fig 37   CAD/CAM-fabricated zirconia abutment on the master cast.

After a further healing period of three months, the composite restoration at tooth 21 was removed and the borders smoothened. The final impression was taken using a custom impression coping, thereby transferring the emergence profile from the clinical situation to the master cast (Fig 34).

The dental technician made a try-in wax-up for the implant-supported crown for tooth 11 and an additional etch piece for tooth 21 (Fig 35). The wax-up try-in demonstrated a relatively flat shape of tooth 11 compared to the contralateral natural tooth 21 (Fig 36).

A custom CAD/CAM-fabricated abutment (Fig 37), stained to mimic the shade of the contralateral tooth (Fig 38), was obtained and a try-in session scheduled.

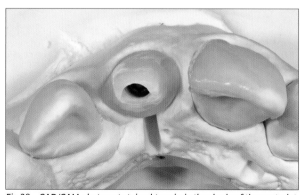

Fig 38   CAD/CAM abutment stained to mimic the shade of the contralateral tooth 21.

At the clinical try-in, the abutment shoulder on the buccal side was found to be placed slightly too far coronally (Fig 39). Subsequently, several try-in appointments were scheduled and the final reconstructions fabricated. For the implant-supported restoration, a zirconia abutment and a cemented lithium disilicate crown was chosen; for the natural tooth, a directly veneered feldspathic reconstruction (Figs 40a-c).

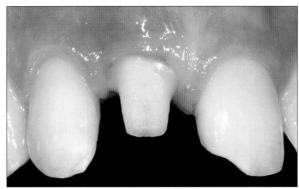

Fig 39　Clinical try-in of an abutment with a shoulder located slightly too far coronally

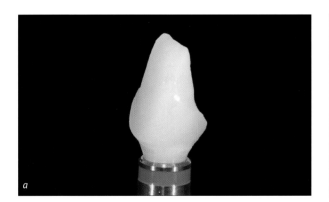

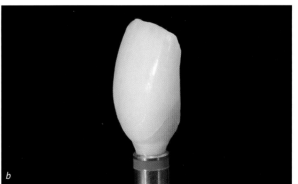

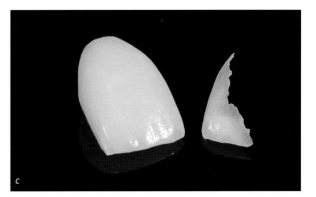

Figs 40a-c　Extraoral view of the final reconstructions: CAD/CAM zirconia abutment on implant 11 (a), lithium disilicate crown on implant 11 (b) and directly veneered feldspathic reconstruction on tooth 21 (c).

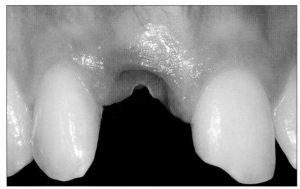

Fig 41   Emergence profile prior to the insertion of final restoration with healthy peri-implant tissues.

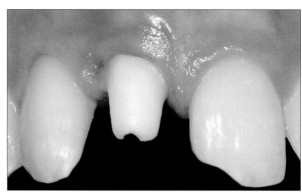

Fig 42   CAD/CAM abutment tightened. PTFE tape and a cotton pellet were placed on top of the screw prior to closing the screw access hole with flowable composite.

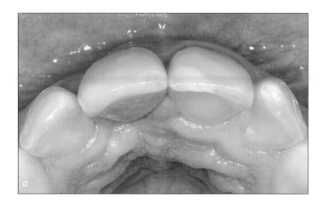

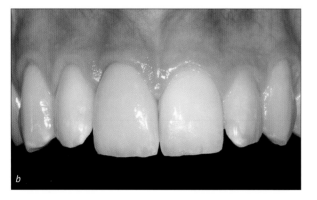

Following the removal of the provisional restoration (Fig 41), the abutment was tightened in place (Fig 42), and both crown 11 and the etch piece 21 were inserted using light-polymerizing flowable resin cement. One week later, the final examination demonstrated periodontal healthy tissues (Figs 43a-c). The corresponding x-ray showed stable marginal bone levels at the level of the implant shoulder (Fig 44).

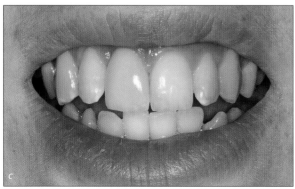

Figs 43a-c   Final view one week after insertion of the final restoration.

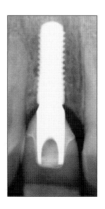

Fig 44   Corresponding x-ray at the follow-up one week after insertion. Marginal bone at the level of the implant shoulder.

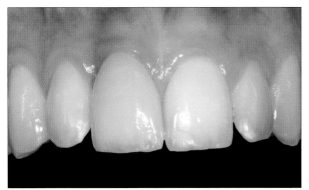

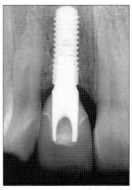

Fig 45   One-year clinical follow-up.

Fig 46   One-year radiological follow-up.

Figures 45 and 46 show the clinical and radiological fol-low-up one year after the insertion of the final restoration.

The limitations at the bone level described earlier did not allow placing the implant in a more palatal position. This resulted in a cemented rather than a screw-retained reconstruction and might slightly increase the risk for a mucosal recession in the long run. Alternatively, primary bone augmentation on the buccal and palatal side would have been necessary. This issue was discussed with the patient, but she refused undergoing an additional surgi-cal procedure.

The vertical and buccal deficits on the soft-tissue level were overcome by using an autologous connective-tissue graft (SCTG). The SCTG provided a further increase in soft-tissue thickness, reducing the risk for recession and optimizing the shade of the peri-implant tissues (Thoma and coworkers 2016a).

In the restorative phase, an individualized zirconia abut-ment was chosen. The abutment was further optimized by staining to mimic the shade of the contralateral tooth. It has been previously shown that all-ceramic reconstruc-tions avoid the grayish discoloration often observed with metal-based reconstructions (Linkevicius and Vaitelis 2015). The veneering material of the all-ceramic crown with a lithium disilicate framework (implant 11) and the minimally invasive reconstruction (tooth 21) were similar.

The prognosis of the case appears to be favorable, as we had provided a large amount of bone on the buccal side of the implant and increased the soft-tissue thickness.

Acknowledgments

Laboratory procedures
Master Dental Technician Pascal Müller – Schönenberger Dentaltechnik AG, Glattbrugg, Switzerland

7.10 Replacement of a Fractured Upper Left Central Incisor: Delayed Placement of a Bone Level Tapered Implant Using a Staged Approach

S. Keith

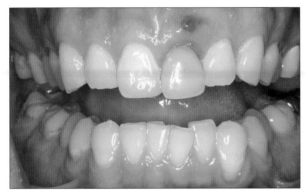

Fig 1   Initial clinical presentation with the fractured tooth 21.

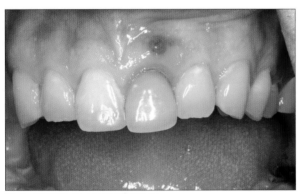

Fig 2   Draining sinus tract at tooth 21.

A 32-year-old male patient was referred to our specialty practice by his general dentist for evaluation and replacement of his failing maxillary left central incisor (tooth 21). This patient presented for care with no significant medical conditions, no known drug allergies, and was not taking any prescription medications. He mentioned the occasional use of over the counter, non-steroidal anti-inflammatories for occasional muscle aches attributed to sporting activities. He did report a history of mild asthma as a child, but no recent episodes of bronchospasm or shortness of breath in the last ten years. He complained of mild discomfort and swelling of the gingival tissue above his front tooth that began approximately 6 weeks prior.

The patient reported that he had been biting into a piece of bread when he felt something crack nearly two months before but that he had not noticed any mobility until about a week before. In addition to the slight mobility, the patient also stated the he had an unpleasant taste aroma emanating from his mouth. He reported that the tooth had originally been subjected to trauma around the age of 15, when he had chipped the central incisor on the edge of a swimming pool. The incisor had subsequently been treated endodontically and restored with composite resin. After the tooth had become darker than the adjacent teeth, his general dentist had found it necessary to restore the incisor with an all-ceramic crown to improve esthetics.

A thorough history and examination revealed no evidence of parafunctional habits or disorders of the temporomandibular joint.

A complete oral examination revealed an Angle class 1 functional malocclusion with mild crowding and slight to moderate incisal wear. Digital palpation of tooth 21 demonstrated class 2 mobility, moderate pain on percussion. and the presence of a draining sinus tract about 4 mm apical to the free gingival margin (Fig 1). The radiographic examination revealed prior endodontic treatment with a composite resin core and all-ceramic crown (Fig 2). There was radiographic evidence of a horizontal root fracture that extended below the osseous crest and associated bone loss on the mesial root surface. Apical palpation of the area elicited discomfort and produced a purulent exudate from the fistula (Fig 3).

The patient stated that he had never been completely satisfied with the appearance of the original restoration. His chief complaint included general discomfort, looseness of his front tooth, oral malodor, and a concern about "the abscess on my gums." He was very concerned about the possibility of replacing his front tooth with a dental implant, since there was an active infection at the site, and wondered whether the result would look natural when the treatment was completed.

Following a complete clinical examination and an evaluation of articulated study casts, the patient was advised of the various treatment options available. He fully understood that the existing fractured central incisor was not restorable and would need to be removed. The site would require a staged approach to the eventual fixed reconstruction with delayed implant placement after tooth removal and site preservation using a bone allograft material to regenerate the site. Once all his questions regarding the phases of treatment and overall treatment time were answered, he agreed to the following treatment plan:

- Tooth 21 was to be surgically removed and the residual extraction defect reconstructed with bone graft regeneration (Hürzeler and coworkers 2006).
- A provisional removable partial denture would be fabricated for delivery at the time of tooth removal and bone grafting.

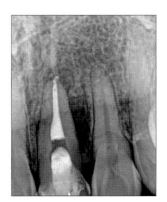

Fig 3 Baseline periapical radiograph.

- Upon completion of healing at the edentulous site, estimated to take 5 to 6 months, a radiographic template would be fabricated for use with the CBCT scan (Chen and Buser 2014).
- Pre-surgical planning software would determine the appropriate implant diameter and length to ideally place a bone-level tapered implant in the site (Klokkevold 2015).
- Following placement of the implant using a non-submerged, unloaded protocol, an implant-level impression would be taken to aid in the fabrication of a screw-retained, fixed provisional restoration for development and maturation of peri-implant mucosal tissues (Santling and coworkers 2015; Elian and coworkers 2017c).
- After an appropriate healing interval with the acrylic-resin provisional restoration, a Zirconia custom abutment and all-ceramic definitive crown would be fabricated, adjusted, and delivered to satisfy the patient's functional and esthetic expectations and to return him to a state of oral health (Zembic and coworkers 2015).

The Esthetic Risk Assessment (ERA) for this patient was completed and revealed a moderate level of surgical and prosthetic expertise required to meet or exceed the demands of this particular patient treatment (Table 1).

Table 1   Esthetic Risk Assessment (ERA)

Esthetic risk factors	Level of risk		
	Low	**Medium**	**High**
Medical status	Healthy, uneventful healing		Compromised healing
Smoking habit	Non-smoker	Light smoker (≤ 10 cigs/day)	Heavy smoker (> 10 cigs/day)
Gingival display at full smile	Low	Medium	High
Width of edentulous span	1 tooth (≥ 7 mm)[1] 1 tooth (≥ 6 mm)[2]	1 tooth (< 7 mm)[1] 1 tooth (< 6 mm)[2]	2 teeth or more
Shape of tooth crowns	Rectangular	Ovoid	Triangular
Restorative status of neighboring teeth	Virgin		Restored
Gingival phenotype	Low-scalloped, thick	Medium-scalloped, medium-thick	High-scalloped, thin
Infection at implant site	None	Chronic	Acute
Soft-tissue anatomy	Soft tissue intact	Inflamed	Soft-tissue defects
Bone level at adjacent teeth	≤ 5 mm to contact point	5.5 to 6.5 mm to contact point	≥ 7 mm to contact point
Facial bone-wall phenotype*	Thick-wall phenotype ≥ 1 mm thickness		Thin-wall phenotype < 1 mm thickness
Bone anatomy of alveolar crest	No bone deficiency	Horizontal bone deficiency	Vertical bone deficiency
Patient's esthetic expectations	Realistic expectations	Moderate expectations	Unrealistic expectations

* If three-dimensional imaging is available with the tooth in place
[1] Standard-diameter implant, regular connection
[2] Narrow-diameter implant, narrow connection

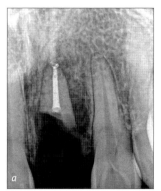
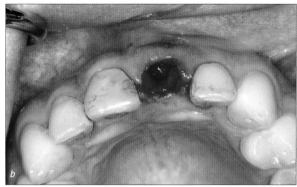

Figs 4a-b   Residual root fragment and debrided site after its removal.

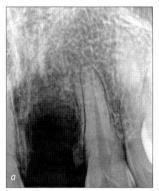
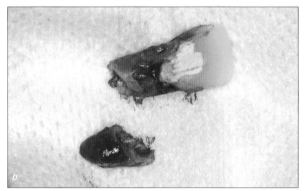

Figs 5a-b   Removed fragments of tooth 21. Oblique root fracture, confirming the need for complete removal.

Treatment began with surgical removal of the failing tooth, reconstruction of the damaged alveolar process, and preparation of the site for implant placement. The patient began a pre-operative course of amoxicillin 500 mg three times a day on the day before the procedure. Under local anesthesia, a minimally invasive approach was taken to severing the periodontal ligament of the retained apical root fragment with periotomes. The fragment was gently luxated with an elevator while preventing damage to the thin remaining buccal plate (Figs 4a-b). The site was thoroughly debrided of residual granulation tissue and irrigated with copious amounts of sterile saline solution. A periapical radiograph confirmed complete removal of the root tip (Figs 5a-b). The socket was then filled with particulate human source bone graft material (Straumann AlloGraft Cortical-Cancellous Mix/LifeNet Health; Straumann USA, Andover, MA, USA) and closed with a resorbable collagen plug (Salvin Dental Specialties, Charlotte, NC, USA) and a 5-0 Vicryl suture (Ethicon, Somerville, NJ, USA) (Figs 6 to 8).

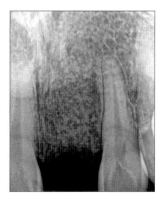

Fig 6   Postoperative radiograph.

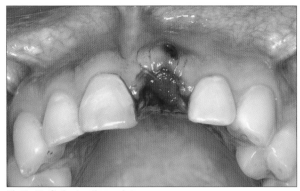

Fig 7 Grafted extraction socket.

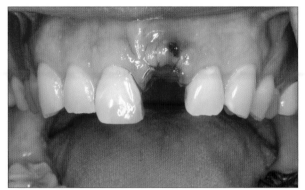

Fig 8 Postoperative view of the site after grafting and removal of the sinus tract.

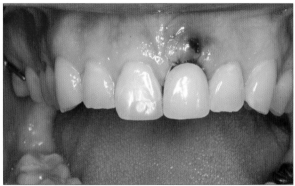

Fig 9 Transitional removable partial denture replacing the missing incisor.

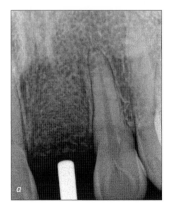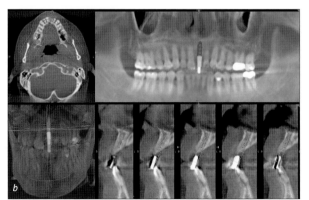

Figs 10a-b Intraoral radiograph and CBCT scan of the edentulous site 21.

A transitional removable partial denture with a pontic was adjusted and delivered for provisional esthetic replacement of the missing central incisor during the healing phase (Fig 9).

The patient was seen for postoperative evaluation at ten days to assess the progress of healing and to remove the sutures. The site was allowed to heal for five months. A second follow-up appointment confirmed tissue healing as anticipated, with good gingival volume and quality.

A preoperative alginate impression was taken to fabricate a presurgical radiographic Higginbottom template for use in planning the anticipated implant position (Fig 10a). A cone-beam computed tomogram (Carestream 146088300 3D; Carestream Health, Rochester, NY, USA) of the patient was taken while the patient was wearing the radiographic template, and the data set loaded was into the software for evaluation and simulation of implant placement (Fig 10b). This pre-operative planning confirmed that the available bone width and volume would allow for the ideal placement of an implant.

The patient was given a preoperative prescription for 21 tablets of amoxicillin 500 mg. The instructions called for one tablet of amoxicillin to be taken orally three times a day for one week, starting on the day before surgery. The patient was given a preoperative oral rinse with chlorhexidine digluconate 0.12% for one minute, and the perioral tissues were disinfected with a topical betadine wipe. The surgical area was anesthetized by local infiltration with 3.6 ml of articaine 4% and epinephrine 1 : 200,000.

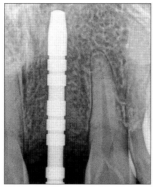

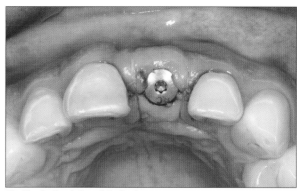

Fig 11   Radiograph   with   2.8-mm radiographic marker in place.

Fig 12   Occlusal view of the implant.

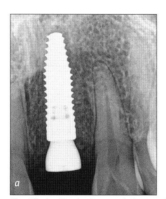

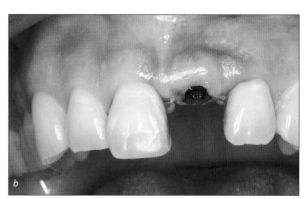

Figs 13a-b   Semi-submerged closure of the implant site and postoperative periapical radiograph.

The edentulous alveolar site was exposed via a crestal incision extending into the sulcus of the adjacent teeth and a full-thickness mucoperiosteal flap elevated. The osteotomy was initiated with a 2.3 mm round bur using the Higginbottom template to guide the entry point into the alveolar ridge. The osteotomy was prepared at 750 rpm with a surgical motor and sterile saline irrigation. The drilling protocol continued through a series of twist drills, beginning at 2.2 mm diameter and progressing through 2.8 mm and to 3.5 mm. Radiographic control images were taken throughout to confirm the proper position and depth of the osteotomy (Fig 11). Upon completion of the osteotomy using a coronal profile drill, the implant (Straumann Bone Level Tapered Roxolid, SLActive, diameter 4.1 mm, length 12 mm; Institut Straumann AG, Basel, Switzerland) was placed with the manual ratchet to confirm an insertion torque in the range of 35 N·cm and excellent primary stability.

The top of the implant was positioned about 1 mm below the surrounding osseous crest and approximately 4 mm below the gingival margin (Fig 12). The soft tissues were reapproximated around the contoured regular CrossFit healing abutment (Institut Straumann AG) and closed with two interrupted 5-0 Vicryl (Ethicon) sutures interproximally (Figs 13a-b).

The transitional removable partial denture was tried in and the tissue surface of the pontic area adjusted to limit contact on the implant healing abutment. The patient was provided with written postoperative instructions and released in good condition. The patient's existing maxillary transitional prosthesis was adjusted to relieve the areas over the implant site. The patient completed the course of amoxicillin 500 mg as described and followed a regimen of twice-daily rinsing with chlorhexidine digluconate 12%.

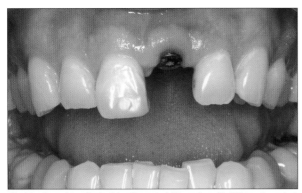

Fig 14   Complete gingival healing at eight weeks with RC healing abutment in place.

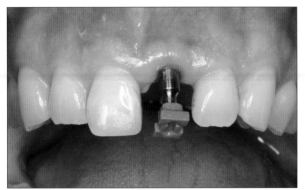

Fig 15   RC Impression coping inserted for the final impression.

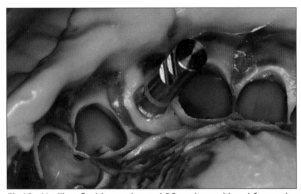

Fig 16   Maxillary final impression and RC analog positioned for pouring the master cast.

The patient was recalled at ten days for a postoperative assessment of the healing process and suture removal. After eight weeks of undisturbed healing (Fig 14), the prosthetic reconstruction phase was initiated. The healing abutment was removed and the internal aspect of the implant prosthetic connection was irrigated with chlorhexidine digluconate 0.12%. An impression was taken in a polyvinyl siloxane material (Take-1; Kerr, Orange, CA, USA) in a custom tray (Figs 15 and 16).

The master cast was poured in a high strength, low expansion die-stone (ResinRock; Whip Mix, Louisville, KY, USA) with a gingival tissue mask (Softissue Moulage; Kerr). The preliminary cast was used by the dental technician to fabricate a screw-retained acrylic resin provisional crown on a temporary titanium cylinder (Institut Straumann AG).

The patient was seen at ten weeks for delivery of the provisional crown to initiate loading of the implant and gingival tissue conditioning. The area was again anesthetized using a local infiltration administration of 3.6 ml of articaine 4% and epinephrine 1 : 200,000.

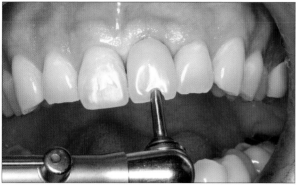

Fig 17   Screw-retained provisional seated at 35 N·cm

After removal of the healing abutment, the screw-retained provisional was tried on the implant, which resulted in gentle blanching of the peri-implant mucosa. After confirmation and adjustment of the interproximal and occlusal contacts, the provisional was polished to a high shine and connected to the implant at 35 N·cm of torque on the abutment screw (Fig 17). The screw access hole was then closed with PTFE tape and light-cured composite resin (Premise A2; Kerr) and a periapical radiograph was taken to confirm complete seating of the provisional restoration and document a baseline of the crestal bone level at the time of implant loading (Figs 18a-b and 19).

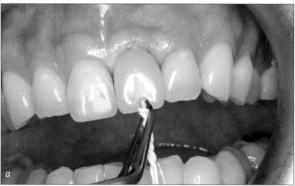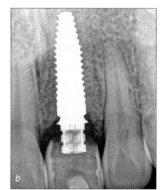

Figs 18a-b   Clinical delivery of the screw-retained provisional and peri-apical radiograph.

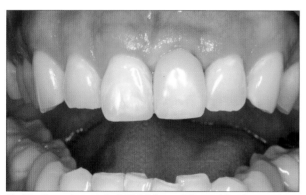

Fig 19   Tissue shape at the initial delivery of the provisional restoration.

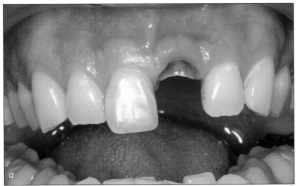

Fig 20   *Removal of the screw-retained provisional after six weeks of tissue conditioning.*

The peri-implant mucosa was allowed to mature around the provisional crown for a period of six weeks. During this time, the patient was able to evaluate the esthetic and functional parameters of tooth shape, incisal edge position, and phonetics. The patient was pleased with the shape and contours of the provisional crown and surrounding mucosal framework. The provisional crown was then removed to confirm soft-tissue contours and to make a final polyvinyl siloxane impression (Take-1; Kerr) (Figs 20 and 21a-b).

The resulting final master cast created a replica of the clinical hard- and soft-tissue contours from which the lab technician would use to design and fabricate the final restoration. This cast was scanned in an optical lab scanner (CARES CS2, Institut Straumann AG) to create a digital Standard Tessellation Language (STL) file. The STL file was uploaded into the CARES Visual Design software to develop a CAD/CAM design for a custom zirconia abutment. The final CARES custom zirconia abutment was milled and delivered to the lab for fabrication of the final all-ceramic restoration.

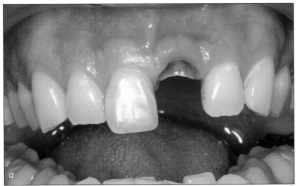
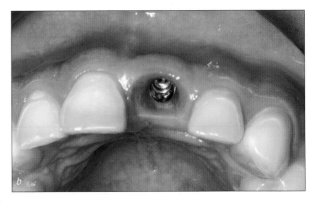

Figs 21a-b   *Clinical appearance of the mature peri-implant transition zone.*

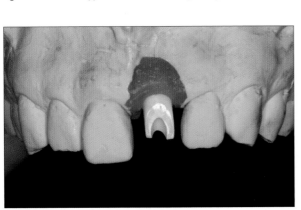

Fig 22   *Master cast with custom zirconia abutment.*

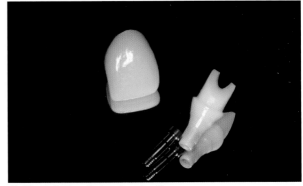

Fig 23   *Definitive all-ceramic restoration.*

The dental lab technician met the patient for a custom shade appointment to determine the correct shade, value, contour and surface texture to match the adjacent unrestored natural dentition. Diagnostic shade photos were recorded for shade verification. The final restoration was fabricated from a pressed lithium disilicate core (IPS e.Max; Ivoclar Vivadent, Schaan, Liechtenstein) with a ceramic veneer. The CARES custom zirconia abutment and final cemented all-ceramic crown were returned to our office for the final try-in and delivery (Figs 24 and 25).

After four weeks to allow for the laboratory fabrication steps, the patient returned to the office for insertion of the definitive restoration. The provisional restoration was accessed through the composite resin in the incisal aspect of the crown and the PTFE tape removed. The provisional was retrieved, and the internal aspect of the implant was thoroughly rinsed with an air/water spray and irrigated with chlorhexidine digluconate 0.12%. The CARES custom zirconia abutment was then inserted into the Regular CrossFit prosthetic connection of the implant (Fig 26). The precisely machined abutment fit intimately with the conical locking interface at the platform switch of this bone-level implant and effectively eliminates microleakage and bacterial movement from the sulcus into the internal aspect of the implant/abutment interface. The implant/abutment passive fit was confirmed with a periapical radiograph (Fig 27).

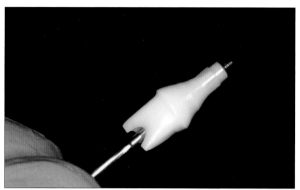

Fig 24   CARES custom zirconia abutment with CrossFit connection.

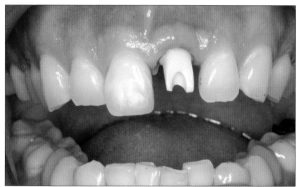

Fig 25   The abutment in situ.

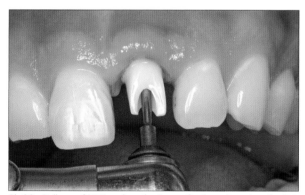

Fig 26   Delivery of 35 N·cm insertion torque for the custom zirconia abutment.

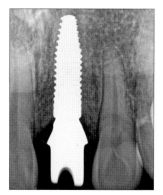

Fig 27   Periapical radiograph.

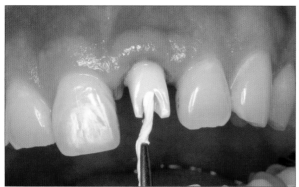

Fig 28   Retrievable obturation of the screw access channel with PTFE tape.

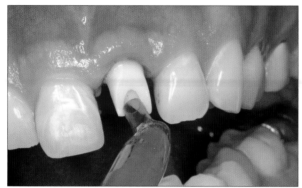

Fig 29   Closing the screw access hole with a light-cured temporary composite.

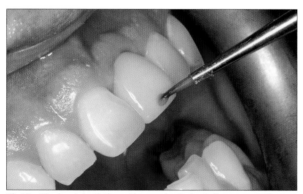

Fig 30   Final custom tinting with ceramic glazing before cementation.

The definitive cemented all-ceramic crown was tried in and the proximal and occlusal contacts evaluated with articulating paper and adjusted as needed. Care was taken to ensure that the restoration did not occlude with the opposing teeth in protrusive movements and that all incisal guidance was carried by the adjacent natural dentition. These occlusal contacts were verified with a computerized digital bite-force sensor system (TekScan; TekScan, South Boston, MA, USA). The prosthesis was evaluated for esthetics and phonetics. After modification with a custom ceramic tint and final glazing in the ceramic furnace, the patient approved the esthetic result. The abutment screw was seated at 35 N·cm of measured torque. The access hole was closed with PTFE tape and Telio CS C&B temporary composite (Ivoclar Vivadent), which was light-cured (Figs 28 to 30).

The area was air-dried and isolated with cotton rolls and the definitive crown cemented with a small amount of resin-reinforced glass-ionomer luting agent (Fuji PLUS; GC America, Alsip, IL, USA) (Fig 31). Careful removal of all excess cement at the restoration/abutment interface was confirmed with an explorer and dental floss to ensure harmonious health of the peri-implant gingival tissues. A post-cementation periapical radiograph was taken to confirm complete removal of cement and establish baseline crestal bone levels (Fig 32). After cementation, alginate impressions of the final crown were taken for the fabrication of a maxillary occlusal guard to be worn during sleep. Home care and oral-hygiene instructions were reviewed with the patient, including the use of an electric toothbrush (Philips Sonicare; Philips, Amsterdam, Netherlands), floss and a water irrigator (WaterPik; Philips) to perform effective plaque removal throughout the entire mouth and in the subgingival area of the implant-supported prosthesis.

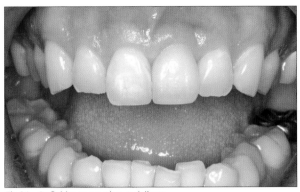

Fig 31   Definitive restoration at delivery.

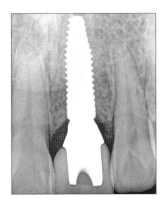

Fig 32   Periapical   radiographs taken after delivery.

The patient was recalled at ten days to reevaluate the gingival response and check the occlusal contacts. The maxillary occlusal guard was adjusted and delivered. Also, a review of oral-hygiene procedures was completed. The patient reported sincere satisfaction with the esthetic and functional outcome of his implant treatment (Fig 33). Further reevaluation took place at six and twelve months, with no complications noted or changes in radiographic bone levels around the implant. After more than two years of service, the patient continued to report satisfaction with his prosthesis and was thrilled with the esthetic outcome (Fig 34). The patient was been referred back to his general dentist for continuing care and regular recall appointments.

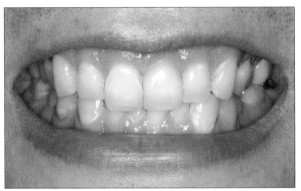

Fig 33   Definitive restoration at full smile.

We think this patient may expect many years of enjoyment and satisfaction from his maxillary anterior single-tooth implant-supported restoration.

Acknowledgments

Laboratory procedures
Mike Sartip, Advanced Dental Lab – Clayton, CA, USA

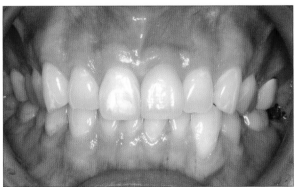

Fig 34   Definitive restoration after more than two years of service.

7.11   Replacement of an Ankylosed Upper Left Central Incisor: Bone Augmentation and Socket Grafting, Late Placement of an RC Bone Level Implant

A. Burgoyne

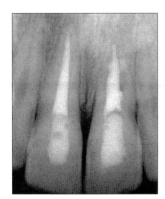

Fig 1   Periapical radiograph of October 2004.

A 15-year-old male patient was referred to us by his pediatric dentist in June 2004 for evaluation of treatment options for his failing tooth 21. The patient had recently seen an endodontist for internal bleaching and been advised that there had been significant resorption and ankylosis. The patient's mother was concerned because the tooth appeared shorter than the adjacent one. His past dental history was significant for trauma (September 2001), where the tooth had been avulsed and reimplanted. Teeth 11 and 21 had been endodontically treated (Fig 1).

The clinical examination revealed that the patient's occlusal function was normal and that the tooth was asymptomatic. The overjet was 3.5 mm, the overbite was 3 mm. The occlusal scheme was a canine-guided posterior disclusion; protrusive contacts were shared by all anterior teeth (Figs 2 and 3).

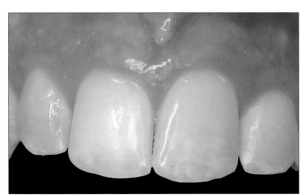

Fig 2   Teeth 11 and 21 at the time the patient was referred.

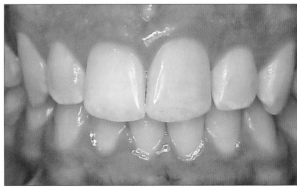

Fig 3   Dentition in terminal occlusion.

It was decided not to initiate treatment at that point but to place the patient on recall to monitor the progression of the resorption. Annual recalls were scheduled through his pediatric dentist, who monitored his dental needs.

In December 2009, the patient decided he wanted to explore definitive treatment for his central incisors. His pediatric dentist had determined that the patient's growth had been complete at age 20 and that he was ready for definitive treatment of tooth 21. At evaluation, that tooth was ankylosed and infraerupted. There was a 1-mm diastema between teeth 12 and 11, a 1.5-mm diastema between teeth 21 and 22, and a 1-mm diastema between teeth 21 and 22 (Figs 4a-e). An esthetic risk assessment was completed as part of the examination (Table 1).

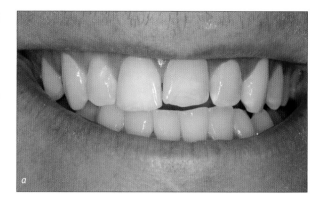

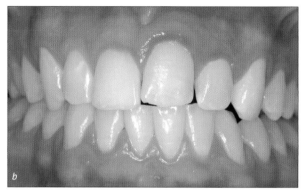

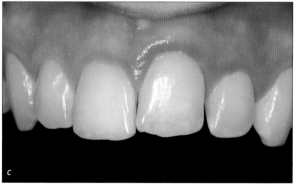

Figs 4a-c   Clinical situation in December 2009. Tooth 21 appeared to be ankylosed and infraerupted.

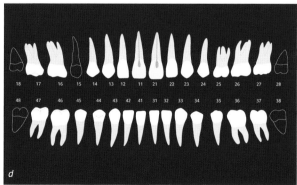

Fig 4d   Dental scheme with the planned treatment for teeth 11 and 21.

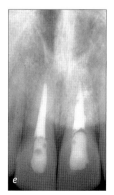

Fig 4e   Periapical radiograph of December 2009 confirming a lack of periodontal ligament around tooth 21, consistent with ankylosis of tooth 21.

Table 1   Esthetic Risk Assessment (ERA)

Esthetic risk factors	Level of risk		
	Low	**Medium**	**High**
Medical status	Healthy, uneventful healing		Compromised healing
Smoking habit	Non-smoker	Light smoker (≤ 10 cigs/day)	Heavy smoker (> 10 cigs/day)
Gingival display at full smile	Low	Medium	High
Width of edentulous span	1 tooth (≥ 7 mm)[1] 1 tooth (≥ 6 mm)[2]	1 tooth (< 7 mm)[1] 1 tooth (< 6 mm)[2]	2 teeth or more
Shape of tooth crowns	Rectangular		Triangular
Restorative status of neighboring teeth	Virgin		Restored
Gingival phenotype	Low-scalloped, thick	Medium-scalloped, medium-thick	High-scalloped, thin
Infection at implant site	None	Chronic	Acute
Soft-tissue anatomy	Soft tissue intact		Soft-tissue defects
Bone level at adjacent teeth	≤ 5 mm to contact point	5.5 to 6.5 mm to contact point	≥ 7 mm to contact point
Facial bone-wall phenotype*	Thick-wall phenotype ≥ 1 mm thickness		Thin-wall phenotype < 1 mm thickness
Bone anatomy of alveolar crest	No bone deficiency	Horizontal bone deficiency	Vertical bone deficiency
Patient's esthetic expectations	Realistic expectations		Unrealistic expectations

* If three-dimensional imaging is available with the tooth in place
[1] Standard-diameter implant, regular connection
[2] Narrow-diameter implant, narrow connection

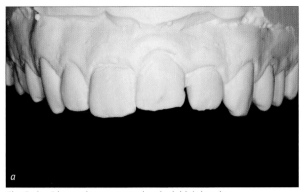

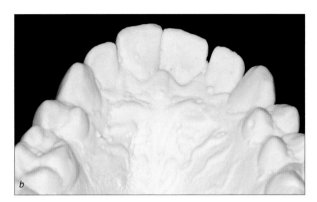

Figs 5a-b   Diagnostic casts capturing the initial situation.

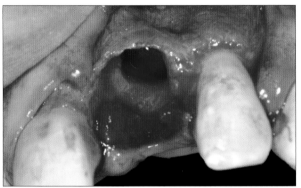

Fig 6   Socket 21 was found to be intact circumferentially. The buccal wall was less than 1 mm thick after the extraction of tooth 21.

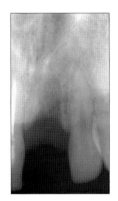

Fig 7   Radiograph after the extraction of tooth 21 showing an intact socket and no root fragments.

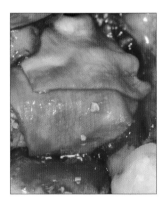

Fig 8   Situation after grafting with Bio-Oss and covering the grafted site with two Bio-Gide membranes.

Diagnostic casts were made to capture the initial situation in December 2009 (Figs 5a-b).

The proposed treatment plan called for an attempt to extrude tooth 21 orthodontically to move the alveolar housing and the free gingival margin further coronally before extracting that tooth. A second option was discussed that would involve removing the crown on tooth 21 and submerging the root to maximize soft-tissue coverage prior to root removal.

The orthodontist felt that extrusion of 21 was not an option and recommended a comprehensive plan. The patient and parent rejected orthodontic therapy and requested treatment involving removal of tooth 21 with subsequent implant placement and restoration.

Therefore, the final treatment plan included the following:

- Extraction of tooth 21
- Bone augmentation with xenografts and autologous bone
- Implant placement
- Additional soft-tissue grafting as needed
- Restoration

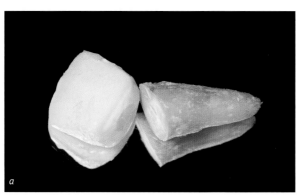
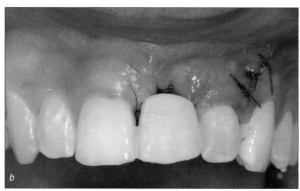

Figs 9a-b   The interim prosthesis included the natural crown of tooth 21, which was bonded to the neighboring teeth.

In accordance with the ITI SAC Guidelines (Dawson and Chen 2009), the patient's treatment was classified as Advanced from a Restorative and Complex from a Surgical standpoint.

In June 2010, tooth 21 was extracted (Figs 6 and 7) and the socket grafted with small particle cancellous granules (Bio-Oss; Geistlich Pharma, Wolhusen, Switzerland)

mixed with autologous bone and covered with a Bio-Gide membrane (Geistlich Pharma) (Fig 8). The initial tooth replacement was the natural crown of the extracted tooth 21, bonded to the adjacent teeth (Figs 9a-b).

Eight days later, the sutures were removed and an adhesively cemented fixed dental prosthesis (FDP) was bonded as the interim restoration (Figs 10a-c).

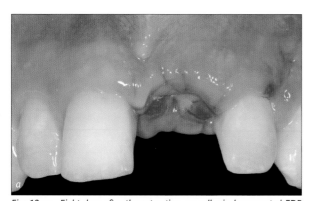
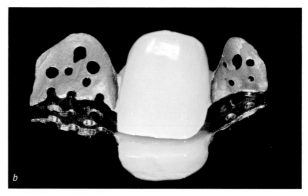

Figs 10a-c   Eight days after the extraction, an adhesively cemented FDP was provided as an interim restoration.

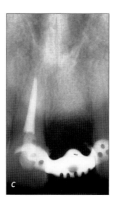

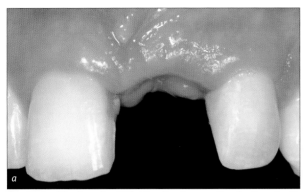

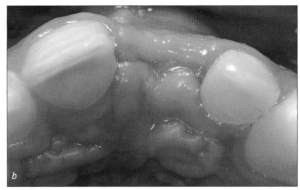

Figs 11a-b   Situation after FDP debonding four months after the extraction of tooth 21.

The FDP debonded once between July 2010 and October 2010, when tooth 11 was prepared for a full-coverage restoration and the FDP removed in favor of a cantilevered pontic to tooth 21 (Figs 11a-b).

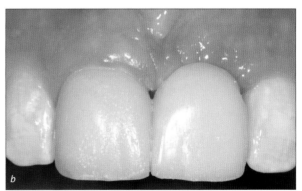

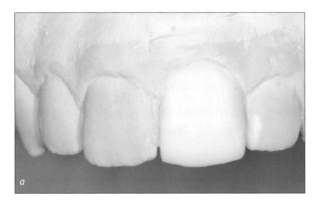

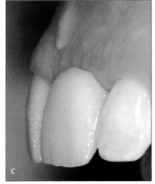

Figs 12a-c   A diagnostic wax-up of tooth 21 was completed. Tooth 11 was prepared for a full-coverage restoration and a provisional cantilevered fixed dental prosthesis was fabricated for 11 and 21 using autopolymerizing methyl methacrylate.

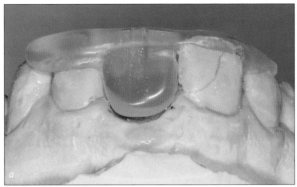

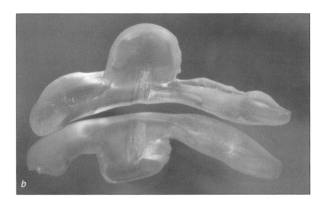

Figs 13a-b   Surgical guide made of Triad.

A surgical guide was made of laboratory composite resin (Triad; Dentsply Sirona, York, PA, USA) representing the predicted contours of tooth 21 (Figs 13a-b).

The implant was placed three weeks later, with the intent of providing an indirect implant retained provisional restoration to assist in guiding the contours of the soft tissue. The implant would be indexed during the surgical procedure for indirect fabrication of the provisional (Figs 15a-c). A bone-level implant (Bone Level RN, diameter 4.1 mm, length 10 mm; Institut Straumann AG, Basel, Switzerland) was placed on the osteotomy at site 21. Autograft material collected during the osteotomy was mixed with Bio-Oss and put aside for contour augmentation after the indexing of the implant position (Figs 14a-f).

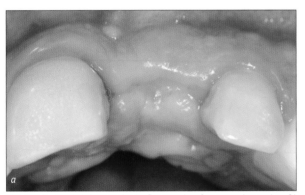

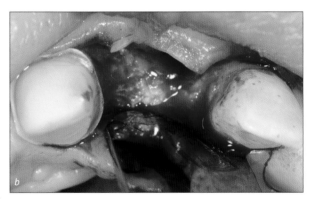

Figs 14a-b   Healed ridge at site 21 five months after extraction and grafting.

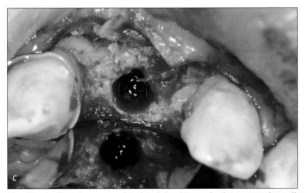

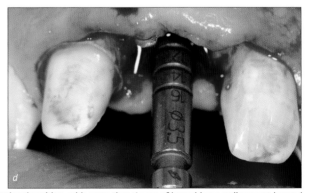

Figs 14c-d   Osteotomy completed to 3.5 × 11 mm in the correct three-dimensional position, with more than 1 mm of buccal bone wall present beyond the osteotomy.

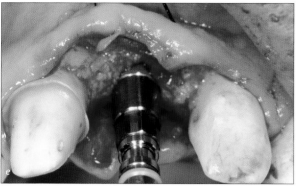

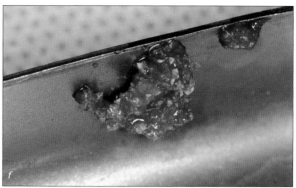

Figs 14e-f   A bone-level implant (Bone Level RN, diameter 4.1 mm, length 10 mm; Institut Straumann AG) in situ. The harvested bone chips were mixed with Bio-Oss for contour grafting on the buccal aspect.

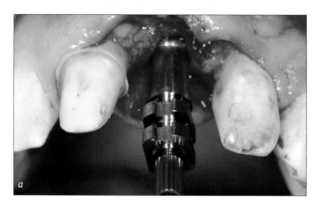

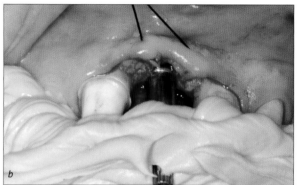

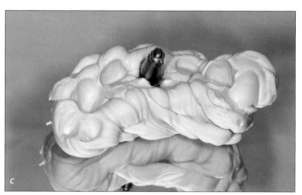

Figs 15a-c   The implant position was indexed using a sterile open-tray impression coping for the RN implant and fast-set registration polyvinyl siloxane (Blu-Mousse; Parkell, Edgewood, NY, USA).

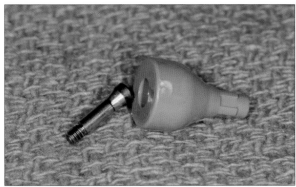

Fig 16   *The gingiva-colored PEEK healing abutment before customization.*

A PEEK healing abutment (Institut Straumann AG) (Fig 16) was chosen to allow customizing of the contours of the healing abutment. The contoured abutment was polished and inserted. The contour augmentation was placed on the buccal aspect of site 21 and the flap closed with 5-0 Vicryl interrupted sutures (Ethicon; Johnson & Johnson Medical, New Brunswick, NJ, USA) (Figs 17a-b and 18).

The provisional cantilevered prosthesis was adjusted to prevent contact with the tissues at site 21 and then seated with a polyurethane provisional cement (Fig 19).

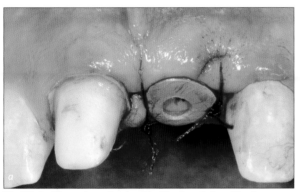
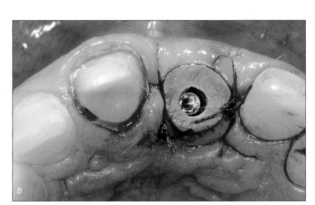

Figs 17a-b   *The contoured and polished healing abutment in situ.*

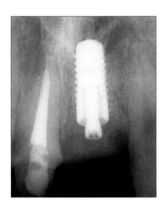

Fig 18   *Periapical control radiograph taken after placing the healing abutment and suturing.*

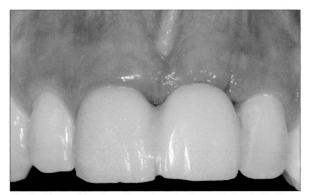

Fig 19   *The provisional cantilevered prosthesis cemented on tooth 11.*

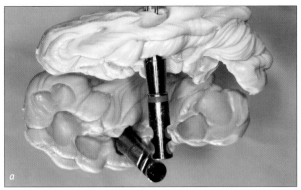

Fig 20a   Implant analog attached to the impression coping.

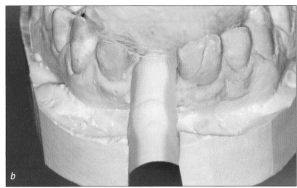

Fig 20b   Stone removed to create room for the implant analog in the cast.

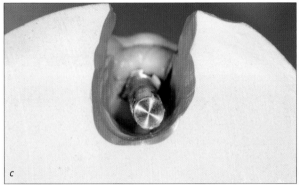

Fig 20c   Assessing the cast to ensure that the analog is not in contact with any stone when the registration is fully seated against the teeth.

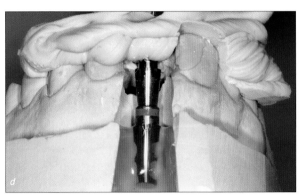

Fig 20d   Triad laboratory composite added and cured.

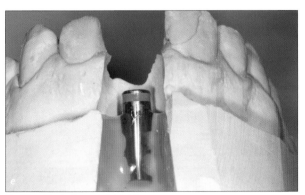

Fig 20e   The index was removed.

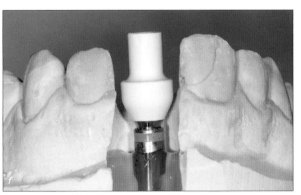

Fig 20f   Temporary abutment placed on the analog.

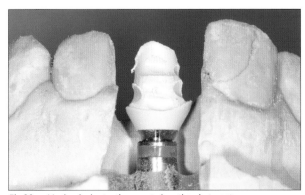

Fig 20g   Mechanical retention created on the abutment.

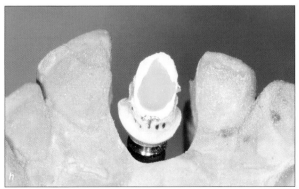

Fig 20h   A screw-retained provisional is desired, so the access is blocked out with a readily visible material that can be removed easily (Play-Doh; Mattel, El Segundo, CA, USA).

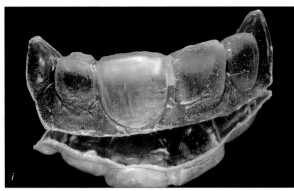

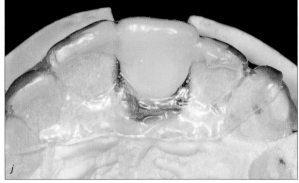

Figs 20i-l   The provisional crown was fabricated using autopolymerizing methyl methacrylate in a matrix and pressure-cured for 10 minutes at 1.4 bar.

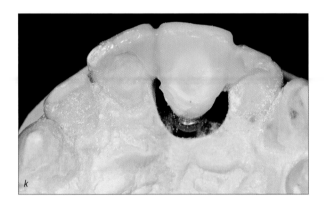

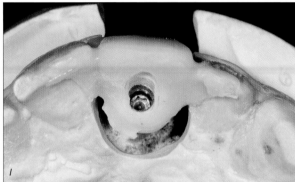

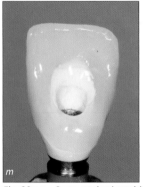

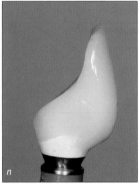

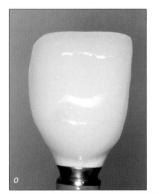

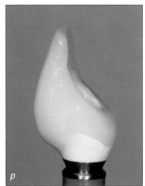

Figs 20m-p   Screw-retained provisional crown before polishing, contoured to provide ideal submucosal support and emergence.

In the laboratory, a Bone Level RN analog (Institut Straumann AG) was retrofitted to an existing model using the surgical index (Figs 20a-e). On this cast, a screw-retained provisional restoration was fabricated using the PEEK temporary abutment (Institut Straumann AG) and autopolymerizing PMMA (Figs 20f-p).

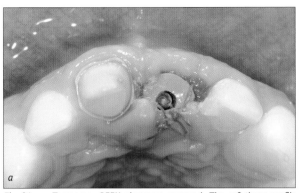
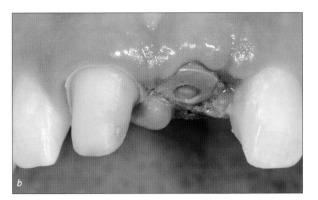

Figs 21a-c   Temporary PEEK abutment removed. The soft-tissue profile was maintained during initial healing.

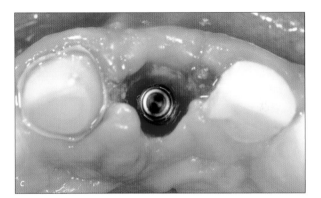

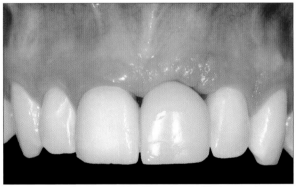

Fig 22   Two weeks after provisional insertion. Modified restoration.

In November 2010, the provisional FDP, sutures, and PEEK temporary abutment were removed. The interrupted sutures had pulled away from the buccal portion of the flap, leading to a loss of the height of the interproximal papilla (Figs 21a-c).

The implant-supported provisional crown was tightened to 15 N·cm and the access closed with PTFE tape and endodontic sealer (Cavit; 3M ESPE, St. Paul, MN, USA). The contours were kept very flat from the implant to the mucosal sulcus on the facial and interproximal surfaces. This concave contour was designed to enhance tissue proliferation in these areas.

The patient was recalled after two and four weeks to make modifications to the contours of the provisional restoration and assess the soft tissue.

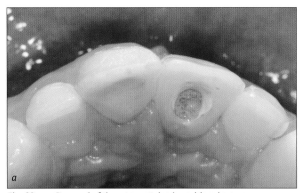

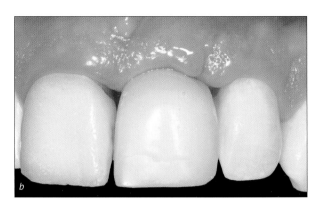

Figs 23a-c   Removal of the screw-retained provisional crown.

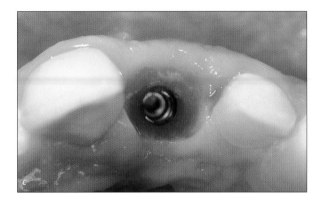

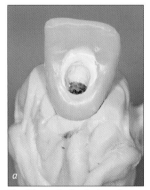
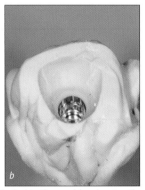
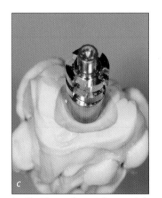
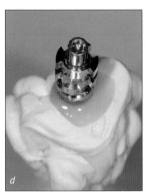

Figs 24a-e   An implant analog was attached to the provisional restoration and a Blu-Mousse impression was taken around the implant provisional. The impression was used for a template to fabricate a customized impression coping. The soft-tissue profile aspect of the impression coping was shaped using a flowable composite.

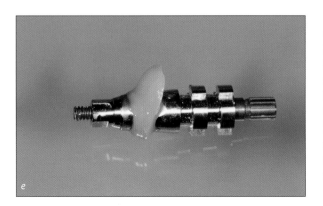

At this point in the management of the provisional restoration, the patient determined that the time constraints associated with his attending university in another city were arduous and wished to complete his restorative therapy. He was advised that the soft-tissue contours were not ideal, but he still wished to finalize treatment. In December 2010, the provisional restoration was removed (Figs 23a-c) and a customized impression coping developed to transfer the contours of the provisional to the master cast (Figs 24a-e).

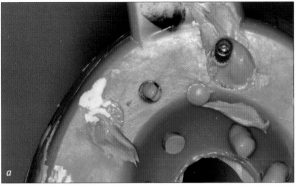
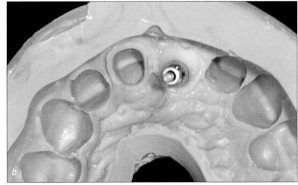

Figs 25a-d   An open-tray polyvinyl siloxane impression was taken using a stock (Coe) tray system. A soft-tissue master cast was made at the laboratory.

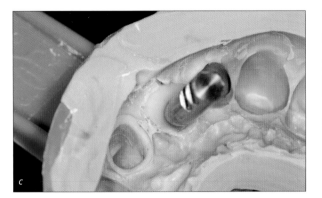
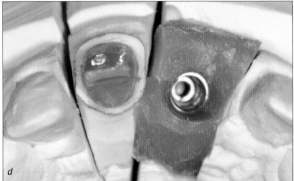

The final impression was taken with a customized open-tray transfer coping, a stock COE tray, and polyvinyl siloxane (Imprint; 3M Espe, St. Paul, MN, USA) (Figs 25a-d).

A pressable-ceramic crown (IPS e.max; Ivoclar Vivadent AG, Schaan, Liechtenstein) was fabricated for tooth 21 and a Straumann CARES zirconia abutment made for the implant-retained crown 21. The material for crown 21 was IPS e.max pressed onto the zirconia abutment, resulting in a screw-retained implant-supported restoration (Figs 26a-d).

The final restorations were delivered in late January of 2011. As with any implant-retained prosthesis in combination with tooth-retained restorations, the implant restoration was seated first (Figs 27a-b to 31). The interproximal contacts were adjusted relative to the implant-retained restoration prior to delivery. After verifying the contacts, esthetics (as per the patient's judgment), and occlusion, the implant-retained crown was tightened to 35 N·cm. The screw head was covered with PTFE tape and sealed with light-cured composite resin.

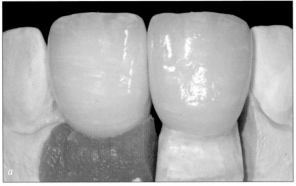

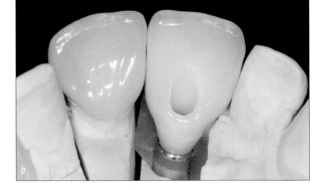

Figs 26a-d   The final restorations on the master cast.

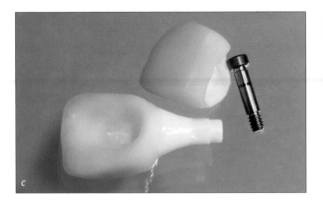

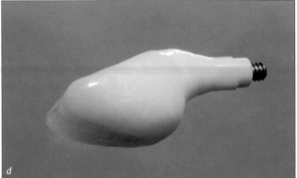

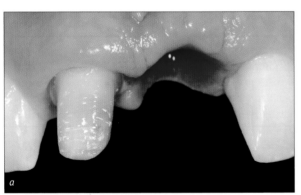

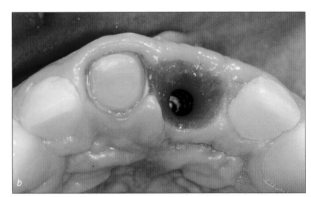

Figs 27a-b   Provisional prostheses removed.

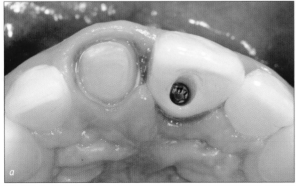

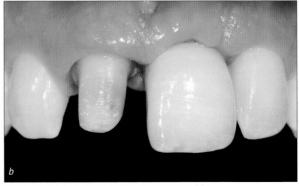

Figs 28a-b   The implant-supported restoration was seated first to ensure proper interproximal contacts between crowns 11 and 21.

A. Burgoyne

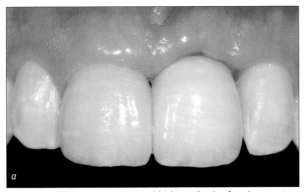

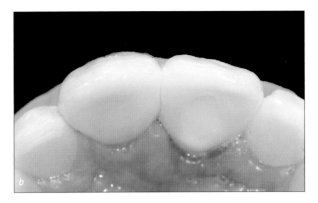

Figs 29a-c   IPS e.max crowns 11 and 21 immediately after placement.

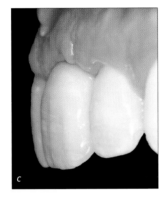

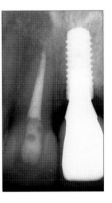

Fig 30   Periapical radiograph after seating the implant- and tooth-supported restorations.

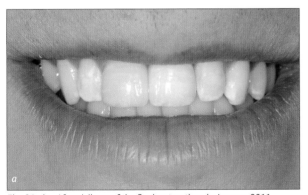

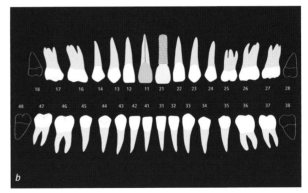

Figs 31a-b   After delivery of the final restorations in January 2011.

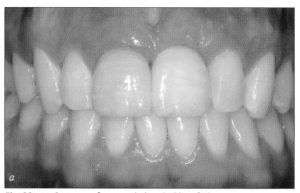

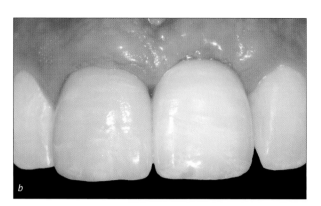

Figs 32a-c   One year after completion. Stable soft tissues.

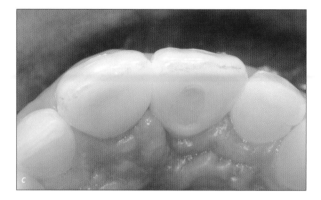

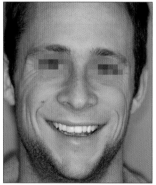

Fig 33   The patient was very satisfied with the esthetic treatment outcome.

The patient was seen for the annual follow-up in December 2011. The soft tissues showed continued improvement relative to the crown contours (Figs 32 and 33). The patient was very happy with the result. Follow-up radiographs were obtained from his general dentist showing the five-year radiographic result (Figs 34a-d).

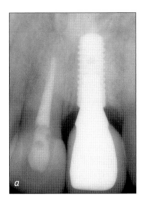
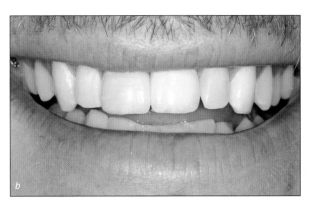
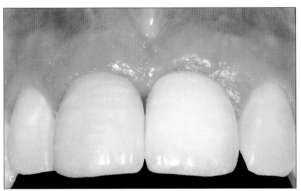
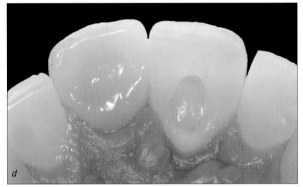

Figs 34a-d   Follow-up periapical radiograph and clinical situation five years after delivery of crowns 11 (tooth-supported) and 21 (implant-supported).

Acknowledgments

Clinical procedures
Dr. Robert Hustwitt, pediatric dentist – Kitchener, ON, Canada

Orthodontic procedures
Dr. Kumi Pather – Kitchener, ON, Canada

Laboratory procedures
Slawek Bilko, ITI Fellow – Toronto, ON, Canada

7.12 Replacement of a Missing Upper Left Central Incisor: Late Placement of an RC Bone Level Implant, CAD/CAM Zirconia Abutment

E. R. Lorenzana, J. Gillespie

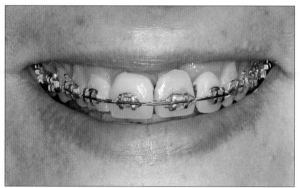

Fig 1 At full smile, the patient presented with a medium to high lip line, exposing the papillae throughout the anterior sextant, but with the upper lip obscuring the gingival margins of the central incisors.

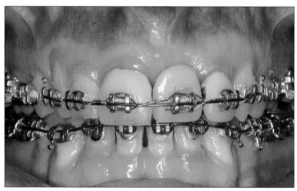

Fig 2 Retracted view of medium phenotype with inconsistent gingival margin positions and a buccal deficiency at the edentulous site.

A healthy 37-year-old female patient was referred for a consultation on the replacement of missing tooth 21 with an implant-supported restoration (Fig 1).

She stated that several years previously the tooth had been traumatically avulsed following a motor vehicle accident. The tooth was replaced with a three-unit fixed partial denture (FPD) immediately afterwards. Over time, she became disillusioned with the FPD and looked for a different option, including orthodontic therapy. She presented still in her orthodontic appliances, with the pontic sectioned free from the FPD but attached to the archwire. Her orthodontist felt that orthodontic treatment had been successfully completed, but nevertheless referred her before removing the appliances in case adjustments were necessary.

A detailed examination of the teeth and periodontium at and around the edentulous space was performed to assess the esthetic risk of implant therapy. The retracted anterior view revealed a mutually protected occlusion, approximately 25% overbite, and a slight midline deviation between the maxillary and mandibular arches (Fig 2).

The observed gingival phenotype was medium-thick, with moderately scalloped papillae, relatively thick tissue, a broad zone of keratinized gingiva, as well as teeth and crowns with a squared-off appearance. The periodontal examination revealed a healthy periodontium with probing depths between 1 to 3 mm throughout the sextant. A buccal bone and soft-tissue volume deficiency was visible at site 21, and there existed a lack of harmonious gingival margin positions in the anterior segment 13 to 23. Measurements of teeth 13, 12 and 22 revealed a 1 : 1 height-to-width ratio, while 13 and 23 displayed an ideal 1.2 : 1 height-to-width ratio.

A cone-beam computed tomography (CBCT) scan was ordered and evaluated. No pathology was noted. The evaluation of the scan included virtual implant placement that revealed adequate bone for implant placement (Fig 3).

However, a cross-sectional view at the root level revealed a buccal deficiency that could have compromised the esthetic outcome of the case, as it relates to recreating the ideal root eminence and emergence profile (Fig 4). This confirmed what was observed clinically at the initial examination.

Following the initial examination and CBCT scan, the collected clinical and radiographic data resulted in the Esthetic Risk Assessment (ERA) presented in Table 1.

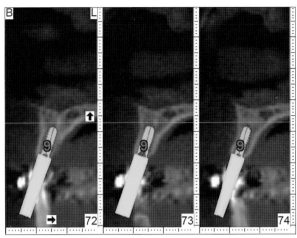

Fig 3   CBCT image with virtual implant placement showing adequate buccolingual bone volume for implant placement.

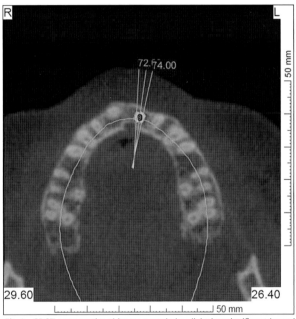

Fig 4   CBCT cross-sectional image revealed a slight but significant buccal deficiency at the edentulous site.

Table 1   *Esthetic Risk Assessment (ERA)*

Esthetic risk factors	Level of risk		
	Low	**Medium**	**High**
Medical status	Healthy, uneventful healing		Compromised healing
Smoking habit	Non-smoker	Light smoker (≤ 10 cigs/day)	Heavy smoker (> 10 cigs/day)
Gingival display at full smile	Low	Medium	High
Width of edentulous span	1 tooth (≥ 7 mm)[1] 1 tooth (≥ 6 mm)[2]	1 tooth (< 7 mm)[1] 1 tooth (< 6 mm)[2]	2 teeth or more
Shape of tooth crowns	Rectangular		Triangular
Restorative status of neighboring teeth	Virgin		Restored
Gingival phenotype	Low-scalloped, thick	Medium-scalloped, medium-thick	High-scalloped, thin
Infection at implant site	None	Chronic	Acute
Soft-tissue anatomy	Soft tissue intact		Soft-tissue defects
Bone level at adjacent teeth	≤ 5 mm to contact point	5.5 to 6.5 mm to contact point	≥ 7 mm to contact point
Facial bone-wall phenotype*	Thick-wall phenotype ≥ 1 mm thickness		Thin-wall phenotype < 1 mm thickness
Bone anatomy of alveolar crest	No bone deficiency	Horizontal bone deficiency	Vertical bone deficiency
Patient's esthetic expectations	Realistic expectations		Unrealistic expectations

* If three-dimensional imaging is available with the tooth in place
[1] Standard-diameter implant, regular connection
[2] Narrow-diameter implant, narrow connection

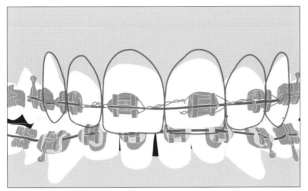

Fig 5   The crown dimension outlines illustrate the desired treatment outcome.

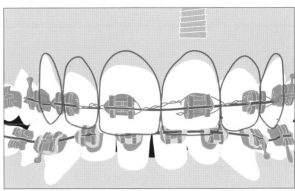

Fig 6   With the treatment illustration as a guide, the implant shoulder could be positioned 3 to 3.5 mm apical to the desired gingival margin.

The patient was presented with several restorative options to replace tooth 21, including replacement of her previous fixed partial denture with a new FPD. In this type of situation, where the abutment teeth require new full-coverage restorations, a fixed partial denture is a reasonable alternative. However, given the patient's previous disappointing experience with her FPD, an implant-supported restoration was her first and only choice. Taking into account all of the factors compiled in the clinical and radiographic examinations and the Esthetic Risk Assessment, as well as the successful completion of her orthodontic treatment, the overall esthetic risk for this patient was considered to be medium. In accordance with the ITI SAC Guidelines (Dawson and Chen 2009), the patient's treatment was classified as Advanced from both a surgical and restorative standpoint.

A comprehensive treatment plan was presented to the patient consisting of implant placement with hard- and soft-tissue augmentation for added buccal contour at site 21, and crown lengthening of teeth 12, 11 and 22. The illustration shows the expected final position of the gingival margins for the entire anterior segment at the completion of treatment (Fig 5).

It was discussed with the patient that crown lengthening would be critical to creating an acceptable esthetic outcome. Furthermore, it was considered essential that she understand that the desired final gingival margin position guides the apicocoronal positioning of the implant. The illustration shows the ideal apicocoronal implant position, allowing 3 to 3.5 mm of distance from the implant shoulder to the desired gingival margin (Fig 6).

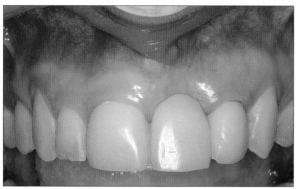

Fig 7 *An acrylic FPD was placed as a provisional following removal of the orthodontic appliance. The pontic was fabricated to the desired final clinical dimensions.*

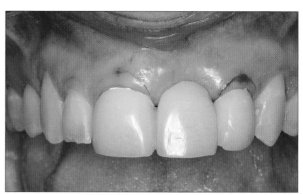

Fig 8 *The desired gingival-margin positions were outlined.*

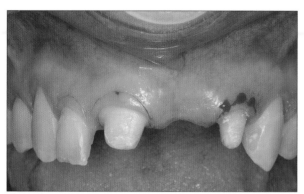

Fig 9 *The provisional FPD was removed to allow completion of the incisions and flap elevation.*

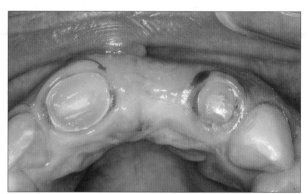

Fig 10 *Occlusal view of the surgical site showing the deficient buccal contour.*

With the treatment plan in place, the orthodontic appliances were removed and a fixed provisional was fabricated by the patient's prosthodontist. The pontic was made to reflect the desired dimensions of the final restoration in order to help guide the final implant position as well as the crown-lengthening procedures on teeth 12, 11, and 21 (Fig 7).

The first step in the surgical procedure was to outline the proposed clinical crown height (Fig 8). The contours were designed to create symmetry throughout the anterior segment. The provisional was removed to allow visualization of the surgical site and completion of the incision (Fig 9). The occlusal view demonstrates the deficiency in buccal contour that could compromise the final esthetic result (Fig 10).

Following flap reflection, the provisional was seated once more to properly evaluate the bone volume and position in relation to the desired implant shoulder position (Fig 11).

The overabundance of bone shown here would have complicated the ideal placement of the implant in relation to the desired emergence profile. 3 to 3.5 mm of space is needed to properly develop the necessary emergence profile. Crown lengthening was performed first on teeth 12, 11, and 22 using rotary and hand instrumentation (Fig 12).

This created the ideal biologic width around the teeth. Osseous recontouring was then accomplished at site 21 to create space for the correct implant depth and mimic the biologic width in the rest of the anterior sextant. The resulting osseous contour not only allows for the proper apicocoronal implant shoulder placement, but also more accurately reflects the natural contours of the alveolar bone around the teeth. Note that the bone at the mesial aspect of teeth 11 and 12 was left intact in order to properly support the interdental papillae.

To further facilitate ideal three-dimensional implant placement in accordance with the prosthodontic plan, a vacuform surgical template was utilized for site preparation (Figs 13 and 14).

In situations where significant modifications have to be made to the recipient site, a surgical guide provides a helpful reference point for correct fixture placement. The template provided guidance in both the orofacial and apicocoronal position, ensuring adequate space for development of the future emergence profile.

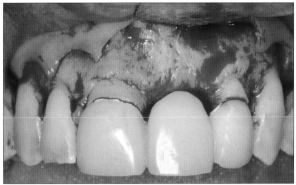

Fig 11   The provisional in place after flap reflection demonstrated an overabundance of bone, given the desired apicocoronal implant position.

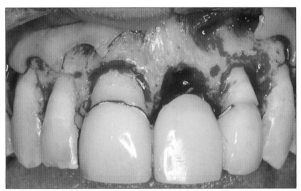

Fig 12   Crown lengthening was performed on teeth 12, 11 and 22. The osseous contour at site 21 mimics the contour of the natural dentition.

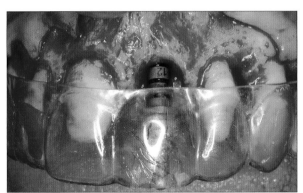

Fig 13   The vacuform template and 2.8-mm diameter depth gauge from the buccal aspect.

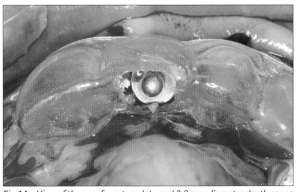

Fig 14   View of the vacuform template and 2.8-mm diameter depth gauge from the occlusal aspect.

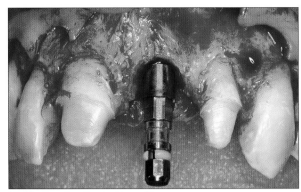

Fig 15 *Bone Level implant in position.*

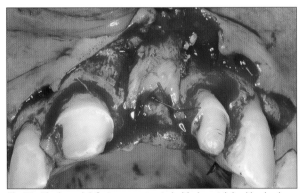

Fig 16 *Occlusal view of the Bone Level implant. It is encased in native bone, yet a buccal defect remains.*

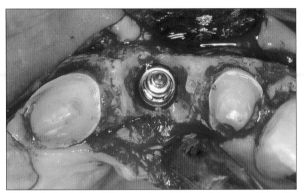

Fig 17 *The buccal defect was augmented with deproteinized bovine bone mineral and a connective-tissue graft.*

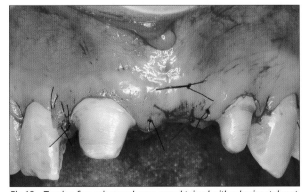

Fig 18 *Tension-free primary closure was obtained with a horizontal mattress suture and single interrupted sutures.*

Upon completion of site preparation, the implant (Bone Level implant, diameter 4.1 mm, length 12 mm, Regular CrossFit SLActive; Institut Straumann AG, Basel, Switzerland) was shown in its ideal three-dimensional position, in accordance with the restorative plan (Fig 15).

The occlusal view of the final implant position showed the implant fully enveloped within the native bone (Fig 16).

However, a buccal defect remained, as previously observed in the CBCT scan. This defect could compromise the final esthetic result if not augmented to more closely resemble the contours of the natural dentition.

Following placement of a healing cap (Bone Level Regular CrossFit, height 2 mm; Institut Straumann AG), a xenograft derived from bovine hydroxyapatite (Bio-Oss, Geistlich, Wolhusen, Switzerland) was placed on the buccal aspect of the socket and covered with an autologous connective-tissue graft harvested with palatal periosteum using a single-incision palatal harvest technique (Lorenzana and Allen 2000) (Fig 17).

The tissue graft was secured with 5-0 chromic gut suture (Ethicon, Pittsburg, PA, USA) coronally and apically over the xenograft.

Flap closure was accomplished using 6-0 nylon suture (Ethilon; Ethicon) (Fig 18). The flap was reapproximated and sutured first at the papillae, followed by a horizontal mattress suture to relieve the tension in the flap. Interrupted sutures were placed to then obtain primary closure of the flap over the implant.

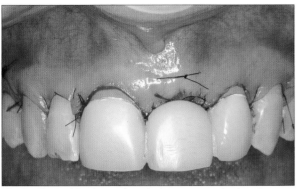

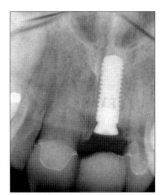

Fig 19 The provisional was adapted prior to cementation in order not to impinge upon the surgical site.

Fig 20 Postoperative radiograph confirming the implant's correct apicocoronal and mesiodistal position, away from vital structures.

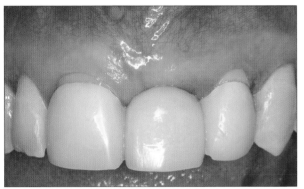

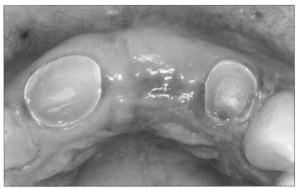

Fig 21 Healing at seven weeks. Re-entry procedures were initiated at this appointment.

Fig 22 Following removal of the provisional, the occlusal view showed abundant soft-tissue volume and keratinized mucosa.

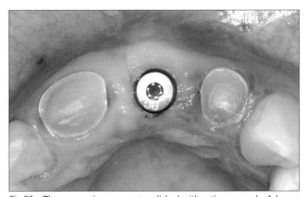

Fig 23 The uncovering was accomplished with a tissue punch. A longer healing cap was placed to allow access to the implant and initiate soft-tissue profile development.

Prior to re-cementing the provisional, the pontic was relieved over the implant site so as not to impinge on the tissues (Fig 19). A periapical radiograph was taken to document the final implant position (Fig 20).

The patient was seen two weeks after surgery for suture removal. Following an uneventful post-operative healing period of seven weeks, the patient was scheduled for re-entry (Fig 21).

Due to the volume of tissue available at the implant site following augmentation, as well as the more than adequate amount of keratinized gingiva present, the implant was uncovered utilizing a tissue punch (Figs 22 and 23). The smaller healing cap was replaced with a longer healing cap to begin the development of the peri-implant soft-tissue profile. Healing was uneventful; four weeks later, the patient was referred to her prosthodontist for the initiation of restorative procedures.

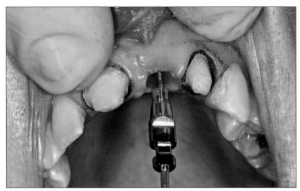

Fig 24   Delivery of the RC impression post.

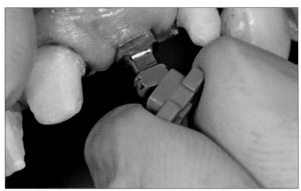

Fig 25   Placement of the polymer impression cap on the impression post.

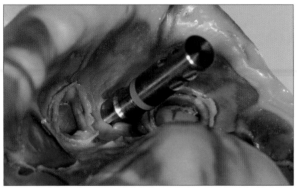

Fig 26   Following the removal of the impression post, it is placed onto the analog and placed back into the impression. The impression can now be poured to fabricate the master cast.

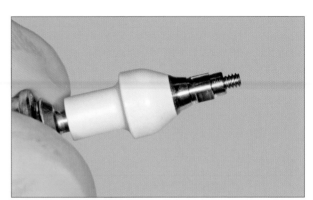

Fig 27   The Bone Level Regular CrossFit (RC) temporary abutment.

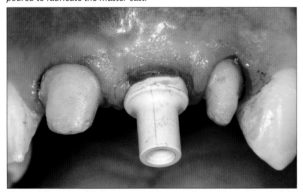

Fig 28   The unmodified temporary abutment is tried in and marked for reduction.

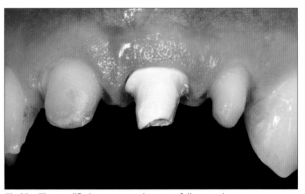

Fig 29   The modified temporary abutment fully seated.

First, a fixture-level impression was taken along with the adjoining preparations by placing a Regular CrossFit (RC) impression post into the implant and tightening the guide screw with an SCS screwdriver (Fig 24). The polymer impression cap was then placed on the impression post and the impression taken (Fig 25). After the impression had set and been removed, the polymer cap remained in the impression. The impression post was removed, attached to a Regular CrossFit analog, and repositioned in the impression tray prior to pouring it in stone (Fig 26).

At this point, the master cast was stored until the peri-implant tissues could be shaped and conditioned with the provisional restoration. Development of the emergence profile began with the modification of a Bone Level Regular CrossFit (RC) temporary abutment (Fig 27). After removal of the healing cap, the unmodified temporary abutment was seated and marked for reduction (Fig 28).

Following reduction, the temporary abutment was seated by turning the screw slowly, allowing time for the tissue to adjust to the pressure exerted by the abutment, until fully seated (Fig 29).

The patient wore the provisional for approximately four weeks until she was satisfied with the soft-tissue contours and overall esthetics (Fig 30). At this point, it was important to transfer the patient's soft-tissue contours to the master cast prior to sending the case to the laboratory. The provisional and temporary abutment were removed. The resulting emergence profile closely mimicked that of the contralateral tooth (Fig 31).

The original soft-tissue model was removed and the temporary abutment placed on the master cast (Fig 32).

Petroleum jelly was applied to the temporary abutment, and the new soft-tissue model was created by applying and forming impression material around the temporary abutment (Figs 33 and 34). The temporary abutment and provisional crown were then repositioned in the patient's mouth, and the case was sent to the laboratory.

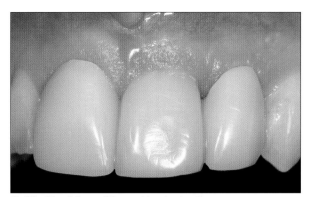

Fig 30   After delivery of the provisional restoration.

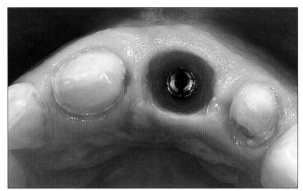

Fig 31   Occlusal view of the peri-implant tissue contours after development of the transition zone. Close similarity to the tissue contours around the contralateral central incisor.

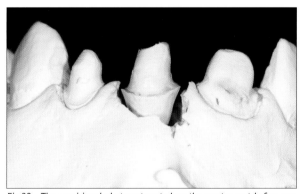

Fig 32   The provisional abutment seated on the master cast before custom soft-tissue modeling.

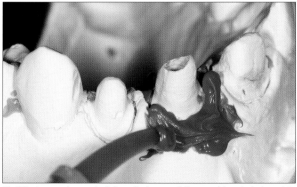

Fig 33   Impression material applied around the provisional abutment to record the transition zone onto the master cast.

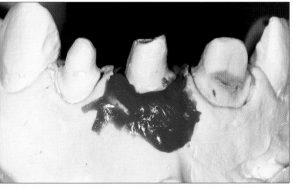

Fig 34   The custom soft-tissue model was now complete and the master cast ready to be delivered to the laboratory.

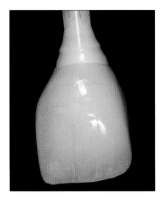

Fig 35   The definitive zirconia abutment and crown.

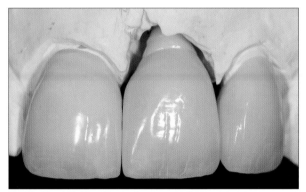

Fig 36   The definitive all-ceramic crowns on the master cast.

The laboratory fabricated a CAD/CAM zirconia abutment, made by first waxing up the abutment contours, then scanning the wax-up for milling of the final abutment. Once completed, an all-ceramic crown was made by building up ceramics over a zirconia core (Fig 35). Two additional crowns were fabricated for teeth 11 and 22 (Fig 36). The custom abutment and crown were returned for final delivery to the patient.

At the delivery visit, the provisional restoration and abutment were removed. The implant and soft tissues were carefully cleaned and irrigated before delivery of the tooth-borne crowns and the custom abutment (Fig 37).

In addition, composite was bonded to tooth 12 in order to restore the contours to match those of tooth 22. Once the fit had been confirmed, the abutment was torqued to 35 N·cm, and the access opening sealed with PTFE tape and composite.

The fit of the final restoration was carefully checked and the occlusion adjusted to a light contact as verified with shimstock prior to cementation. The restoration was cemented, and any excess was carefully removed following the final set (Fig 38). On the day of delivery, the shape, color, contour, and translucency of the restorations appeared to integrate harmoniously with the natural dentition. However, it was evident that following the restorative procedures, additional tissue healing and maturation was necessary prior to achieving the desired final esthetic result.

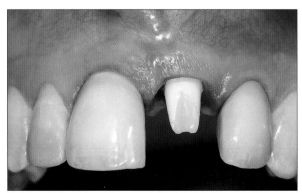

Fig 37   After insertion of the zirconia abutment, torqued to 35 N·cm and sealed with PTFE tape and composite.

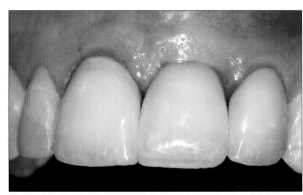

Fig 38   The final implant-supported restoration on the day of delivery.

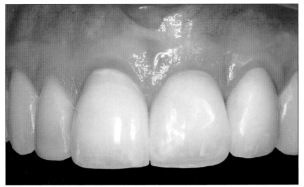

Fig 39 Retracted anterior view at one year after delivery. Symmetric gingival contours in harmony with the restorations across the anterior sextant.

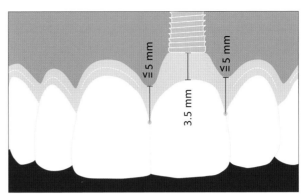

Fig 40 A stable soft-tissue level could be expected due to the ideal relationship between the bone crest, implant shoulder and contact points.

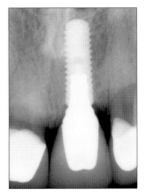

Fig 41 Periapical radiograph at one year.

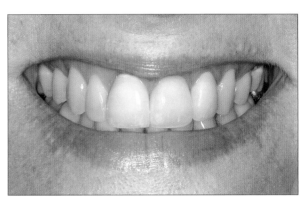

Fig 42 Full smile at one year after delivery, demonstrating a stable, pleasing esthetic result.

The one-year photograph documents the final harmonious perio-prosthetic integration of the restorations and the gingival tissues that comprises a stable esthetic treatment outcome (Fig 39).

The contours of the marginal gingiva were symmetrical throughout the anterior sextant and in concert with the restorative contours of the restorations and natural dentition. The papillae completely filled the interdental spaces, a testament to the pre-operative planning of the apicocoronal implant position and surgical execution of the necessary osseous recontouring (Fig 40).

The one-year postoperative radiograph demonstrated stable bone levels around the implant, with the appropriate interdental bone position in relation to the interdental contacts that supported the papillae at the mesial and distal aspects of the implant fixture (Fig 41).

Finally, the one-year smile reflected the realization of the patient's vision and her satisfaction with the final esthetic result (Fig 42).

Acknowledgments

Orthodontic procedures
Dr. Brad D. Bruchmiller, South Texas Orthodontics – San Antonio, TX, USA

Laboratory procedures
Nuance Dental Ceramics, Inc. – Mansfield, TX, USA

7.13 Replacement of a Missing Upper Left Central Incisor: Late Placement of an RC Bone Level Implant and Adjacent Tooth Restoration

A. Hamilton

A healthy 38-year-old male patient was referred for replacement of a failing tooth-supported cantilever fixed dental prosthesis on teeth 11 and 21 (Figs 1 to 5). The patient reported a history of trauma at 13 years of age that had resulted in the subsequent loss of tooth 11, as well as endodontic treatment of the adjacent abutment tooth 21. A metal-ceramic cantilever fixed dental prosthesis replacing tooth 11 had been provided by his general dentist several years after the loss of the tooth, with tooth 21 as the sole abutment. At the time of initial presentation, this restoration had been in service for over 20 years.

The patient's primary complaint was poor esthetics of his bridge, in particular the dark discolored margin around abutment tooth 21. Throughout the examination, the patient was observed to have a "guarded smile" and appeared to be very self-conscious about the esthetics of his teeth (Fig 1). However, on several brief occasions his full smile displayed 1 to 2 mm of gingiva. Further esthetic assessment revealed incongruent shapes, contours, and colors of the maxillary central incisors, which were not in harmony with his natural teeth. An Esthetic Risk Assessment (ERA) was completed as part of the examination and discussed in the informed-consent process (Table 1).

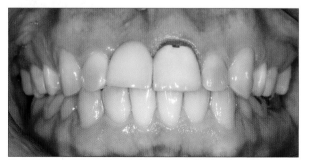

Fig 1   "Guarded" smile—the patient had become self-conscious of the appearance of his front teeth.

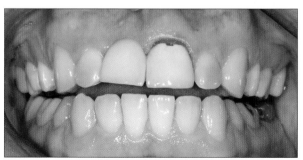

Fig 2   Lip line in repose.

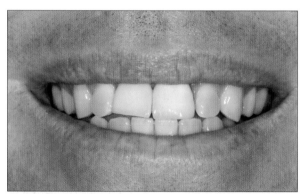

Fig 3   Retracted view with recession and dark discoloration of the gingival margin around tooth 21.

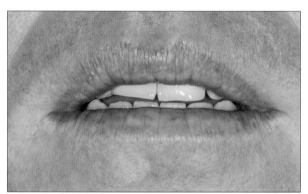

Fig 4   Retracted view with the teeth slightly apart, highlighting the uneven incisal edge angulations and lengths between teeth 11 and 21.

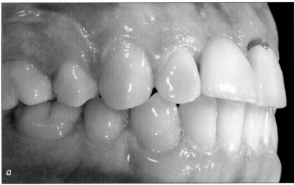

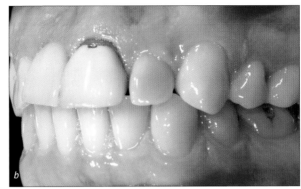

Figs 5a-b   Left and right lateral views. Angle class I occlusal relationship with moderate wear facets on the canines. Absence of a root eminence is also noted above pontic 11 compared to tooth 21.

An occlusal evaluation revealed an Angle class I canine and molar relationship with a slight discrepancy between the maxillary and mandibular midlines, mutually protected occlusion, and approximately 15% of vertical overlap (Figs 3 to 5). Wear facets on the maxillary and mandibular canines indicated some degree of parafunctional activity. Protrusive contacts were only present on tooth 21.

The examination of the initial periapical radiograph displayed favorable proximal bone levels of the adjacent teeth and adequate vertical bone height in the edentulous space. A very wide root-canal restoration was present in tooth 21, with compromised radicular dentine thickness (Fig 6). The incisive canal was also prominent, prompting further assessment with three-dimensional imaging (Fig 7).

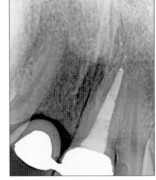

Fig 6   Periapical radiograph provided by an endodontist following endodontic retreatment of tooth 21. Prominent nasopalatine canal.

A multi-slice CT scan was requested as part of the preoperative planning process (Fig 7). As tooth 11 had been missing for many years, extensive bone loss was expected. Fortunately, as visible in slices 34 and 35, the bone supply was sufficient for implant placement, although a slight labial horizontal deficiency would require some form of contour augmentation. The proximity of the incisive canal was noted during the radiographic evaluation and was taken into consideration during implant planning and surgery.

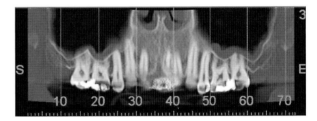

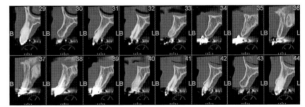

Fig 7   Preoperative CT scan for three-dimensional visualization of the bone in the edentulous site and adjacent anatomical structures.

Table 1   Esthetic Risk Assessment (ERA)

Esthetic risk factors	Level of risk		
	Low	**Medium**	**High**
Medical status	Healthy, uneventful healing		Compromised healing
Smoking habit	Non-smoker	Light smoker (≤ 10 cigs/day)	Heavy smoker (> 10 cigs/day)
Gingival display at full smile	Low	Medium	High
Width of edentulous span	1 tooth (≥ 7 mm)[1] 1 tooth (≥ 6 mm)[2]	1 tooth (< 7 mm)[1] 1 tooth (< 6 mm)[2]	2 teeth or more
Shape of tooth crowns	Rectangular		Triangular
Restorative status of neighboring teeth	Virgin		Restored
Gingival phenotype	Low-scalloped, thick	Medium-scalloped, medium-thick	High-scalloped, thin
Infection at implant site	None	Chronic	Acute
Soft-tissue anatomy	Soft tissue intact		Soft-tissue defects
Bone level at adjacent teeth	≤ 5 mm to contact point	5.5 to 6.5 mm to contact point	≥ 7 mm to contact point
Facial bone-wall phenotype*	Thick-wall phenotype ≥ 1 mm thickness		Thin-wall phenotype < 1 mm thickness
Bone anatomy of alveolar crest	No bone deficiency	Horizontal bone deficiency	Vertical bone deficiency
Patient's esthetic expectations	Realistic expectations	Moderate expectations	Unrealistic expectations

* If three-dimensional imaging is available with the tooth in place
[1] Standard-diameter implant, regular connection
[2] Narrow-diameter implant, narrow connection

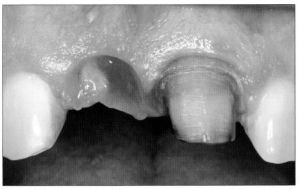

Fig 8   Following removal of the defective metal-ceramic bridge, the darkness of the core of abutment tooth 21 became apparent.

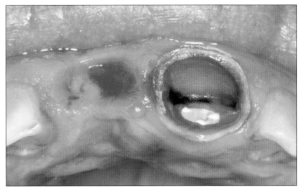

Fig 9   Occlusal view. Horizontal deficiency and associated concavity at the proposed implant site 11, as opposed to the root eminence present at site 21.

Removal of the existing cantilever bridge revealed a very dark core of the abutment tooth 21 (Fig 8). To minimize further tooth preparation, which would be required to block out the discoloration, non-vital internal bleaching was to be performed prior to the final restoration with an all-ceramic crown. A slight labial horizontal concavity over the area of the proposed implant site 11 required some form of grafting to create a natural convex soft-tissue contour and profile (Fig 9).

Following comprehensive evaluation, several key factors were taken into consideration when deciding on a new fixed tooth-supported dental prosthesis versus a stand-alone implant replacement and tooth-supported crown:

- Long-term survival of the previous cantilever metal-ceramic fixed dental prosthesis
- Compromised structural integrity of abutment tooth 21
- Favorable anatomical environment for implant replacement
- Patient's functional and esthetic expectations

After discussing the risks and benefits of both treatment options, the patient decided on an implant. The following treatment plan was agreed upon:

- Implant placement with simultaneous contour augmentation using guided bone regeneration (GBR) in a two-stage surgical approach
- Fixed tooth-supported cantilevered provisional fixed dental prosthesis
- Internal non-vital bleaching of tooth 21
- Second stage uncovering surgery following four months of healing
- Soft-tissue conditioning with a provisional implant crown
- Final restoration with a metal-ceramic abutment and all-ceramic crowns four to six months later

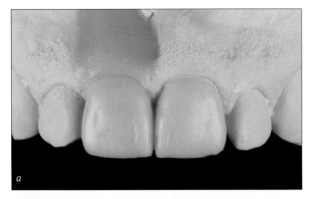

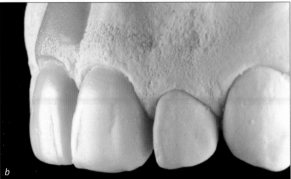

Figs 10a-b Diagnostic wax-up performed as part of the esthetic assessment, surgical implant planning and subsequent fabrication of a provisional restoration. Soft-tissue wax-up of the defect to restore the natural gingival form.

A diagnostic wax-up was performed as part of the implant planning process, to serve as a blueprint for the implant position and tooth reduction (Figs 10a-b). A silicone index made on the diagnostic wax-up was used to fabricate a duplicate provisional bridge in bisacryl composite (Protemp; 3M ESPE, St. Paul, MI, USA), to be used as a basic surgical guide (Fig 11). A hole was cut into the palatal aspect of the pontic of the provisional, a marking was made on the labial aspect, and the cervical aspect was trimmed precisely to the planned mucosal margin. This technique provided the necessary information to assist with ideal three-dimensional positioning of the implant.

Implant surgery was performed under local anesthesia with preoperative antibiotic prophylaxis (Amoxicillin 2 g p. o. one hour before surgery) and a 0.12% chlorhexidine mouthwash (Curasept ADS; Curaden Healthcare, Saronno, Italy). A midcrestal incision was made in the edentulous area, with vertical relieving incisions on the distal line angles of both adjacent teeth to create a trapezoidal flap. This flap design provided ideal access for visualization of the bone during osteotomy preparation, implant placement, and simultaneous bone grafting. However, alternative flap designs could have been considered to minimize scarring from the releasing incisions, which are visible in the result. The elevation of a full thickness mucoperiosteal flap was followed by placement of a silk retraction suture, used to delicately tether the free end of the flap to the lip for the duration of the surgery.

The osteotomy was prepared following the manufacturer's drilling protocol and a bone level implant was placed with good primary stability (Straumann Bone Level RC SLA, diameter 4.1 mm, length 10 mm; Institut Straumann AG, Basel, Switzerland) (Fig 12). The final implant position was verified again with the surgical guide, ensuring the vertical position of the implant/abutment connection was 3 mm below the proposed mucosal margin. To avoid the incisive canal, the implant was placed with a slight mesiolabial inclination, which necessitated a cement-retained restoration.

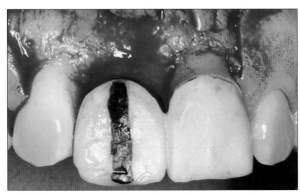

Fig 11 Reflection of a full-thickness mucoperiosteal flap and positioning of a surgical implant guide.

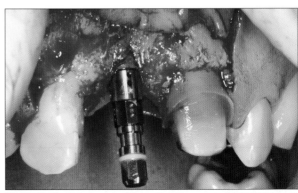

Fig 12 Implant placement with small dehiscence and thin labial bone, as expected.

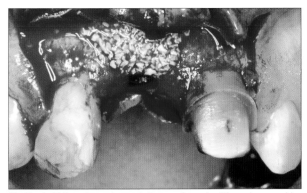

Fig 13   Labial contour augmentation performed with a slow-resorbing deproteinized bovine bone mineral xenograft.

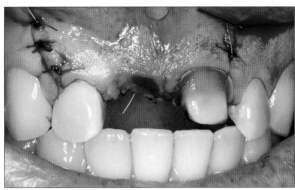

Fig 14   Wound closure with 4-0 monofilament nylon simple interrupted sutures.

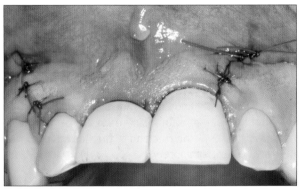

Fig 15   A fixed cantilever tooth-supported provisional restoration was used throughout the healing phase.

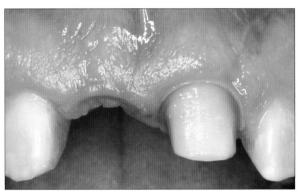

Fig 16   After three months healing. Commencement of non-vital internal bleaching.

Simultaneous labial contour augmentation was performed with a slow resorbing deproteinized bovine bone mineral xenograft (Bio-Oss; Geistlich Pharma, Wolhusen, Switzerland) (Fig 13). A 1-mm cover screw was placed to allow for a two-stage surgical approach, and the graft was covered with a non-crosslinked porcine-derived resorbable collagen membrane (Bio-Guide; Geistlich Pharma) following the principles of guided bone regeneration (Buser 1993).

Surgery was completed by primary wound closure, achieved with interrupted monofilament sutures and a

reverse-cutting needle (Dyloc; Dynek, Adelaide, Australia) (Fig 14). A cantilever fixed provisional bridge was provided during healing, which allowed for optimal pressure-free healing and met the patient's functional and esthetic requirements during this treatment phase (Fig 15).

At the three-month follow-up, the mucosa exhibited excellent healing, with minor scarring visible where the vertical releasing incisions had been made. Internal non-vital bleaching of tooth 21 was commenced with sodium perborate and saline (Rotstein and coworkers

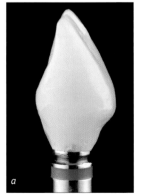
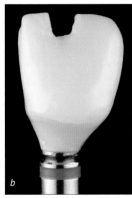
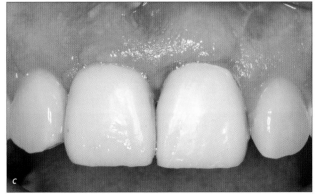

Figs 17a-c   Implant-supported screw-retained provisional crown placed following second-stage reentry to shape the transition zone.

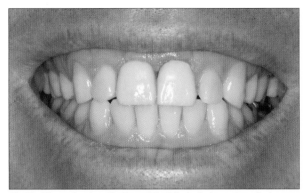

Fig 18 The patient's smile showed the full gingival margin as he became more confident about the appearance of his teeth.

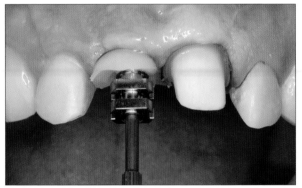

Fig 19 Open-tray pick-up impression taken with the custom impression coping.

1991) placed into the residual pulp chamber under rubber-dam protection. A significant improvement in shade was evident after the first application (Fig 16), and the process was repeated three times, each for one week.

A minimal second-stage procedure was performed with a small midcrestal incision above the implant. An implant-supported screw-retained provisional crown was fabricated intraorally with a titanium provisional abutment (RC titanium provisional abutment; Institut Straumann AG) and bisacryl composite (Protemp; 3M ESPE), with a separate provisional crown on the adjacent tooth (Figs 17a-c and 18). This allowed for the development of the emergence profile and the shaping of the transition zone prior to the final impressions.

Following a three-month period of soft-tissue maturation with the provisional restoration, an open-tray impression using a customized impression coping technique conveyed the emergence profiles to the laboratory technician (Figs 19 and 20). This allowed the technician to recreate the established transition zone in the final restoration and also documented the location of the mucosal margin to ensure the cement margin was not placed too far submucosally.

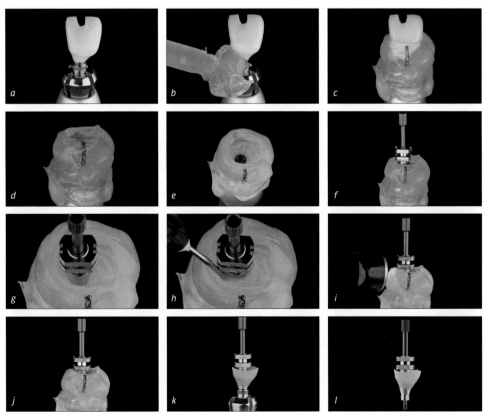

Figs 20a-l Fabrication of a custom implant impression coping. The provisional was placed into a laboratory analog holder, and an index was made of the emergence profile from the provisional implant restoration with clear silicone impression or bite registration material, and a line drawn to correspond to the labial surface (a-c). This was then removed and an impression coping inserted, where a gap was clearly visible between the index and the coping (c-g). This gap was filled with flowable composite resin and light-cured (h-i). The impression coping was removed from the silicone with the replicated emergence profile attached (j-l).

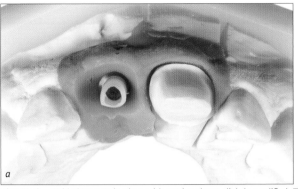
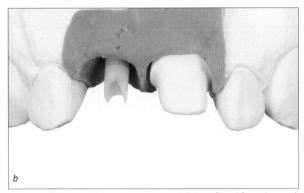

Figs 21a-b Gold abutment in place with waxing sleeve slightly modified. The contours of the transition zone were accurately transferred from the provisional restoration to the soft-tissue replica on the cast.

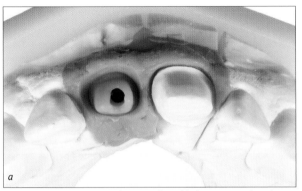
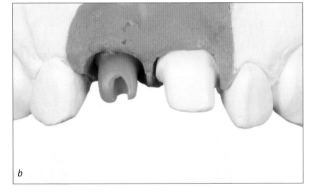

Figs 22a-b Abutment waxed up onto the gold abutment, ready to be cast.

A machined "cast-to" gold abutment (RC Gold abutment; Institut Straumann AG) was customized with the lost-wax technique and veneered with feldspathic ceramics (IPS d.SIGN; Ivoclar Vivadent, Schaan, Liechtenstein) to create a strong, durable and esthetic abutment that matched the core of the adjacent natural tooth (Figs 21 to 23). Lithium disilicate (e.max; Ivoclar Vivadent) crowns were then fabricated for both central incisors (Figs 23 and 24).

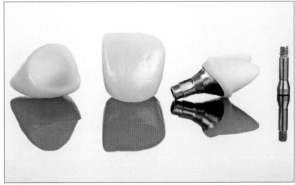

Fig 23 The abutment was cast in gold with a ceramic add-on to create a tooth-colored core for the fabrication of all-ceramic crowns.

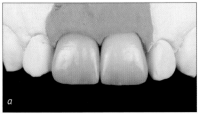
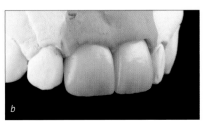
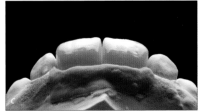

Figs 24a-c The final contours of the crowns were assessed on the cast, which displayed ideal contours and natural surface texture.

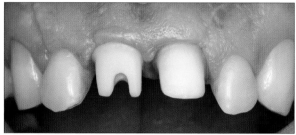

Fig 25 Abutment inserted with the screw tightened to 35 N·cm. No blanching of the tissue is present as the final restoration replicates the emergence profile of the provisional restoration.

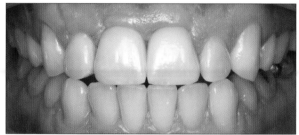

Fig 26 Retracted view on the day of cementation.

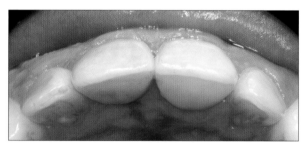

Fig 27 Occlusal view of the final crowns. Good soft-tissue volume and a slight convexity created by the contour augmentation.

During insertion of the definitive abutment, no blanching of the soft tissues was visible, as the emergence profile conformed closely to the shape of the provisional restoration (Fig 25). The crown margins ran less than 0.5 mm submucosally on the labial and conformed to the scallop of the tissue. Once the fit, contacts, contours, and esthetics of the final restorations had been confirmed, the abutment screw was tightened to 35 N·cm. PTFE tape was placed to protect the abutment screw, and the screw access hole was slightly underfilled with composite resin to match the optical characteristics of the abutment. A significant improvement in the core color of tooth 21 following internal bleaching was visible, which facilitated an ideal color match for the central incisor restorations. Both lithium disilicate crowns were bonded in place with resin cement (Variolink; Ivoclar Vivadent) according to manufacturer instructions. A practice cementation technique, as described by Wadhwani and coworkers 2009, was utilized for the implant crown to minimize the cement excess.

The restorations appeared to be in harmony with the patient's dentofacial esthetics. He was very happy with the final esthetic and functional outcomes of treatment (Figs 26 to 28). The labial tissue profile was symmetrical with the adjacent natural tooth, with the bone graft recreating the desired convex tissue contours (Fig 27). The patient was ready to smile much more following the treatment, with full display of the mucosal margin (Fig 28).

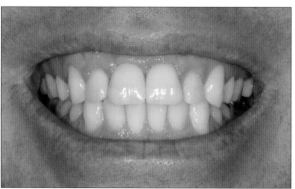

Fig 28 Full smile on the day of delivery.

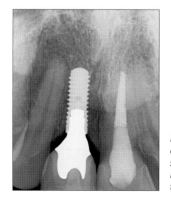

Fig 29 Periapical radiograph taken on the day of delivery demonstrating favorable proximal bone levels on the implant and adjacent teeth.

The patient was seen after two weeks to evaluate the peri-implant tissues for signs of inflammation or residual cement. The occlusion was re-evaluated to ensure light shimstock pull through, with even contact on both maxillary central incisors in mandibular protrusion. Oral hygiene procedures were reviewed with the patient, including a demonstration on flossing techniques. The patient was then scheduled for yearly maintenance visits.

The patient returned for a review twelve months after delivery of the final restorations (Figs 30 to 34). The clinical evaluation showed excellent periodontal and peri-implant health around the restorations. Excellent esthetics had been maintained, with no visible recession or exposure of the crown margins with symmetrical gingival/mucosa margins of the adjacent restorations on the central incisor teeth. Further papillary maturation and fill was evident around the implant-supported restoration 11. Periodontal probing depths were less than 3 mm, and there was no bleeding on probing.

This case report demonstrates the successful application of scientific principles and clinical techniques to provide an optimal esthetic and functional outcome for the replacement of a single missing maxillary central incisor.

Acknowledgments

Laboratory Procedures and Photography
MDT Szabolcs Hant – Core Dental Ceramics, Perth, WA, Australia

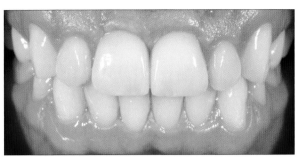

Fig 30   Retracted view at twelve months. Signs of tissue maturation.

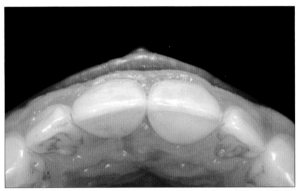

Fig 31   Occlusal view at twelve months. Minimal loss of tissue volume around the implant.

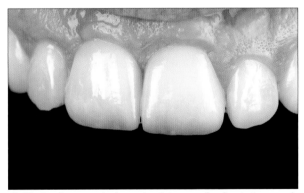

Fig 32   Excellent reproduction and maintenance of surface texture was visible in the all-ceramic restorations when compared with the natural teeth.

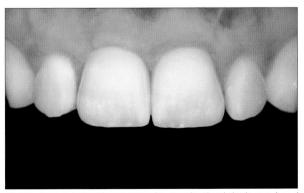

Fig 33   Cross-polarized image at twelve months. Good shade match and stability following internal bleaching.

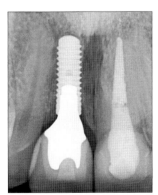

Fig 34   Periapical radiograph at twelve months.

7.14 Replacement of a Fractured Upper Left Central Incisor: Early Placement of a Monotype Zirconia Implant, Semi-submerged Transmucosal Healing

M. Gahlert

The present case involved the placement of a mono-type ceramic implant with concurrent guided bone re-generation using transgingival semi-submerged healing. Various studies have described the successful outcome of this procedure around transmucosal titanium im-plants (Brägger and coworkers 1996; Hermann and co-workers 2000; Jung 2004b; Cordaro and coworkers 2012). In addition, even typical intraosseous bone defects aris-ing around titanium implants as a result of peri-implant infections have successfully been treated using guided bone regeneration in combination with transmucosal healing (Mombelli and coworkers 2015). Advantages of monotype ceramic implants include the absence of sub-mucosal microgaps, reduced plaque affinity compared to titanium (Scarano and coworkers 2004), and an im-mensely rigid overall implant body.

A 31-year old woman was referred to our clinic with an inflammation of the gingiva at tooth 21. On the day of the examination, a panoramic radiograph was taken.

The anamnesis of the patient revealed that 18 years pre-viously, tooth 21 had received endodontic treatment as a result of trauma. Eight weeks previously, the patient had noticed initial signs of an inflammatory soft-tissue reaction (pain, bleeding) around tooth 21. The patient consulted her attending dentist and was subsequently referred to our clinic. The gingival display of the patient during speaking and laughing was remarkable (Figs 1 and 2).

After the clinical and radiographic examination, the di-agnosis of a longitudinal fracture of tooth 21 was made. The patient was informed about her surgical treatment options, which including an esthetic risk assessment (Martin and coworkers 2006).

Treatment plan
As a first step, prior to tooth extraction, a temporary replacement for tooth 21 was made in the dental lab (Fig 3).

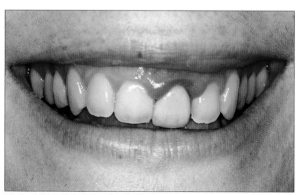

Fig 1 *Initial clinical situation in October 2011.*

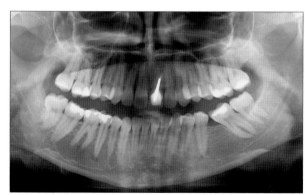

Fig 2 *Panoramic radiograph.*

Impressions of the upper and lower jaw were necessary for preparing diagnostic casts and for manufacturing the template and a translucent surgical stent.

The second step was the extraction of tooth 21, including curettage of the inflamed tissue in the alveolar socket. Here it was important to check the anatomical condition of the alveolar bone to determine how much bone had been destroyed by the local inflammation. During the extraction, an esthetic risk management can be performed.

Based on the treatment guidelines in connection with esthetic outcomes following immediate placement in the anterior maxilla as presented at the 5th ITI Consensus Conference (Morton and coworkers 2014), the following conditions should be met to achieve predictable esthetic outcomes in connection with immediate implant placement:

- Intact socket walls
- Thickness of the facial bone wall of at least 1 mm
- Thick soft tissue
- No acute infection at the planned implantation site
- Availability of bone apical and palatal to the socket to provide primary stability

The patient was informed about two bone augmentation options: augmentation of the buccal bone defect prior to implant placement or implant placement with simultaneous bone augmentation as a "one-step" procedure.

In this patient, who had high esthetic expectations, the likelihood of the facial bone wall being very thin or even damaged was great due to the acute infection at site 21. It was decided to perform early implant placement six weeks after the extraction with simultaneous bone augmentation. The patient's thin gingival phenotype and the acute infection at the future implant site contributed to this decision.

An esthetic risk assessment (Table 1) was performed.

The patient had previously been informed of the possibility of a completely metal-free rehabilitation by her attending dentist. She was therefore interested in ceramic implants. She was informed about the new-generation zirconium dioxide (ZrO_2, zirconia) monotype ceramic implants with a microrough surface (Bormann and coworkers 2011; Gahlert and coworkers 2012) and all-ceramic restorations. Various clinical outcomes were demonstrated to the patient by showing her different documented cases and long-term data on success and survival rates of zirconia implants (Oliva and coworkers 2010; Gahlert and coworkers 2013) The patient was

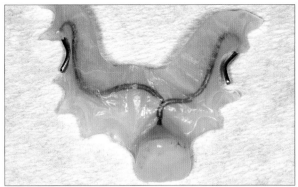

Fig 3 *Esthetic template with clamps stabilized on the palatal side of the teeth.*

offered participation in a prospective multicenter study about replacing single-tooth gaps using monotype all-ceramic implants (Gahlert and coworkers 2016) and consented to participate in this clinical trial to evaluate the new implant material (zirconium-dioxide ceramic) and design (one-piece monotype implant without an internal connection). The patient agreed to sign the treatment contract to join the clinical study in order to get the metal-free reconstruction. Additionally, she received a financial estimate for the surgical and prosthetic treatment. A timetable of the entire esthetic rehabilitation was set up as follows:

- Tooth extraction, followed by a healing period of 6 weeks
- Implant placement and simultaneous augmentation of bone defect, followed by a healing period of 3 months (one step procedure) *OR*
- Bone augmentation, followed by a healing period of 3 months, followed by implant placement and an unloaded healing period of 8 weeks ("two-step procedure"), x-ray control
- Surgical uncovering of the implant shoulder and fabrication of a chairside provisional tooth using prefabricated parts combined with the composite tooth of the template; impression-taking for the laboratory-made provisional restoration, followed by a healing period of one to two weeks
- Reevaluation of the peri-implant mucosa and provisional cementation of the finished lab-produced provisional restoration; waiting time for the development of red esthetics (optional; between two and eight weeks)
- Final impression-taking and a patient visit to the dental technician, followed by the fabrication of the definitive all-ceramic crown (normally two to four weeks, including the try-in)
- Cementation of the restoration, standardized peri-apical radiograph, beginning of maintenance period

Table 1   Esthetic Risk Assessment (ERA)

Esthetic risk factors	Level of risk		
	Low	**Medium**	**High**
Medical status	Healthy, uneventful healing		Compromised healing
Smoking habit	Non-smoker	Light smoker (≤ 10 cigs/day)	Heavy smoker (> 10 cigs/day)
Gingival display at full smile	Low	Medium	High
Width of edentulous span	1 tooth (≥ 7 mm)[1] 1 tooth (≥ 6 mm)[2]	1 tooth (< 7 mm)[1] 1 tooth (< 6 mm)[2]	2 teeth or more
Shape of tooth crowns	Rectangular		Triangular
Restorative status of neighboring teeth	Virgin		Restored
Gingival phenotype	Low-scalloped, thick	Medium-scalloped, medium-thick	High-scalloped, thin
Infection at implant site	None	Chronic	Acute
Soft-tissue anatomy	Soft tissue intact		Soft-tissue defects
Bone level at adjacent teeth	≤ 5 mm to contact point	5.5 to 6.5 mm to contact point	≥ 7 mm to contact point
Facial bone-wall phenotype*	Thick-wall phenotype ≥ 1 mm thickness		Thin-wall phenotype < 1 mm thickness
Bone anatomy of alveolar crest	No bone deficiency	Horizontal bone deficiency	Vertical bone deficiency
Patient's esthetic expectations	Realistic expectations		Unrealistic expectations

* If three-dimensional imaging is available with the tooth in place
[1] Standard-diameter implant, regular connection
[2] Narrow-diameter implant, narrow connection

The surgical protocol was in accordance with the concept of "early implant placement with soft-tissue healing" (Buser and coworkers 2008a; Buser and coworkers 2008b) and was explained to the patient. The treatment began with the extraction of tooth 21. After the extraction, the diagnosis of a longitudinal fracture was confirmed. During the curettage of the granulation tissue, the resorption of the buccal bone wall was evident. Finally, the gingiva around the extraction socket was adapted with two sutures. No bone substitute material or socket-preservation techniques were used. The previously manufactured template was adapted to the gap. Again, the patient was repeatedly informed about the necessary bone augmentation during implant placement.

The clinical situation six weeks later showed the healed keratinized gingival epithelium and no signs of inflammation (Figs 4 and 5a-b).

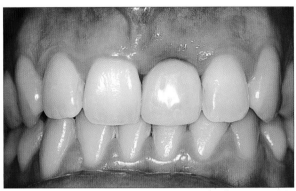

Fig 4   Clinical situation with template six weeks after extraction of the tooth.

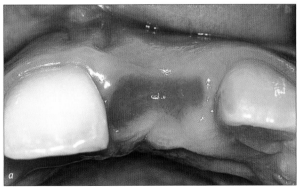
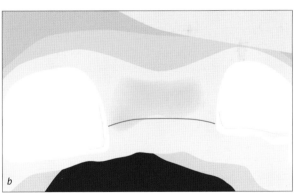

Figs 5a-b   Healed gingiva at the gap site 21 (Fig 5a) and incision design (Fig 5b). The crestal incision was placed in the center of the tooth gap at a distance of 1 mm from the palatal side of the gap to facilitate thickening of the buccal soft tissues.

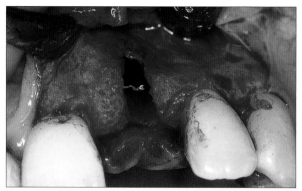

Fig 6 Bone defect after preparing the mucoperiostal flap and degranulation of soft tissue.

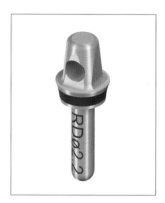

Fig 7 Position indicator with 4-mm abutment.

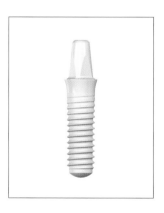

Fig 8a All-ceramic monotype implant 4.1 mm in diameter and with a 4-mm abutment height (Institut Straumann AG).

The patient had no pain in the bone area around the extraction socket. Following the administration of local anesthesia at sites 11, 21, 22, and 23, both on the buccal and palatal sides (Ultracain D-S forte 1 : 100,000; Sanofi), a marginal incision was made in at sites 11, 22, and 23. The crestal incision at site 21 was placed in the center of the gap at a distance of 1 mm from the palatal side of the gap to facilitate thickening of the soft tissue on the buccal side. A mucoperiostal flap was prepared and the residual granulation tissue was eliminated. The bone defect of the buccal side was evident, but the alveolar crest was otherwise sufficient for implant placement (Fig 6).

The surgical stent for correct three-dimensional implant placement was positioned and the preparation of the osteotomy was begun. After using the pilot drill, a position indicator (Institut Straumann AG, Basel, Switzerland) was inserted to control the correct angle of the implant axis and to choose the adequate abutment height (4.0 or 5.5 mm) of the monotype ceramic implant (Fig 7).

The 4-mm abutment had the right height in terms of intermaxillary distance and relative to the final all-ceramic restoration. The countersink marked the final step of the osteotomy preparation. To check the correct final position of the implant shoulder (1 mm further apically than the cementoenamel junction of the neighboring teeth), a position indicator was used, again. Following to that, a taper was used to prepare the implant bed for the bone-level threads of the ceramic implant. A monotype ceramic implant (Institut Straumann AG, Basel, Switzerland) with a length of 10 mm, an abutment height of 4 mm, a diameter of 4.1 mm, and a microrough surface (Röhling and coworkers 2014) was placed (Figs 8, 9, and 10a-b).

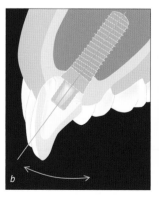

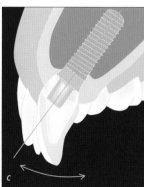

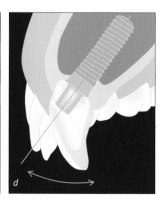

Figs 8b-d Prosthetic flexibility of the crown using the 4-mm abutment in relation to the inclination of the implant position.

However, the surgical handling of a monotype implant in a prosthetically driven position is not easy at all and requires detailed planning and surgical experience. Thus, a surgical stent is recommended in every case.

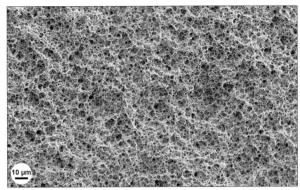

Fig 9   Microrough ZLA-surface (Institut Straumann AG).

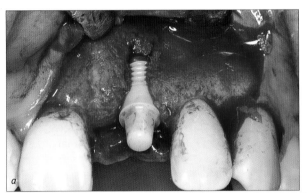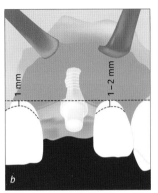

Figs 10a-b   (a) Insertion of the all-ceramic implant in correct three dimensional position and correct position of the implant shoulder 1 mm under the enamel-cement junction of the neighboring teeth. (b) Correct position of the implant shoulder 1 to 2 mm apical to the cementoenamel junction of the neighboring teeth but in a supracrestal position.

During osteotomy preparation, autologous bone was collected from the implant bed. The exposed implant surface was covered with these bone chips, and a collagen membrane (Bio-Gide; Geistlich, Wolhusen, Switzerland) was used to cover this particulate bone material (Figs 11 and 12). When it comes to contour augmentation in esthetic sites, the ITI recommends covering the layer of autologous bone chips that is used to cover the defect with a second layer of a bone substitute with a low-substitution rate to optimize the contour of the alveolar crest and to stabilize it over the long term. In this case it was decided to use only autologous bone because the patient refused the use of any allogeneic, xenogeneic, or synthetic bone substitute materials. In the long term, this may affect the volume stability and thus the contour of the alveolar crest.

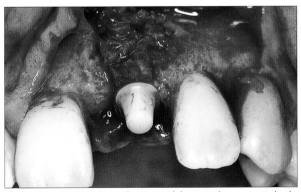

Fig 11   Harvested autologous bone material was used to augment the dehiscence area of the implant.

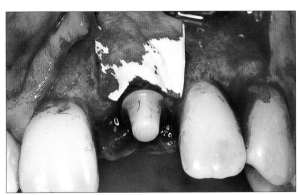

Fig 12   Collagen membrane covering the augmented dehiscence defect.

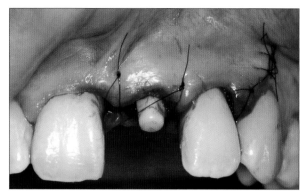

Fig 13   6-0 sutures adapted to the wound. Augmentation took place in semi-submerged transmucosal healing mode.

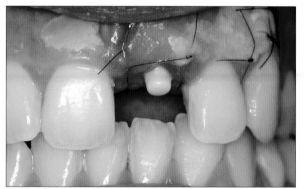

Fig 14   Normal postoperative situation 7 days later with some scabs on the gingiva.

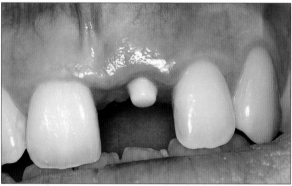

Fig 15   Normal soft-tissue conditions three months later with favorable mucosal leve.l

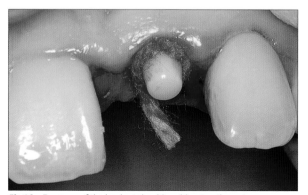

Fig 16   Exposure of the implant shoulder with retraction sutures.

The wound was closed with 6-0 sutures and the tooth of the template was ground hollow to avoid premature contact with the all-ceramic implant abutment (Fig 13).

Fit checker (GC Europe, Leuven, Belgium) was used to ensure that the reduced composite tooth of the template had no contact with the transmucosal abutment of the monotype implant. The patient received instructions for the postoperative period. After seven days, when the sutures were removed, no clinical signs of inflammation were noticed (Fig 14).

The clinical situation three months later showed non-irritant peri-implant mucosal conditions. The delayed immediate placement of a monotype ceramic implant in combination with a simultaneously augmentation with autologous bone using semi-submerged transmucosal healing did not result in any problems in the postoperative healing phase (Fig 15).

At the chairside-provisional visit, the patient received local infiltration anesthesia on the buccal and palatal sides. The peri-implant mucosa was displaced from the implant shoulder by a retraction cord between the peri-implant mucosa and the implant shoulder (Fig 16).

A prefabricated composite or PEEK cap (Institut Straumann AG) was snapped onto the implant shoulder and was shortened and prepared by a red diamond (Figs 17 and 18).

After separating the hollowed tooth from the template, the provisional was adapted to the prepared composite/PEEK cap. The gap between the cap and the hollowed provisional was filled with a two-component composite material (Structur 3; Voco, Cuxhaven, Germany) and subsequently polymerized. After the induration period, the half-finished chairside provisional was removed from the abutment. During the final adaptation of the provisional to the peri-implant soft tissue, a prefabricated healing cap was snapped onto the implant abutment to keep the mucosa displaced from the shoulder.

To take an impression for a laboratory-made provisional is optional at this point. However, taking an impression with a custom impression tray at a later time point is advisable because the shape of the peri-implant mucosa will have changed. The finished chairside provisional was snapped onto the implant shoulder and secured with temporary cement (Figs 19 and 20).

The peri-implant mucosa was clinically reevaluated two weeks later.

The chairside provisional began to shape the papillae on the mesial and distal sides of the ceramic implant (Fig 21).

In this special case, a custom provisional restoration made by the dental technician, was used to create perfect peri-implant red esthetics. The provisional replaced the chairside provisional until the mucosa around the ceramic implant was in perfect shape for the final impression.

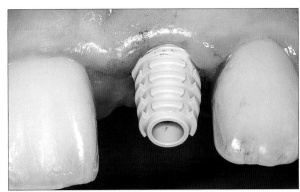

Fig 17   Composite/PEEK cap for a chairside provisional snapped onto the shoulder of the implant.

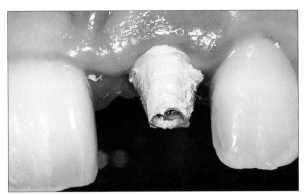

Fig 18   Prepared cap.

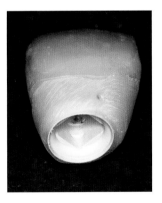

Fig 19   Finished chairside provisional.

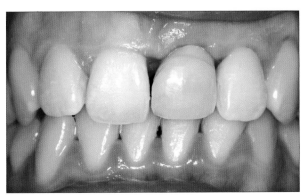

Fig 20   Chairside provisional 21 in situ.

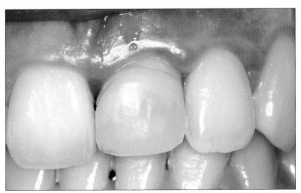

Fig 21   Chairside provisional 21 two weeks later. Regeneration of the distal and mesial papilla.

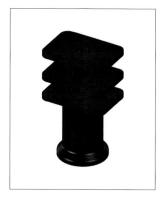

Fig 22   *Prefabricated impression cap.*

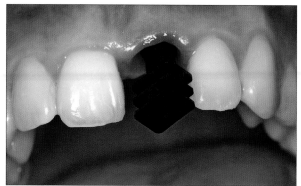

Fig 23   *Impression cap snapped onto the implant shoulder.*

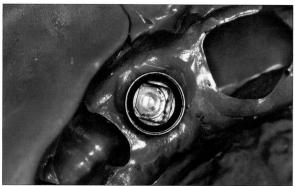

Fig 24   *Impression cap fixed in the hardened impression material.*

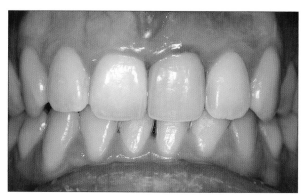

Fig 25   *Provisional tooth 21, manufactured in the dental lab.*

The provisional was removed from the abutment with a clamp. After cleaning the abutment, a prefabricated impression cap (Institut Straumann AG) was snapped onto the implant abutment and shoulder (Figs 22 and 23).

A laboratory-made custom tray was used to take an exact dental impression (Impregum; 3M Espe, Neuss, Germany) (Fig 24).

The color and shape of this provisional restoration was chosen by the dental technician at the lab. Three days later, the provisional restoration replaced the chairside provisional and remained in place until the peri-implant red esthetics were perfect (Fig 25).

Relining—the addition of material to the external surface of the provisional restoration to shape the emergence contours—is optional for dynamically compressing the papillae and creating a perfect esthetic result (Wittneben and coworkers 2013).

The red esthetics was reevaluated six weeks later. The peri-implant mucosa showed perfect contours, so the final dental impression was taken (same procedure as previously). The patient wore the provisional restoration as before until the final crown was ready. Close communication between dental technician, dentist and patient with regard to the design of the final restoration is required to achieve an esthetic result that corresponds to the patient's esthetic imagination.

Once the all-ceramic crown had been delivered from the dental lab, the definitive cementation took place. To avoid excess cement, cementation followed a strict protocol (Table 2).

Table 2   *Cementation protocol*

Recommended cement: Ketac Cem
Apply only as much cement as necessary to the inside area of the crown, using a small dental brush.
Press down crown during curing
Use Superfloss to remove excess cement; watch out for the contact point while removing Superfloss
Perform x-ray check

The crown was cemented with glass-ionomer cement (Ketac Cem; 3M Espe). A small dental brush applied a thin layer of cement to the inside of the crown, avoiding to fill it completely. The crown was then placed onto the ceramic abutment. During the initial setting oif the cement, the crown was actively pressed down by hand. A special dental floss (Superfloss; Oral B) removed residual cement on the mesial and distal side of the crown. A standardized periapical radiograph was taken to check the fit of the restoration and to document the radiographic status for subsequent follow-ups (Figs 26 and 27).

The patient was instructed to use a specific "red-to-white" brushing technique to actively stimulate the gingiva for further papillary regeneration at the implant site.

In the context of the one-year prospective long-term study in which the patient participated, the success and survival rates of the ceramic implants were 97.6% (Gahlert and coworkers 2016). Three-year follow-up data was collected in this study and submitted for publication.

After four years of loading, another standardized periapical radiograph and a smile-line photo were taken (Figs 28 and 29).

The use of a monotype ceramic implant made of zirconia is a favorable option for a highly biocompatible and metal free treatment.

The present treatment resulted in a beautiful esthetic outcome, even though the initial clinical situation had been highly demanding.

Ceramic implants made of zirconia have opened a new chapter in implant dentistry and give dentists, dental technicians, and researchers the chance to generate new perceptions within the field of implantology.

Acknowledgments

Laboratory procedures
Otto Prandtner, MDT – Munich, Germany

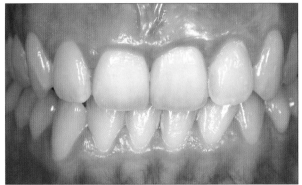

Fig 26   Clinical status one week after cementation of the all-ceramic crown 21 (July 2012).

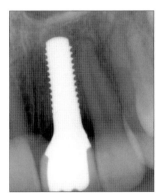

Fig 27   Standardized   periapical radiograph control.

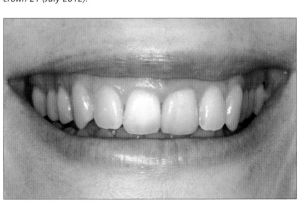

Fig 28   Clinical status in August 2016, confirming stability of the peri-implant soft tissue after four years of loading.

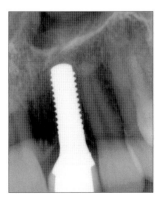

Fig 29   Periapical radiograph taken in November 2016 at five years after implant placement.

8 Esthetic Complications

V. Chappuis, W. Martin, D. Buser

8.1   Causes of Esthetic Complications

Handling esthetic complications is a challenge for any clinician. Unesthetic treatment outcomes will not only affect the patient emotionally but are also difficult to remedy in most situations. Implant-supported rehabilitations are predictable and survival rates of > 90% have been reported in the literature (Adell and coworkers 1990; Lindquist and coworkers 1996; Wennström and coworkers 2005; Buser and coworkers 2012; Chappuis and coworkers 2013). However, surviving implants are not necessarily successful.

Different criteria for implant success have been applied in the literature (Albrektsson and coworkers 1986; Buser and coworkers 1990; van Steenberghe 1997; Karoussis and coworkers 2004). Essentially, success has been related to acceptable radiographic bone levels and the absence of complications. But in esthetically sensitive situations, these osseointegration-oriented success criteria are not sufficient, as they only describe implant function and the stability of the peri-implant bone based on two-dimensional radiographs.

Smith and Zarb extended the criteria for success by emphasizing that a successful implant must have an adequately esthetic appearance (1989). An esthetic restoration should resemble the natural tooth or teeth in all aspects and imitate their natural appearance in terms of color, form, texture, size, and optical properties (Smith and Zarb 1989; Belser and coworkers 2004).

Esthetic success in the anterior maxilla involves many clinical parameters but is principally related to the peri-implant mucosal architecture in direct comparison to the contralateral natural tooth (Cooper 2008). Implant-supported restorations in the esthetic zone need to be evaluated objectively, selectively assessing the peri-implant soft-tissue architecture and its associated restoration(s) (Belser and coworkers 2004).

In 2005, the Pink Esthetic Score (PES) was introduced to assess the peri-implant soft tissue based on seven objective variables (Fürhauser and coworkers 2005). Various indices, or sets of criteria, have been defined to render esthetic success measurable in a standardized way, criteria designed to yield objective descriptions of individual parameters of the soft- and hard-tissue architecture (Fürhauser and coworkers 2005; Jemt 1997; Meijer and coworkers 2005; Belser and coworkers 2009). Today, the most commonly used indices are the Pink Esthetic Score (PES), which evaluates the soft-tissue architecture surrounding the implant, and the White Esthetic Score (WES), which analyzes the restored tooth in terms of form, color, and surface texture (Chen and Buser 2014).

While substantial improvements and innovations in implant dentistry have occurred in recent years, the complication rates remain high (Cooper 2008). There are several reasons why the numbers have been so high in recent years. First, the number of implants placed has increased significantly over the past 10 to 15 years. The number increased from 49.9% in 2002 to 60.8% in 2006, showing an increase of 21.8% in only 4 years (American Dental Association 2008). Second, the high complication rate may also be related to the increased number of implants placed in compromised patients or at compromised sites with inadequate bone or soft-tissue volume, or using more aggressive protocols (van Steenberghe 2003).

Causes for implant complications have been classified as biological, mechanical, technical, or esthetic (Pjetursson and coworkers 2004; Jung and coworkers 2012; Chrcanovic and coworkers 2014; Froum 2010):

Biological complications are mostly patient-related, but can also be multifactorial, such as a susceptibility to peri-implantitis, inadequate oral hygiene, or cement residue. Reducing these risks requires good patient compliance and an intensive maintenance program (Klinge and Meyle 2012).

Technical complications are mostly related to materials and the design of components, such as the loosening of retaining screws or abutments, fracture of components and reconstructive materials, or loss of retention of cemented prostheses. Unlike biologic complications, technical complications can be solved by adjustment in most cases (Salvi and Brägger 2009).

Mechanical complications are related to implant fracture, in turn ultimately leading to implant loss. Due to the development of a solid screw design and new, stronger titanium alloys, implant fractures have become a rare complication. The annual rate of implant fractures has fallen from 0.3% in older studies to 0.08% more recently (based on five-year studies of complication rates; Pjetursson and coworkers 2014).

Esthetic complications can be related to one of the above parameters or may be influenced by multiple factors. A systematic review revealed a cumulative esthetic five-year complication rate of 7.1% (3.6%–13.6%) in implant-supported single crowns in the anterior maxilla (Jung and coworkers 2012). In addition, esthetic complications can be the caused iatrogenically by misjudging the preoperative risk, selecting an inappropriate treatment approach, inaccuracy in 3D implant positioning, or inappropriate implant dimensions.

8.1.1 Incorrect 3D Implant Position

The optimal placement of the implant shoulder in the correct 3D position still remains one of the most significant factors relating to esthetic failures, irrespective of the selected implant design ("bone-level" or "tissue-level" design; Pjetursson and coworkers 2014; Evans and Chen 2008). If an implant is not placed within the comfort zones, bone remodeling occurs around the implant shoulder in order to reestablish biologic width following restoration (Chen and Buser 2009; Berglundh and Lindhe 1996). This biological phenomenon, caused by microleakage due to the microgap at the implant/abutment interface, is observed around the most commonly used implant brands and is often termed a "bone saucer." In general, this "saucer" has a horizontal dimension of 1 to 1.5 mm and a vertical dimension of 1 to 3 mm, depending on the implant/abutment interface design, the implant brand, and the position of the microgap in relation to the bone crest.

Efforts have been made to reduce this implant/abutment microleakage by introducing a platform-switching interface in combination with a modified internal connection (Broggini and coworkers 2006; Maeda and coworkers 2007). Even though some success in reducing the bone-saucer effect at the implant shoulder level has been observed clinically after a follow-up period of five to nine years (Chappuis and coworkers 2015), systematic reviews remain inconclusive, in particular with respect to long-term data and the multifactorial cause of peri-implant bone loss (Abrahamsson and Berglundh 2009; Atieh and coworkers 2010; Annibali and coworkers 2012; Romanos and Javed 2014; Strietzel and coworkers 2014).

Correct 3D implant positioning is related to the concepts of comfort zone and danger zone, which take the biologic width into account and still apply today, even if a modern implant design is selected (Buser and coworkers 2004).

Mesiodistal malpositioning occurs if an implant is placed too close to the neighboring tooth (≤ 1 mm). This poses a risk of vertical bone loss at the adjacent tooth with a subsequently reduction in papillary height due to healing-induced crestal bone remodeling (Esposito and coworkers 1993) (Figs 1a-f).

Orofacial malpositioning, too far to the facial and outside the bony envelope, results to insufficient facial bone supporting the soft tissues, with facial recession as a consequence. If an implant is placed to palatal it may not lead to an esthetic failure, unless it is placed too shallow, which can result in ridge-lapped restoration causing more difficulty for the patient to maintain good plaque control (Figs 2a-f).

Coronoapical malpositioning is not just a problem if the implant is placed too far coronally, resulting in a visible implant shoulder, but also if the implant is inserted too far apically. Apical malpositioning favors facial recession due to bone remodeling following abutment connection. Angulation problems with an excessive facial inclination yields a shoulder position that is also too far facially, which is associated with facial bone loss and mucosal recession (Figs 3a-e).

Angulation malpositioning, especially with an inclination that is too far to the facial, leads to a shoulder position that is also too far to the facial, which is associated with facial bone loss and mucosal recession (Figs 4a-d).

In summary, if the implant shoulder is misplaced and the comfort zones are not respected, remodeling will cause unavoidable bone loss, leading to facial recession or insufficient papillary height (Figs 1 to 4; Dr. W. Martin).

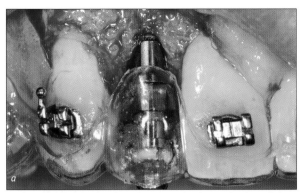

Fig 1a   Frontal retracted view of the dental implant at the time of placement. Slight mesial positioning towards the root of tooth 11.

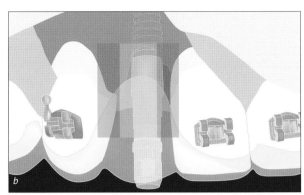

Fig 1b   Placement of the implant outside the mesiodistal comfort zone.

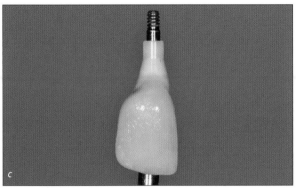

Fig 1c   Facial view of the final restoration (Zirconia CARES abutment with ceramic veneer). Constricted emergence profile from the mesial aspect.

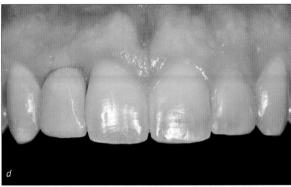

Fig 1d   Frontal retracted view of implant restoration 12 at the one-year follow-up visit. Mucosal margin deficiency on the mesial aspect.

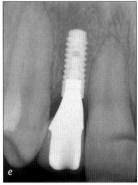

Fig 1e   Periapical radiograph of implant 12 at one year. Limited interdental bone mesial to the implant.

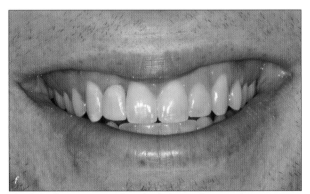

Fig 1f   Smile at one year. Disruption in harmonious margin contours.

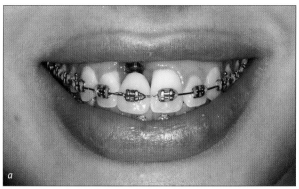

Fig 2a   The smile highlights the facial position of the implant and subsequent tissue loss on teeth 12 and 21, as well as facial to implant 11.

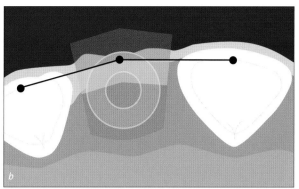

Fig 2b   Position of the implant outside the orofacial comfort zone.

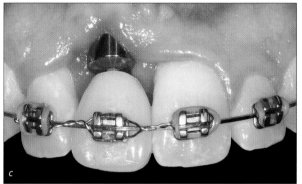

Fig 2c   Frontal retracted view of implant 11 with evident mucosal tissue recession as well as deficiencies on the adjacent teeth.

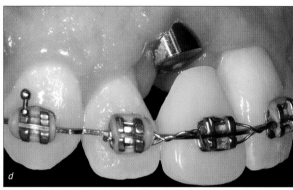

Fig 2d   Lateral retracted view. Facial angulation and position of the implant in relation to the adjacent teeth.

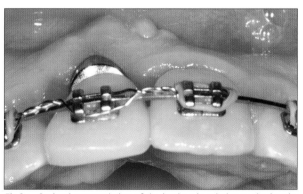

Fig 2e   Occlusal retracted view of the implant in relation to the interim restoration. Facial positioning of the implant.

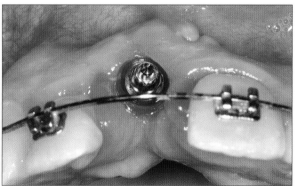

Fig 2f   Occlusal retracted view of the implant and its facial position in relation to the adjacent teeth.

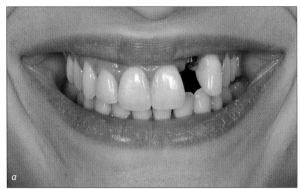

Fig 3a   The smile highlights the coronoapical positioning of the implant and the deficiency in the supporting tissues.

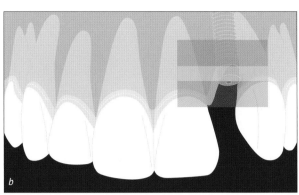

Fig 3b   The implant is positioned slightly apical to the coronoapical comfort zone.

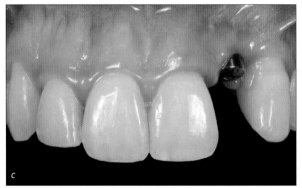

Fig 3c   Frontal retracted view of implant 22. Position of the implant and corresponding deficiency of the peri-implant tissue support.

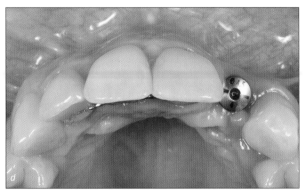

Fig 3d   Occlusal retracted view of implant 22. Acceptable orofacial position.

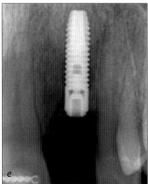

Fig 3e   Periapical radiograph. Position of the implant relative to the adjacent teeth and the available bone for tissue support.

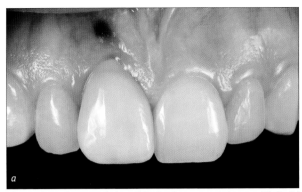

Fig 4a   Frontal retracted view of the implant-supported crown 11. Facial mucosal recession.

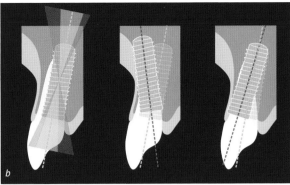

Fig 4b   Axial angulation of a dental implant and the corresponding comfort and danger zones and the potential influence on peri-implant tissues.

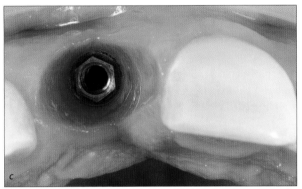

Fig 4c   Occlusal retracted view of the implant 11. Facial position of the implant platform in relation to tooth 12.

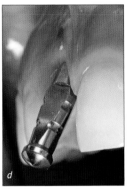

Fig 4d   Lateral retracted view of implant 11. Facial axial angulation in relationship to the adjacent teeth.

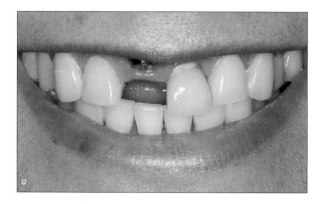

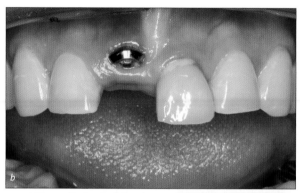

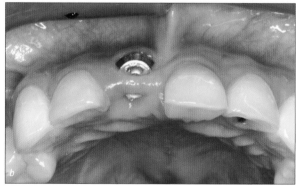

Figs 5a-c   Oversized implant diameter in the esthetic zone leading to facial bone loss.

8.1.2   Implant Selection

Esthetic complications can also be triggered by improper implant selection. Oversized implant platforms that are too large for a given site carry a risk of violating the comfort zone not only in the mesiodistal but also in the orofacial dimension (Figs 5a-c, Dr. W. Martin and Figs 6a-d). As a consequence, a more facial position of the implant shoulder, outside the bony envelope, will impair the esthetic outcome. Replacement of a missing lateral incisor is a particularly demanding situation. As a general recommendation, a regular implant platform with a diameter of 4 to 5 mm is recommended in maxillary central incisor, canine, and premolar sites, whereas in mandibular central incisor sites and all lateral incisor sites, narrow-diameter implants (NDI) with diameters of 3 to 3.5 mm are preferred.

A recent systematic review on NDI implants demonstrated good clinical results in such situations (Klein and coworkers 2014). However, NDIs should not be placed if a correct restoration-driven 3D implant position is not feasible; in these cases, bone augmentation is necessary. Despite the better mechanical properties of implants made of titanium alloys compared with commercially pure titanium implants, NDIs should be used with caution in borderline cases, under strict adherence to the ITI Consensus Guidelines (Klein and coworkers 2014).

In the past, the root-shaped implant design was utilized in the esthetic zone to provide support and to reduce the distance from the implant surface to the facial bone wall, in order to limit dimensional changes and to improve primary stability in post-extraction sites (Botticelli and coworkers 2006). However, experimental studies have revealed that the facial bone wall cannot be maintained, irrespective of the implant design (Araújo and coworkers 2005a; Caneva and coworkers 2010; Favero and coworkers 2013; Alharbi and coworkers 2015). In contrast, the root-shaped implant design resulted in significantly more bone loss on the facial aspect than cylindrical implant designs (Caneva and coworkers 2010). The hypothesis is that the root-shaped design can compress the surrounding bone wall, especially on the facial aspect, interfering with vascularization and promoting bone loss (Figs 6a-d; Dr. V. Chappuis).

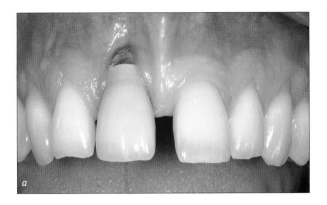
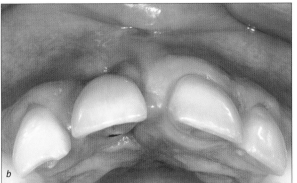
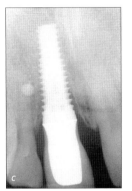
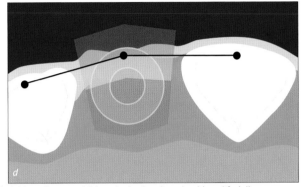

Figs 6a-d   Root-shaped implant with oversized implant diameter leading to facial bone loss. In addition, the implant is malpositioned facially.

8.1.3 Insufficient Facial Bone Wall

Sufficient facial bone-wall height and thickness is the key to achieving pleasing esthetics. Circumferential anchorage of the implant within the alveolar bone is an important prerequisite not only for long-term function but also for an esthetic successful treatment outcome.

Clinical and experimental studies have revealed that a facial bone-wall thickness of 2 mm or more is needed to maintain its dimensions (Spray and coworkers 2000; Qahash and coworkers 2008). If the facial bone wall is insufficient in height and thickness at the time of implant insertion, simultaneous bone augmentation is necessary to regenerate the facial bone architecture (Figs 7a-d; Dr. V. Chappuis).

In the anterior maxilla, the facial bone wall is frequently very thin by nature (Braut and coworkers 2011; Januário and coworkers 2011) and needs to be augmented to maintain its contour so it can support the soft-tissue architecture over time. The best-documented surgical techniques for predictably regenerating sites deficient in bone is guided bone regeneration, using a barrier membrane and appropriate bone fillers (Aghaloo and Moy 2007). The combination of a collagen membrane, and autologous bone chips, and Bio-Oss particles provides good regenerative outcomes with high long-term PES scores (Buser and coworkers 2013a; Buser and coworkers 2013b).

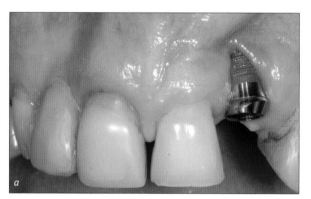
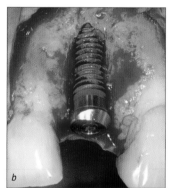
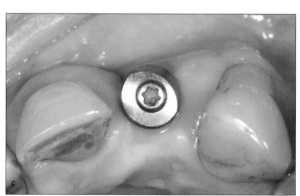
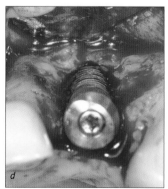

Figs 7a-d   Failure of the facial bone to regenerate after an implant was placed immediately after tooth extraction, leading to mucosal recession on the facial aspect (a, b). No bone regeneration occurred on the facial aspect of the implant (c, d). In addition, the implant is malpositioned facially.

8.1.4 Esthetic Failure Due to Late Facial Growth

Craniofacial growth and subsequent implant infraposition is a well-documented problem in single-tooth implant patients (Forsberg 1979; Bishara and coworkers 1994; Andersson and coworkers 2013; Zitzmann and coworkers 2015). While the study of Bernard and coworkers (2004) examining vertical changes in the anterior maxilla after a mean observation rate of 4.2 years found no differences in the "young adult" group (15.5 to 21 years), the "mature adult" group (40 to 55 years) exhibited vertical changes of between 0.12 and 1.86 mm (Bernard and coworkers 2004). It was also documented that for patients with a short or long face type, further growth—especially the ongoing eruption of adjacent teeth—creates a serious risk even after the age of 20 (Heij and coworkers 2006).

A long-term observational study examined the effect of infraposition of single-tooth implants in esthetic sites after 17 to 19 years in 57 patients (Andersson and coworkers 2013). Limited infraposition (< 0.5 mm) was observed in 50% of patients, whereas 35% revealed infraposition of > 1 mm. Infraposition was slightly more frequent in females and in patients with a "long-face" appearance.

A recent study examined 35 patients with a mean age of 29.3 ± 9.9 years after a follow-up of three years. The authors observed a higher submersion rate in the second and third decades of life than in the fourth and fifth (Schwartz-Arad and Bichacho 2015). Although adolescent growth ceases by the late teens, it is well known that the nasomaxillary complex still undergoes slow growth in adulthood, the so-called late facial growth (Forsberg and coworkers 1991; Akgul and Toygar 2002; Albert and coworkers 2007; Machtei and coworkers 2008; Roccuzzo and coworkers 2002; Schwartz-Arad and Bichacho 2015). However, the timeframe for late facial growth can vary widely with age, especially in the case of long or short facial types (Heij and coworkers 2006). In addition, the risks related to continuous tooth eruption in adulthood should also be considered.

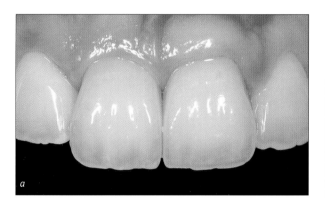
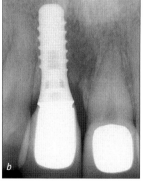
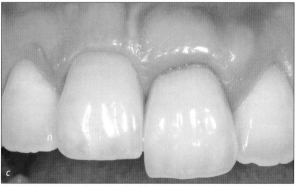
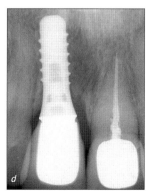

Figs 8a-d   This female patient had been 21 years old at the time of implant placement (a-b). At the 11-year follow-up at the age of 32, infraposition of the implant crown of 2.5 mm is observed (c-d). Interestingly, the patient was not particularly disturbed by the infraposition of the implant crown.

In summary, the issues related to late facial growth before implant placement should be explained to the patient. In particular, patients with known risk factors such as short or long face, young age, high smile line, or high esthetic expectations should be informed about the potential need for future restorative corrections. It is currently not possible to predict with absolute certainty which patients are prone to late residual growth or what the extent of these adult craniofacial changes might be (Froum 2010) (Figs 8a-d; Dr. V. Chappuis).

8.1.5 Esthetic Failure Due to Implants and Third-party Implant Components Lacking Scientific Validation

Clinicians are cautioned to purchase implants from manufacturers who follow good manufacturing practices in keeping with International Organization for Standardization (ISO) or US Food and Drug Administration (FDA) standards. Defects in raw materials and in the manufacturing process may certainly manifest themselves, so clinicians should be diligent in maintaining records of product lot numbers and patients records to ensure an appropriate response (Figs 9a-d; Dr. V. Chappuis).

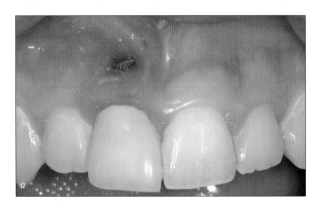
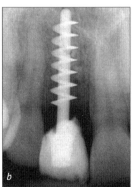
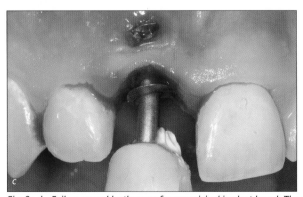
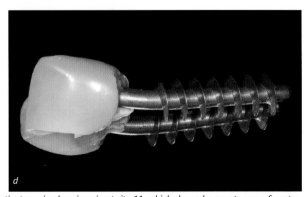

Figs 9a-d   Failure caused by the use of a non-original implant brand. The patient was in chronic pain at site 11, which showed a spontaneous fenestration on the facial aspect, exposing an implant thread (a). The periapical radiograph shows a peri-implant defect in the crestal area (b). Due to lack of osseointegration, the implant could be easily unscrewed (c). The removed implant including remnants of the cement overfill of the composite crown (d).

Special consideration should be given to the selection of abutments for implants in the esthetic zone. The use of validated abutments (original abutments) by the manufacturer of the implant system will insure that the fit of the implant connection will be precise and limit (rotational) movement during function, reducing the risk of screw loosening or abutment fracture (Hamilton and coworkers 2013, Gigandet and coworkers 2014). If non-validated (non-original) abutments are used, the fit of the abutment and the design of the abutment screw may cause a rotational misfit during function, which can lead to fracture of the abutment and failure of the restoration. Zirconia abutments in particular require a precise fit on the implants, and any misfit will increase the risk for abutment fracture (Sui and coworkers 2014), which in turn can lead to esthetic failure, such that the restoration has to be refabricated (Figs 10a-b; Dr. W. Martin).

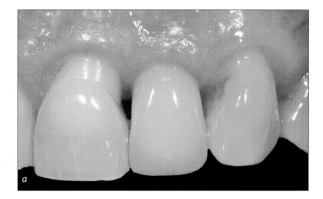

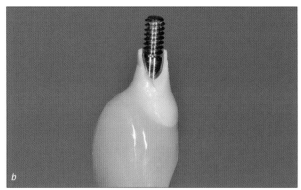

Figs 10a-b   Fracture of a non-validated zirconia abutment 6 months after being connected to implant 22.

8.2 Management of Esthetic Complications

With an estimated two million new implants inserted worldwide every year, and tens of millions of implants currently in service, the estimated number of implants that are failing annually is likely to be in the range of 200,000 to 250,000 (Machtei and coworkers 2008). Failed implant sites present a challenging therapeutic dilemma to the clinician: on the one hand, the alveolar bone at these sites is usually further reduced, making it less than ideal for subsequent implant placement. On the other hand, implant therapy will often be the only treatment option that will allow a fixed prosthetic reconstruction (which is frequently the treatment of choice for many of our patients). Since failures are often preceded by complications at various levels of the treatment, early detection of any complications amenable to rescue therapies may reverse the fate of the implant. A further dilemma is that replaced implants reveal lower survival rates than reported for pristine sites (Machtei and coworkers 2008).

8.2.1 Decision Criteria for Salvaging Esthetic Implants

The first prerequisite for salvaging an esthetically compromised implant is the correct 3D position within the comfort zones. The second prerequisite is sufficient bone support, which will secure the long-term survival of the restoration. If the two prerequisites are met, the following options for salvaging an esthetically compromised implant can be considered: soft-tissue re-augmentation, bone re-augmentation, segmented osteotomy, and prosthetic options.

In order to decide if a failing implant can be salvaged, a 3D CBCT is preferred for assessing the peri-implant conditions, the 3D implant position, the remaining bone, and the integrity of the adjacent teeth. If the salvaging

of a failing implant appears questionable, early implant removal in esthetic sites is more likely to preserve the alveolar ridge, leaving more options for future treatments. Postponed implant removal may result in a severely deficient residual ridge at the failed implant site and may also jeopardize neighboring implants/teeth.

Soft-tissue re-augmentation. Correction of facial recessions can be attempted in sites presenting a shallow isolated buccal gingival recession. While the coverage of facial recessions around teeth is well documented (Roccuzzo and coworkers 2002; Cairo and coworkers 2008; Chambrone and coworkers 2009; Tatakis and coworkers 2015), coverage around implants is only poorly understood. A prospective case-series study examined a coronally advanced flap in combination with a connective-tissue graft in order to cover recessions around implants. Although the authors found a significant improvement in the soft-tissue situation with a reduction in soft-tissue dehiscences of 66% after 6 months, complete coverage of the recession around the implant was not achievable (Burkhardt and coworkers 2008). Recession coverage using a connective-tissue graft from the tuberosity, which was subsequently deepithelialized, resulted in a mean coverage of 89.6% and in complete coverage in 56.3% of cases after 1 year (Roccuzzo and coworkers 2014). A slightly modified technique used a combined surgical-prosthetic approach using a coronally advanced flap with a connective-tissue graft and a new restoration (Zucchelli and coworkers 2013). The results revealed complete coverage in 75% of treated sites. In summary, there is a need to improve the technique of recession coverage in order to achieve not only better esthetics for the patient, but also a stable long-term result regarding the augmented soft tissue around the implants (Figs 11a-j; clinical images courtesy of Dr. Stephen Chen of Balwyn, Australia).

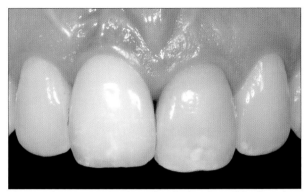

Fig 11a Eleven years after immediate flapless (type 1) implant placement, further dentoalveolar growth has resulted in an incisal-edge discrepancy between implant crown 11 and the adjacent natural tooth 21. The facial mucosa appears thin. The scarring derives from the previous apical surgery that was performed before the tooth was lost. The patient was seeking a replacement crown to improve the appearance.

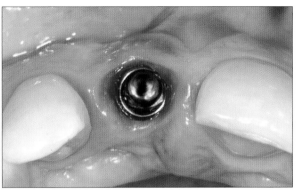

Fig 11b Occlusal view after removal of the crown. Remodeling on the facial aspect of the ridge. The facial mucosa is thin. It was necessary to provide treatment to increase the volume of soft tissue on the facial aspect before providing a new crown.

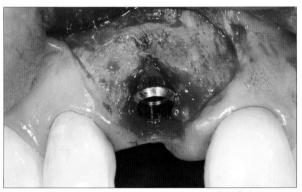

Fig 11c After flap elevation, a V-shaped dehiscence of the facial bone was seen, exposing the rough part of the implant.

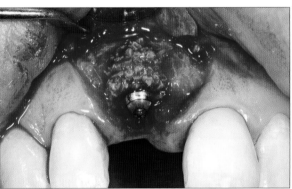

Fig 11d A combination of autologous bone chips and DBBM was grafted onto the dehiscence and the facial surface of the bone.

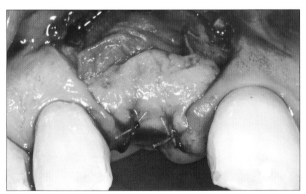

Fig 11e The graft was protected with a resorbable collagen membrane. A connective-tissue graft was harvested from the palate and place at the coronal aspect of the implant over the membrane. Two sutures were used to secure the graft.

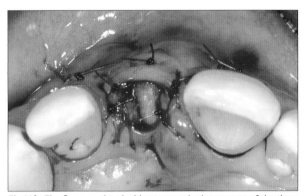

Fig 11f The flap was closed without coronal advancement of the tissue to avoid displacing the mucogingival junction and the scarred portion of the mucosa coronally. The connective-tissue graft can be seen above the crest of the ridge.

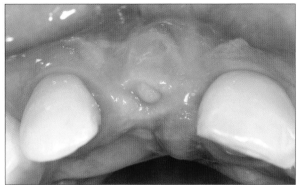

Fig 11g   After ten weeks, the graft had healed and been incorporated into the surrounding tissues with complete re-epithelialization.

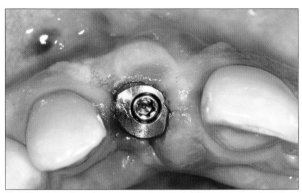

Fig 11h   A healing abutment was attached following removal of tissue above the top of the implant.

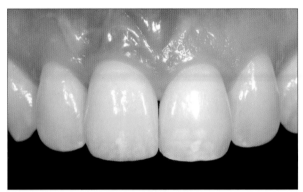

Fig 11i   A new implant crown was fabricated.

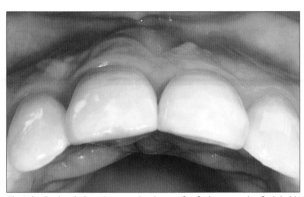

Fig 11j   Occlusal view. Increased volume of soft tissue on the facial side of the implant.

Bone re-augmentation. The literature on bone regeneration around ailing implants is very scarce and limited to case reports (AlGhamdi 2012). Continuous bone loss is a consequence of peri-implantitis or excess cement in most cases. A recent consensus report suggested that the incidence of peri-implantitis was around 28% to 56% (Lindhe and Meyle 2008). Longitudinal studies have shown that peri-implant health at sites affected by peri-implantitis may not be easy to reestablish, especially in cases that develop disease early (Charalampakis and coworkers 2011). Surgical resective therapy has been described as one option in the treatment of peri-implantitis (Land and Berglundh 2011). This approach predictably reduces pocket depths around the implant, but at the same time it results in a marked exposure of the implant surface. To limit deficient esthetic outcomes, other authors have evaluated the efficacy of regenerative surgical procedures (Roos-Jansåker and coworkers 2007; Matarassi and coworkers 2014). The effectiveness of regenerative treatment following peri-implantitis is significantly influenced by the peri-implant defect morphology, with beneficial results obtained in circumferential intrabony defects (Schwarz and coworkers 2010).

Segmented osteotomy. Segmented osteotomy can be considered in cases with implant malposition. However, achieving pleasing esthetics requires not only sufficient bone support on the facial crest but also a sufficient distance from the neighboring root if a segmented osteotomy is taken into consideration. Limited case reports are available for this possibility to reposition misplaced implants in a correct prosthetic position by segmented osteotomy (da Cunha and coworkers 2011; Kassolis and coworkers 2003; Stacchi and coworkers 2008). Segmented osteotomy is a complex procedure, and the available literature is limited to case reports. Therefore, this treatment option should be chosen with caution.

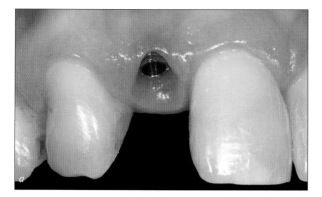
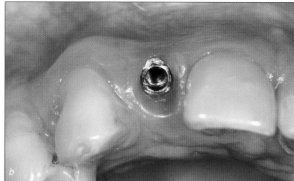

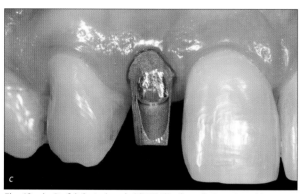
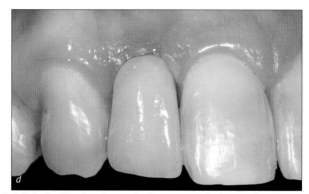

Figs 12a-d   Prefabricated angled (25°) titanium abutment used to correct a facially inclined implant that resulted in a compromised restorative outcome due to a lack of restorative space.

Prosthetic options to improve esthetics. In clinical situations that result in implants in non-favorable positions or angulations or in areas with inadequate mucogingival contours, various prosthetic techniques and materials are utilized to achieve an acceptable esthetic outcome. These restorative procedures are often initiated to make implant removal and re-treatment unnecessary, salvaging a compromised treatment. A common clinical scenario is when the implant is placed in a shallow coronoapical position with a facial angulation. This situation will require an angled abutment to correct the axis of inclination, which if severe (> 20°) can lead to unfavorable compressive and tensile stress on the surrounding crestal cortical bone (Sadrimanesh and coworkers 2012). Therefore, attempts should be made to minimize occlusal load on the restoration. The choice of abutment material is often limited to a metal alloy (gold or titanium) rather than zirconia, as the abutment is often thinned in an effort to correct the angulation and could fracture (Thulasidas and coworkers 2015). Restorative space is also compromised in the orofacial dimension and will limit the technician in the choice of materials to develop a proper emergence profile, depth and translucency in the definitive restoration (Figs 12a-d; Dr. W. Martin).

If mucogingival defects are present before or after implant placement, a proper diagnosis is a key factor in determining the available surgical or prosthetic options. Traditionally, diagnostic casts that highlight the hard- and soft-tissue defects in white and pink wax can be used by the clinician to determine the treatment approach in addition to educating the patient on the procedures necessary for rehabilitation (Fig 13; Dr. W. Martin).

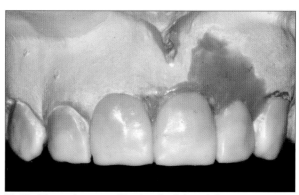

Fig 13   Diagnostic wax-up of hard- and soft-tissue defects.

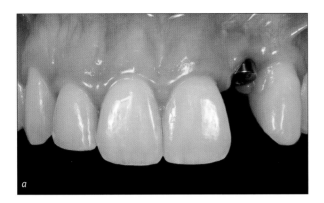

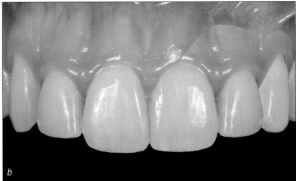

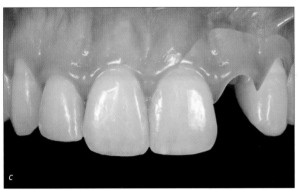

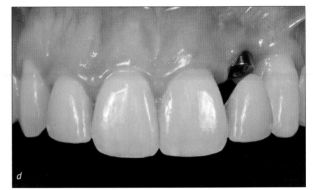

Figs 14a-d   Digital mock-up of hard- and soft-tissue defects around implant 22.

The availability of software programs (Adobe Photoshop, Adobe Systems, San Jose, CA, USA) can make the diagnostic procedure more effective through the use of sectional copying of the ideal contralateral side, followed by the masking of layers that isolate the pink and white deficiencies (Figs 14a-d; Dr. W. Martin).

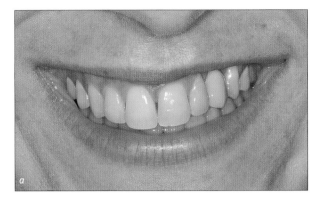
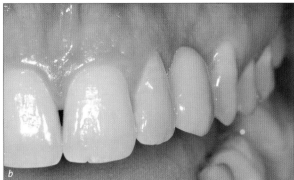
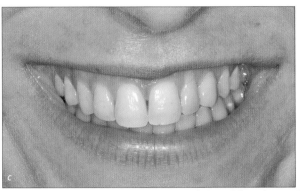
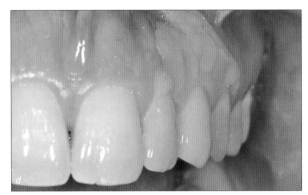

Figs 15a-d   Intraoral assessment of hard- and soft-tissue defect using a PVS material.

If a mucogingival defect remains after implant placement and restoration, an intraoral assessment can be performed with a polyvinyl siloxane material placed in the defect and allowed to fully set under lip pressure (Figs 15a-d; Dr. W. Martin).

This technique will create ideal contours that can be appreciated immediately, as patients often confuse the mucogingival defects with a restoration they interpret as overcontoured.

The presence of a mucogingival defect after implant placement should first be addressed with surgical options to improve contours. Here the restorative clinician will assist the surgeon by fabricating an undercontoured provisional restoration to minimize pressure on the grafted area. Once healing is complete, the provisional restoration can be modified to provide ideal emergence contours, and shaping of the tissue in the transition zone can be initiated (Figs 16a-o; Dr. W. Martin).

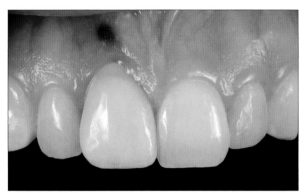

Fig 16a   Implant crown 11 with a facial mucogingival defect and amalgam tattoo.

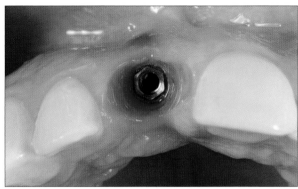

Fig 16b   Occlusal view of the facial mucogingival defect after crown and abutment removal.

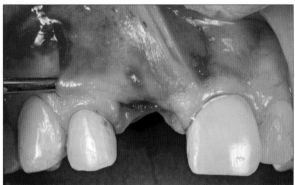

Fig 16c   Lateral approach for a split-thickness pouch for a connective-tissue graft

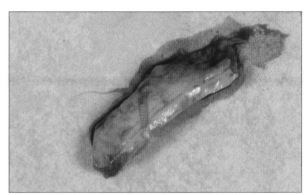

Fig 16d   Connective-tissue graft harvested from the palate.

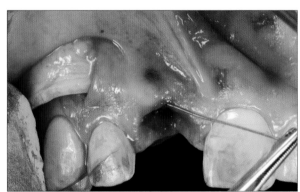

Fig 16e   Subepithelial placement of the connective-tissue graft with the help of a suture through the peri-implant mucosa.

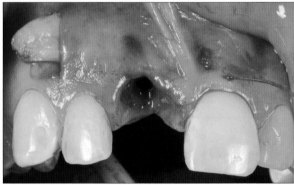

Fig 16f   Still placing of the connective-tissue graft with the suture drawn to the lateral base of the pouch.

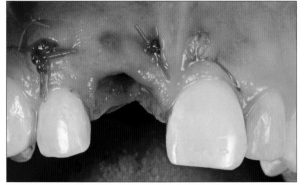

Fig 16g   Facial view of the sutures used to stabilize the connective-tissue graft.

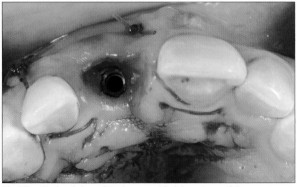

Fig 16h   Occlusal view of the improved facial contours of the mucosa.

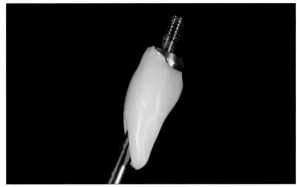

Fig 16i   An undercontoured screw-retained provisional to encourage coronal tissue placement.

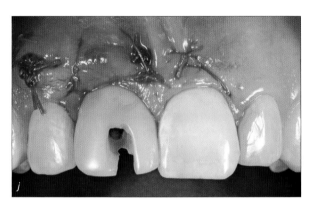

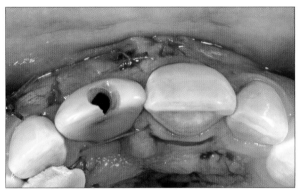

Figs 16j-k   Facial and occlusal view of the provisional in place before sealing the access hole.

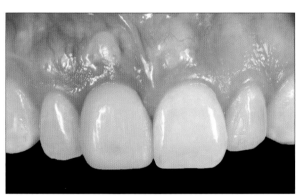

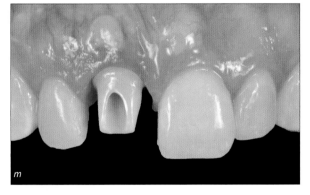

Fig 16i   After 8 weeks of healing and after removing the amalgam tattoo, a new screw-retained provisional was placed that implemented the ideal contours.

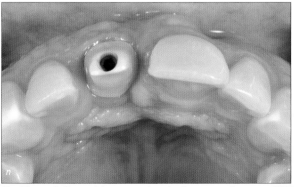

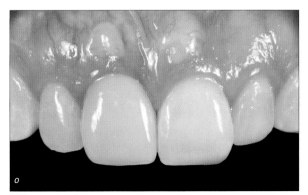

Figs 16m-o   Delivery of the custom zirconia abutment and cemented lithium disilicate restoration.

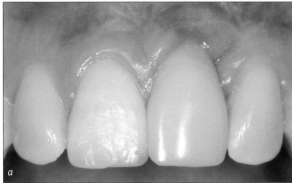 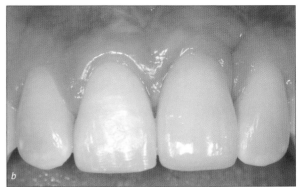

Figs 17a-b   A mucogingival defect masked with pink ceramics, extending into the distal interdental aspect and creating a "double-papilla" situation.

If surgical procedures would be ineffective or are not desired, prosthetic alternatives can be a suitable effort to maintain esthetic symmetry. Prosthetic materials (ceramics, composite, and acrylic resin) used to mask the mucogingival defect have varying benefits and shortcomings in terms of fabrication, application, and longevity (Goodacre 1990; Duncan and Swift 1994; Hannon and coworkers 1994; Costello 1995; Zalkind and Hochman 1997; Greene 1998; Priest and Lindke 1998; Botha and Gluckman 1999; Jacques and coworkers 1999; Cura and coworkers 2002; Haj-Ali and Walker 2002; Barzilay and Irene 2003; Garcia and Verrett 2004; Capa 2007; Kamalakidis and coworkers 2007; Cascione and coworkers 2008; Mankoo 2008; Coachman and coworkers 2009; Kim and coworkers 2009a; Salama and coworkers 2009; Coachman and coworkers 2010; Kim and coworkers 2010; Alani and coworkers 2011). Selecting the right material for a given clinical situation is a key component in achieving mucosal symmetry with the final restoration and the surrounding dentition. Traditionally, gingiva-colored ceramics have been incorporated into implant restorations to mask these defects; more recently, there have been reports on the use of these ceramics on zirconia abutments within the submucosal contours in thin-tissue phenotype patients (< 2 mm thickness) that resulted in improved esthetic outcomes (Thoma and coworkers 2016c).

Gingiva-colored ceramics has advantages in terms of color stability, surface porosity, and durability, but can be technique-sensitive and will require accurate shade communication with shade tabs specific to the ceramic system being used (Wang and coworkers 2013). In addition, meticulous treatment planning and mock-ups of the tissue replacement are recommended to communicate the desired contours to the technician.

If the defect is known prior to implant placement, the Pink Power Concept (PPC) has been described as a structured implant/restorative strategy for the treatment of multi-unit gaps in the esthetic zone (Vailati and Belser 2011). Key components of this approach evaluate the smile line and its influence on the degree, position, and contours of the artificial gingiva.

Patient education is paramount in these situations, the focus being on the best possible combination of esthetic outcomes and cleansability.

A region of particular interest is the mucogingival defect adjacent to the natural tooth, where pink ceramics should be applied mainly at the zenith of the restoration and should not extend into the interdental embrasure, where it may limit access for efficient oral hygiene and potentially result in a "double-papilla" situation (Vailati and Belser 2011) (Figs 17a-b; Dr. W. Martin).

Most importantly, an adequately designed PPC restoration has to provide an optimum combination of esthetic excellence and cleansability by creating the illusion of a harmoniously scalloped mucosal contour with papillae, eliminating or significantly reducing any black triangles and reestablishing the normal length-to-width ratios of the anatomical tooth crowns (Vailati and Belser 2011) (Figs 18a-h; clinical images courtesy of Prof. Urs Belser, Bern, Switzerland).

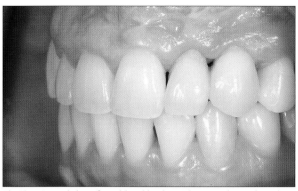

Fig 18a   Lateral view of provisional in place. There are three minor short-comings from an esthetic point of view: (1) short papilla between 22 and 23, (2) apically located emergence of the ovate pontic 22 from the alveolar mucosa, (3) black embrasure between 21 and 22.

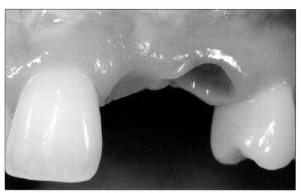

Fig 18b   After provisional shaping, the edentulous ridge exhibited harmoniously configured soft tissue on both implant 23 and the concave contact area for the ovate pontic 22. The remaining mucogingival defect will require replacement with pink ceramics in the final restoration.

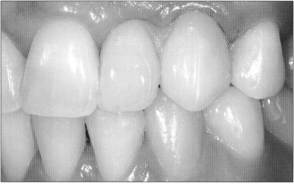

Fig 18c   Initial placement of the definitive restoration with the gingiva-colored ceramics between 22 and 23. Minor modifications are needed to improve the contours for esthetics and hygienic access.

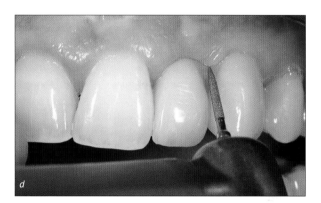

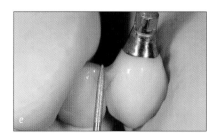

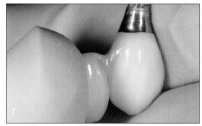

Figs 18d-f   Intra- and extraoral contouring with a fine-grained, flame-shaped diamond bur to create an entirely convex profile.

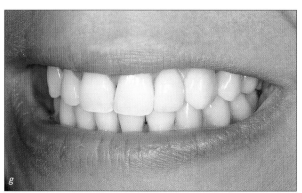

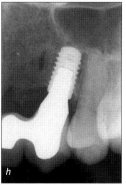

Figs 18g-h   Final view showing the filled embrasure 22/23 with gingiva-colored ceramics (g). Periapical radiograph at two years (h).

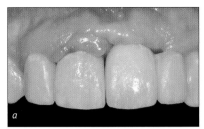 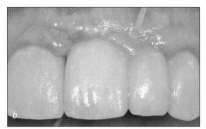 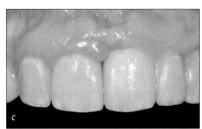

Figs 19a-c   Masking a mucogingival defect in the embrasure distal to implant 21 with composite resin.

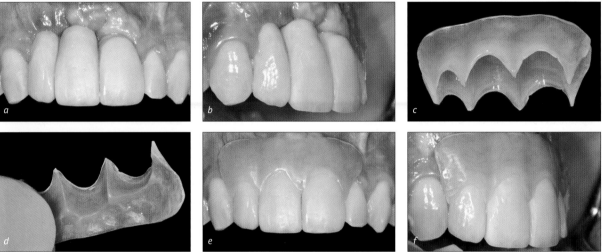

Figs 20a-f   Masking a mucogingival defect facial and apical to implants 11 and 21 with a removable acrylic-resin prosthesis.

Gingiva-colored composite resin has the advantage over ceramics that it can be controlled by the clinician through application, modification, and repair, but can be deficient in long-term esthetics because color stability is limited, often necessitating removal and replacement over time (Figs 19a-c; Dr. W. Martin).

Particular attention should be focused on the color of the composite material, as most materials have too much chroma and are too reddish. The goal of the shade selection should be to obtain a rather pale gingiva-like color that will blend into its environment discreetly (Vailati and Belser 2011). Custom shade tabs with combinations of base colors and modifiers will aid in creating more life-like color matches. In managing a mucogingival defect, moisture control and bonding to the restoration is critical to reduce delamination and staining. Access for plaque control remains critical and, when possible, retrievable restorations are recommended.

Acrylic resin should be restricted to situations where a large mucogingival defect is present that extends beyond the border of the mucosal margin(s) of the restoration.

These situations will require the acrylic resin to be utilized as a removable prosthesis that will gain its retention through mucostatic and embrasure extensions (Figs 20a-f; Dr. W. Martin). Acrylic resin is an inexpensive way to mask a large mucogingival defect, but it has moderate color stability and can be easily misplaced by the patient, necessitating a remake. It might be considered to provide the patient with multiple masking prostheses right at the outset.

For more in-depth information on vertical tissue deficiencies, please check out the ITI Online Academy's congress lecture "Prosthetic Solutions for Vertical Tissue Deficiencies" by Dr. Urs C. Belser (charges apply). See what else the Online Academy has to offer at **academy.iti.org**

8.2.2   Criteria for Implant Removal

Even though no clear guidelines exist for deciding when an implant should be removed, the following factors should be included in the decision-making process for removal of a failing implant.

a.   Esthetic failures
b.   Implant mobility
c.   Peri-implantitis
d.   Implant fracture
e.   Implant malposition
f.   Pain
g.   Local pathology
h.   Psychological problems
i.   Damage to the prosthetic interface
j.   Obsolete components/implants

In addition, it may be advisable to remove the failing implant before advanced bone loss has occurred to facilitate its replacement without the need for extensive reconstructive procedures or potential damage to the adjacent teeth.

Implant mobility or implant fracture are unmistakable signs of implant failure. In affected sites, all parts of the implant should be immediately removed to prevent further bone loss. A mobile implant with near-complete bone loss can be removed with a rotating counterclockwise driver with a countertorque ratchet, forceps with counterclockwise rotation, and minimum luxating movements to minimize damage to the surrounding tissues. However, implant removal may also be well indicated if the implant is non-mobile, namely due to incorrect placement or infection of the grafted site, or advanced peri-implantitis. In cases with an immobile implant, surgical removal is required.

Tools for implant removal. In the majority of cases when an esthetic complication has occurred, implant removal is the most effective approach, with subsequent augmentation and new implant placement. During implant removal, it is of paramount importance to avoid additional damage to the remaining bone and neighboring dentition. Since in most esthetic failure cases the facial bone wall will be compromised, maintenance of the palatal bone wall —an essential bony structure for any future implant treatment—is decisive. Trephine burs can cause much damage to the surrounding bone and should be avoided. Implants can be removed by small fissure burs, performing a careful osteotomy in the buccal and interproximal regions to weaken osseointegration, such that the implant can be removed by forceps.

Piezosurgery. Today, there are very fine piezosurgery tools to sever bone at the bone-to-implant interface. They provide better intraoperative control during cutting than to high-speed burs (Vercellotti 2000) (Figs 21a-b; Dr. V. Chappuis).

Removal torque systems. Major progress in removal tools has brought the advent of implant-removal torque systems. Reverse-torque ratcheting is the least invasive techniques for implant removal without damaging the surrounding structures. An intact implant connection with a corresponding adapter is needed to engage the implant and apply reverse-torque until the implant becomes mobile (Figs 21c-d; Dr. V. Chappuis).

Reverse screw systems. The reverse-screw technique is a second option, especially when the connection is damaged (Anitua and Orive 2012). It provides counterclockwise rotation relatively easily, utilizing a reverse screw attached to a ratchet. Extraction torques range from 20 to 80 N·cm. When the maximum torque of 200 N·cm is reached, small fissure burs or piezosurgery can be used in order to weaken the osseointegration. Care must always be taken in the case of narrow-diameter implants in dense cortical bone, which can easily fracture (Figs 21e-k; Dr. V. Chappuis).

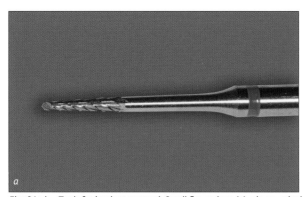
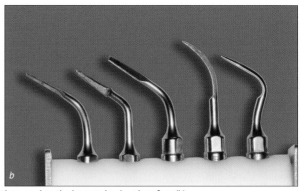

Figs 21a-b   Tools for implant removal. Small fissure burs (a); piezosurgical tools to weaken the bone-to-implant interface (b).

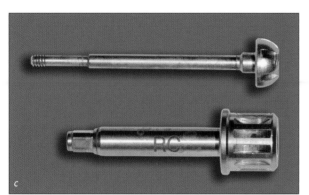
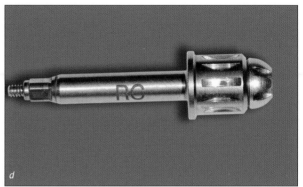

Figs 21c-d   More tools for implant removal. Reverse torque device, a tool from the implant manufacturer that fits into the internal connection (c, below). After mounting, the reverse-torque device is secured with a screw on the implant (c, above; d). The ratchet can be used in a counterclockwise direction.

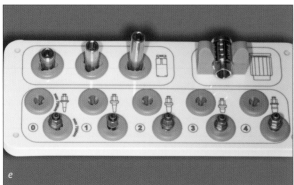
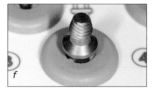
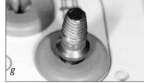
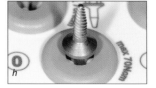
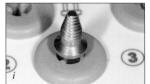

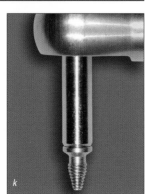

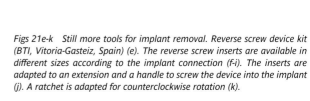

Figs 21e-k   Still more tools for implant removal. Reverse screw device kit (BTI, Vitoria-Gasteiz, Spain) (e). The reverse screw inserts are available in different sizes according to the implant connection (f-i). The inserts are adapted to an extension and a handle to screw the device into the implant (j). A ratchet is adapted for counterclockwise rotation (k).

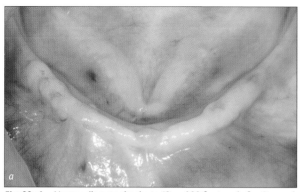 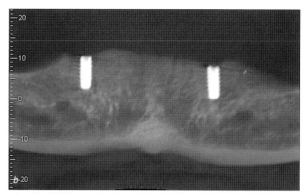

Figs 22a-b   Narrow-diameter implants 43 and 33 fractured after 2 years in function. The CBCT reveals a close relation to the mental foramen. Placement of a longer implant is not an option due to anatomical considerations.

Immediate reimplantation can be considered if sufficient bone volume is available. Preferably, no infection should be present at the implant site; a low-risk patient profile would be desirable. Immediate replacement with a larger-diameter dental implant has been suggested as an option for immediate implant replacement (Evian and Cutler 1995). In esthetic sites, this option has to be considered with care, since a larger-implant diameter may well interfere with the correct 3D implant position, leading to facial malposition due to the wider implant diameter. In addition, a wider diameter may lead to a more unfavorable bone wall defect morphology, which is more challenging in terms of predictable bone regeneration. Another option for immediate implant replacement is the use of a longer implant, if the residual bone volume and the anatomy as such allow this approach (Figs 22a-j; Dr. V. Chappuis).

In summary, immediate reimplantation is rarely feasible at esthetic sites due to anatomic limitations.

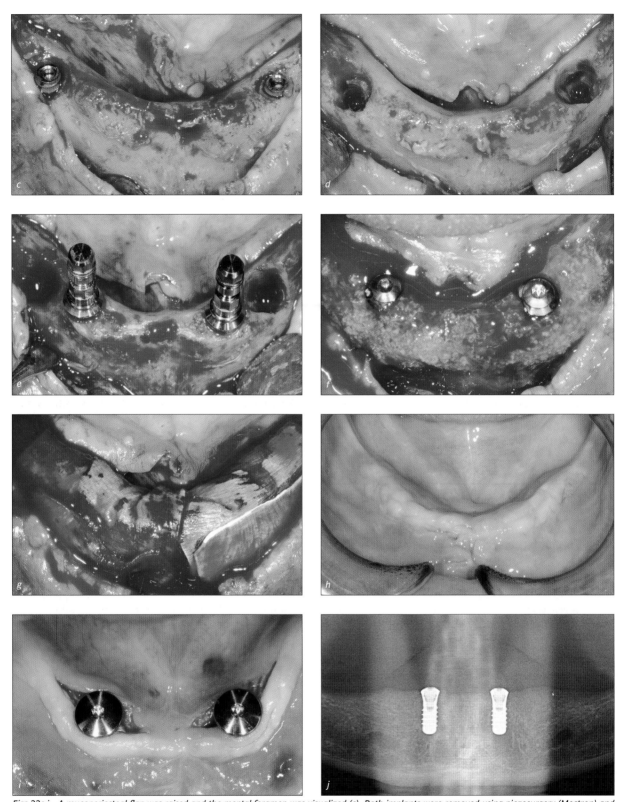

Figs 22c-j   A mucoperiosteal flap was raised and the mental foramen was visualized (c). Both implants were removed using piezosurgery (Mectron) and the reverse screw techniques (BTI) (d). Two new implants were placed (SP Roxolid, diameter 4.1 mm, length 10 mm; Institut Straumann AG, Basel, Switzerland) (e). The defects were grafted with autologous bone chips, DBBM (Bio-Oss; Geistlich Pharma, Wolhusen, Switzerland) and collagen membrane (Bio-Gide) using contour augmentation (f-g). After ten weeks of healing, at abutment connection, the soft tissues presented healthy and an ISQ value of 82 was measured (i). The postoperative radiograph showed a good alignment of the newly placed implants and sufficient distance from the mental foramen (j).

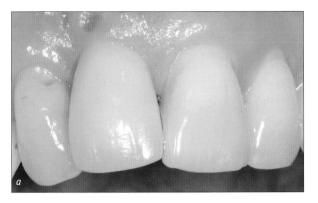
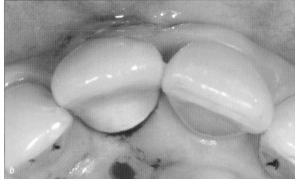
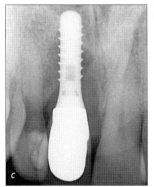
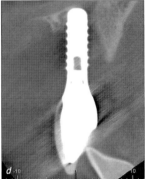
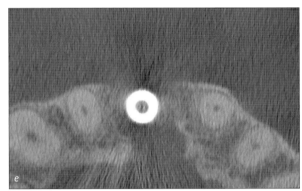

Figs 23a-e   21 years after implant placement, the patient presented with recurring pain and bleeding at site 11. Clinically bleeding on probing was observed. A pocket depth of 10 mm was measured with suppuration (a-b). The periapical radiograph reveals significant bone loss up to the 4th implant thread (c). A CBCT was taken to decide whether regeneration of the peri-implant defect is an option or whether implant removal is indicated. The CBCT revealed a complete loss of the facial bone wall and significant vertical bone loss on the palatal bone wall in combination with a cratering defect perforating incisal canal (d-e). It was decided to remove the implant.

The literature on treatment outcomes of immediate implant replacements in esthetic sites is very scare and no clinical guidelines are available so far on implants placed in previously failed sites. Some clinical data demonstrated that the short-term survival rate of dental implants (71%–83%) was lower compared with earlier reports for implants placed in pristine bone sites (Grossmann and Levin 2007), whereas recent studies showed higher survival rates between 85-94% (Mardinger and coworkers 2012; Wang and coworkers 2015). More predictable survival rates of 94% after an observation period of 5.8 years were obtained by using moderately rough implant surfaces combined with bone augmentation in low-risk patient profiles (Wang and coworkers 2015). However, the available literature is very limited. Further clinical studies, with more extensive clinical cases and a longer follow-up period, are required to obtain sufficient evidence on this procedure.

Delayed reimplantation should always be considered if a severe infection is present or if the residual bone volume does not allow the correct placement of an implant with adequate dimensions. To reduce further bone loss following implant removal, simultaneous ridge preservation or staged ridge augmentation techniques can be applied (Darby and coworkers 2009; Vignoletti and coworkers 2012; McAllister and Haghighat 2007) (Figs 23 and 24). If an implant cannot be replaced immediately after its removal, consideration should be given to reconstructing the site to allow a replacement later (Fig 25). It should be noted, however, that the literature concerning bone augmentation after implant removal is very limited as well. Site reconstruction should follow the established principles of GBR and socket grafting (Figs 23a-e to 30a-n; Dr. V. Chappuis; see also Chapter 5; prosthetic restoration by Dr. Ramona Buser, Department of Reconstructive Dentistry and Gerodontology, University of Bern, Switzerland).

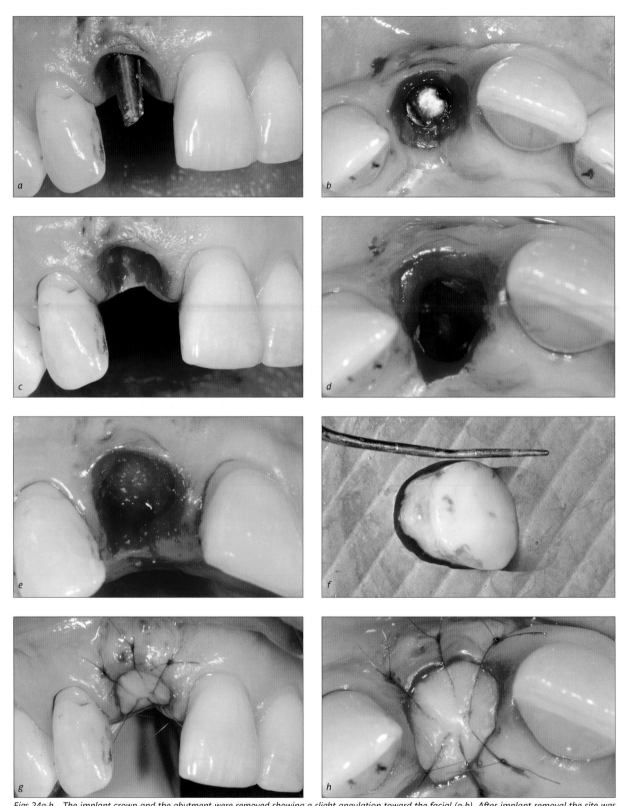

Figs 24a-h   The implant crown and the abutment were removed showing a slight angulation toward the facial (a-b). After implant removal the site was carefully cleaned and rinsed (c-d). Bio-Oss Collagen (Geistlich Pharma) was placed into the wound to preserve as much bone as possible (e). In order to optimize the regenerative outcome, a free gingival graft was harvested from the palate using a punch (f). The graft was adapted to the surgical site and sutured with 7-0 Seralon (Serag-Wiesner, Naila, Germany) (g-h).

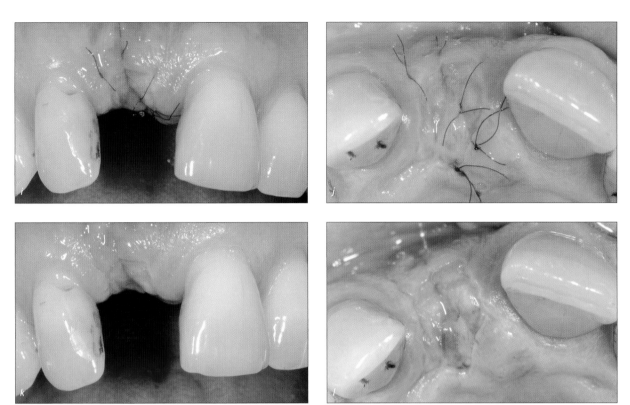

Figs 24i-l   After two weeks, the site had healed uneventfully. The free gingival graft nicely integrated with the surrounding soft tissues.

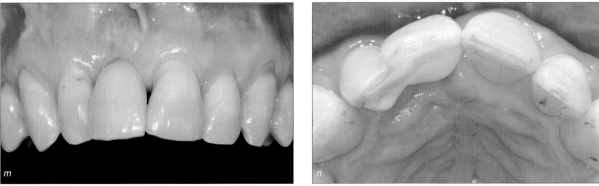

Figs 24m-n   Due to the significant bone defect and the patient's wish not to reduce smoking, a resin-bonded fixed dental prosthesis was provided.

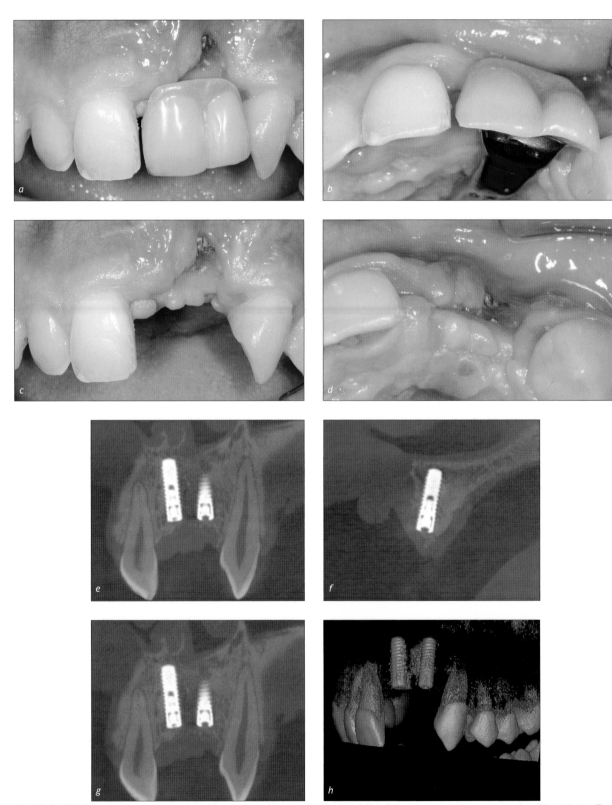

Figs 25a-h This 21-year-old patient presented with esthetic and regenerative implant failure following staged ridge augmentation. The patient suffered from chronic pain in the anterior maxilla. A large vertical and horizontal bone- and soft-tissue defect was visible. The site showed signs of chronic infection and biomaterial leaking from the previously grafted site. An orthodontic implant on the palate served as a fixed provisional (a-d). The CBCT revealed insufficient bone regeneration of the previously grafted site. In addition, the two NDI were placed too far apically (e-h). Implant removal was planned. Due to the infection of the implant site and the large soft-tissue defect exhibiting significant scar tissue, delayed reimplantation was chosen.

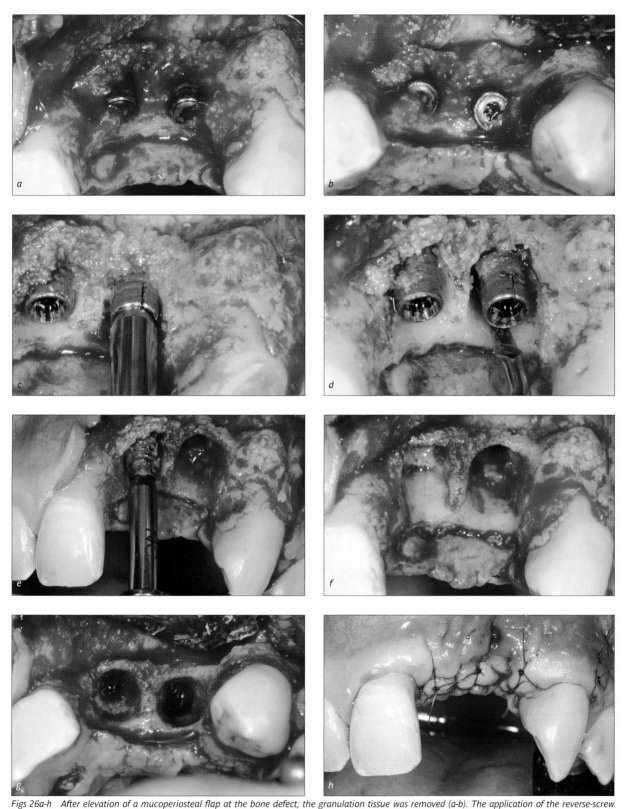

Figs 26a-h   After elevation of a mucoperiosteal flap at the bone defect, the granulation tissue was removed (a-b). The application of the reverse-screw system (BTI) caused a longitudinal fracture of the implant (c-g). Due to the significant infection of the site, grafting was delayed to a second-stage surgery. After implant removal, a collagen sponge was inserted to improve soft-tissue healing (Collagen Tissue cone, Baxter, Deerfield, IL, USA) and the wound margins were adapted (h).

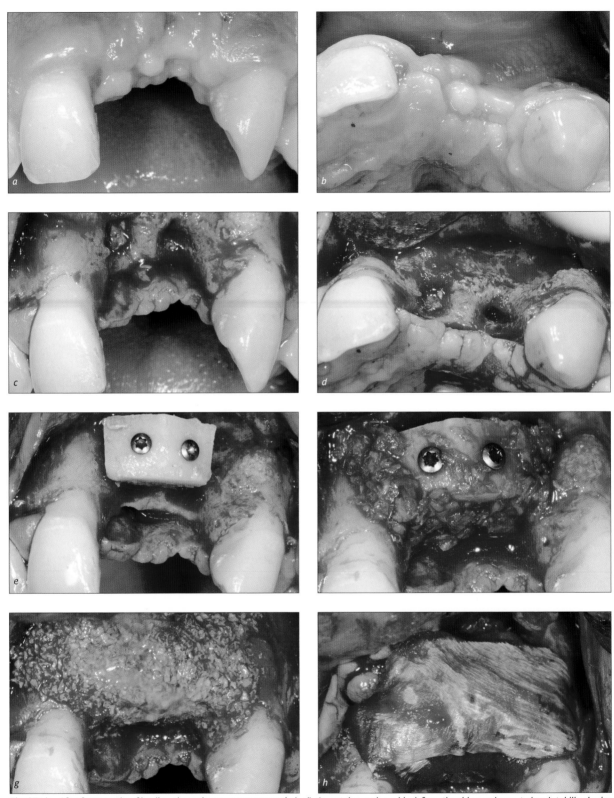

Figs 27a-h   After four months of healing, the patient was asymptomatic (a-d). An autologous bone block from the chin was harvested and stabilized using two traction screws (Medartis, Basel, Switzerland) (e). The voids between the recipient site and the block were filled with autologous bone chips (f). In order to minimize postsurgical graft resorption, the autologous bone was protected by DBBM (Bio-Oss) and a double layer of a collagen membrane (Bio-Gide) (g-h).

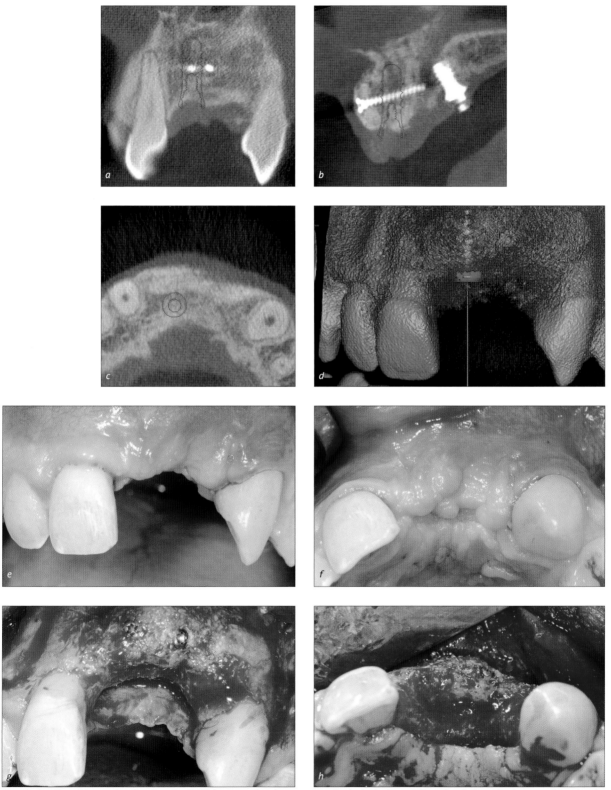

Figs 28a-h   After eight months of healing, the CBCT shown excellent bone regeneration in the horizontal dimension. Only one implant was planned at site 21 to optimize the esthetic outcome. An STL implant design was chosen to compensate for the vertical deficiency (SP, diameter 4.1 mm, length 10 mm; Institut Straumann AG) (a-d). The soft tissue showed improved keratinization and integrity at reentry (e-f). After flap elevation, the grafted site revealed no signs of resorption, since the fixation screws were well covered by bone (g-h).

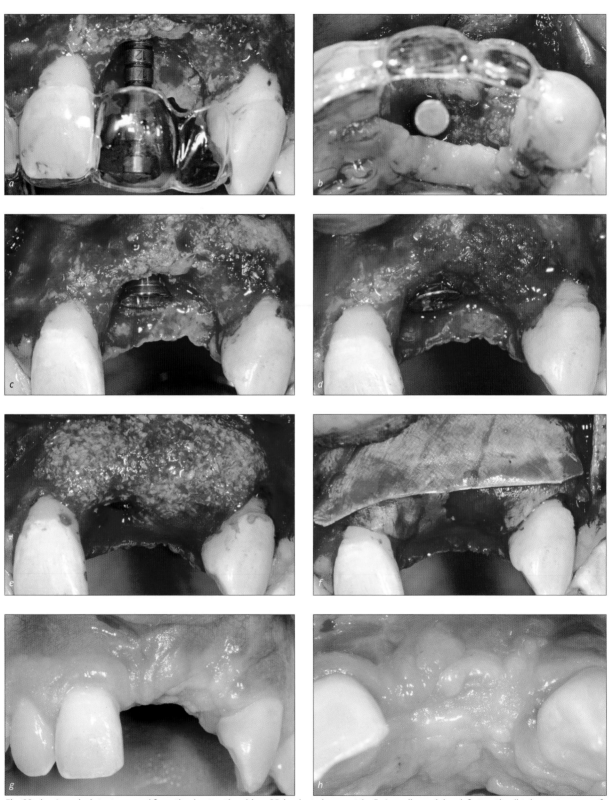

Figs 29a-h   A surgical stent was used for optimal restoration-driven 3D implant placement (a-d). A small remaining defect on the distal aspect was regrafted using autologous bone, DBBM (Bio-Oss), and Collagen Membrane (Bio-Gide) (c-f). At abutment connection, the site showed uneventful healing (g-h).

For more in-depth information on complications, please check out the ITI Online Academy's congress lecture "Biological and Technical Complications in Implant Dentistry" by Dr. Lisa J. A. Heitz-Mayfield (charges apply). See what else the Online Academy has to offer at **academy.iti.org**

For more in-depth information on how to manage esthetic failures, please check out the ITI Online Academy's congress lecture "Surgical Treatment of Esthetic Disasters" by Dr. Waldemar Daudt Polido (charges apply). See what else the Online Academy has to offer at **academy.iti.org**

9 <u>Conclusions</u>

W. Martin, V. Chappuis

The main objective of this volume of the ITI Treatment Guide is to comprehensively address the current therapeutic modalities and materials used in the treatment of patients requiring single-tooth replacement in the esthetic zone. The authors' goal is to provide state-of-the-art knowledge on both the surgical and restorative procedures to achieve predictable esthetic results.

Single-tooth replacement in the esthetic zone is categorized as an "advanced" or "complex" treatment in the ITI SAC Classification. Therefore, these treatments should be performed by experienced clinicians. A detailed esthetic risk assessment (ERA) and treatment planning prior to implant surgery is the key to achieving predictable esthetic results. The ERA is a tool used to isolate factors that could jeopardize a successful esthetic outcome. In addition, the surgical and prosthetic considerations in this Volume 10 of the ITI Treatment Guide provide the experienced clinician with therapeutic approaches that optimize functional and esthetic outcomes from a long-term perspective. Finally, the clinician will gain insights into how to analyze and handle esthetic complications.

The educational content is based on clinical recommendations by the ITI Consensus Conferences, evidence-based concepts, and derived practical procedures, specifically addressing the following topics:

1. Preoperative patient assessment based upon the SAC Classification and treatment planning using the esthetic parameters of the ERA and digital technology

Patient care begins with a detailed systematic assessment of the individual esthetic risk of a given clinical situation. This assessment includes the evaluation of patient-related general and local risk factors and their influence on the potential to achieve esthetic outcomes. The incorporation of modern technology such as cone-beam computed tomography (CBCT) in conjunction with implant planning software that highlights the planned restorative outcome will help develop an accurate plan for the surgical treatment approach. Communicating the esthetic risk to the patient ahead of time is critical for determining whether his or her expectations can be met or whether alternative treatment approaches should be explored. Of particular importance is the direct association between the complexity of a case and the importance of adhering to evidence-based treatment approaches, which is highlighted within this Treatment Guide in the form of case presentations.

2. Selection of bone grafts, biomaterials, membranes and available biologics (such as growth factors, enamel matrix proteins, or autologous platelet concentrates)

Clinical experience and a knowledge of grafting materials and adjuncts is a key to creating a stable foundation for a successful esthetic outcome. Understanding the osteogenic and osteoconductive capacity of biomaterials and available biologics is a prerequisite for successful bone regeneration. In addition, the defect morphology significantly influences the regenerative potential of the applied biomaterials, membranes, and biologics and should be taken into consideration in comprehensive treatment planning.

3. Understanding the current knowledge about post-extraction dimensional hard- and soft-tissue modifications in the esthetic zone and how they influence clinical practice; understanding the indications for ridge preservation and soft-tissue enhancement

To achieve an esthetically successful outcome, regenerating the natural hard- and soft-tissue architecture of the natural dentition is of primary concern. The healing process following tooth extraction and its related dimensional hard- and soft-tissue alterations has become an important research topic. A key prerequisite for esthetic outcomes in the anterior maxilla is an adequate three-dimensional osseous volume of the alveolar ridge, including an intact facial bone wall of sufficient thickness and height in combination with correct restoration-driven implant positioning. Deficiencies of the facial bone anatomy have a negative impact on esthetics and are a critical causative factor for esthetic implant complications and failures. Therefore, clinicians need to understand the physiological dimensional changes in the ridge after tooth extraction and implant placement in the anterior maxilla. Based on this knowledge, the clinician can decide on the most suitable treatment protocol, the proper timing, and the selection of the most appropriate biomaterials for successful treatment outcomes.

4. Surgical step-by-step management, selecting the appropriate implant design, length, and diameter to optimize treatment outcomes

Recent advances in implant biomaterials, implant design, and surface technology require extensive knowledge about indications for their use and proper handling. New titanium alloys have been developed with the goal to improve mechanical properties, not only to minimize the risk of implant fracture but also to expand the indications for narrow-diameter implants (NDI) in sites with limited bone volume. In order to enhance its strength, titanium can be alloyed with other elements, such as aluminum, vanadium, or zirconium. Although the same surface modifications (by sandblasting and acid-etching) can be applied to commercially pure titanium (SLActive) and some titanium alloy implants, it is possible that these new implant materials may end up with different surface characteristics (e.g., in terms of roughness, hydrophilicity, and wettability).

More recently, yttria-stabilized zirconia as a new dental implant material was brought to the market. Similar to the development of titanium implants, one- and two-piece zirconia implants have been developed. Ceramic implants made of zirconia appear to be a highly interesting biomaterial for medical applications, and zirconia implants have been proposed as a possible alternative to titanium implants. However, as of today, zirconia implants in dentistry have demonstrated less favorable clinical survival and success rates than titanium implants. Well-conducted long-term studies are urgently needed to permit a meaningful assessment of the survival or success rates of zirconia implants and recommendations on their use compared to titanium.

5. Prosthetic considerations, techniques and materials to maximize soft-tissue contours, restoration design, material selection and optical properties with a focus on guidelines related to the recommended clinical and laboratory step-by-step procedures.

The restorative phase of implant rehabilitation is of equal importance, as the application of sound, evidence-based clinical and laboratory protocols is critical to create a restoration the mimics the adjacent teeth in terms of shade, contours, and optical properties. In particular, the shaping of the transition zone with properly contoured provisional restorations (preferably screw-retained) and the capturing of these tissues (customized impression copings) are key aspects of communicating a restorative design to the laboratory technician. The introduction of CAD/CAM technology to aid in the fabrication of customized abutments, frameworks and esthetic restorative materials (lithium disilicate and zirconia) have enhanced the opportunities to create these esthetic restorations.

6. Analysis and management of surgical and prosthetic complications found in areas of esthetic importance.

When implant-supported restorations would result in esthetic compromise, careful evaluation of the cause is necessary. Subsequent surgical and prosthetic options to improve the result should be discussed and weighted against removal of the implant. The patient should be very well informed, prior to the initiation of care, of the compromised esthetic result and any additional surgical procedures needed to increase the soft- and hard-tissue volume, as these procedures are not as predictable once implants are in place. In some situations, prosthetic materials (gingival porcelains, composites and acrylic resins) could aid in successfully masking tissue defects when designed to maintain access to hygiene while providing an acceptable esthetic outcome.

10 <u>References</u>

References have been listed in the order of (1) the first or only author's last name and (2) the year of publication. Identical short references are distinguished in the text by lowercase letters, which if used are given in parentheses at the end of the respective entry in this list of references.

Abduo J, Lyons K, Bennani V, Waddell N, Swain M. Fit of screw-retained fixed implant frameworks fabricated by different methods: a systematic review. Int J Prosthod. **2011** May – Jun; 24(3): 207 – 220.

Abrahamsson I, Berglundh T, Glantz PO, Lindhe J. The mucosal attachment at different abutments. An experimental study in dogs. J Clin Periodontol. **1998** Sep; 25(9): 721 – 727.

Abrahamsson I, Berglundh T. Effects of different implant surfaces and designs on marginal bone-level alterations: a review. Clin Oral Implants Res. **2009** Sep; 20 (Suppl 4): 207 – 215.

Adell R, Lekholm U, Rockler B, Brånemark PI. A 15-year study of osseointegrated implants in the treatment of the edentulous jaw. Int J Oral Surg. **1981** Dec; 10(6): 387 – 416.

Adell R, Eriksson B, Lekholm U, Brånemark PI, Jemt T. Long-term follow-up study of osseointegrated implants in the treatment of totally edentulous jaws. Int J Oral Maxillofac Implants. **1990** Winter: 5(4):347 – 359.

Adibrad M, Shahabuei M, Sahabi M. Significance of the width of keratinized mucosa on the health status of the supporting tissue around implants supporting overdentures. J Oral Implantol. **2009**; 35(5): 232 – 237.

Agar JR, Cameron SM, Hughbanks JC, Parker MH. Cement removal from restorations luted to titanium abutments with simulated subgingival margins. J Prosthet Dent. **1998** Jul; 78(1): 43 – 47.

Aghaloo TL, Moy PK. Which hard tissue augmentation techniques are the most successful in furnishing bony support for implant placement? Int J Oral Maxillofac Implants. **2007**; 22 (Suppl): 49 – 70.

Akcalı A, Schneider D, Ünlü F, Bıcakcı N, Köse T, Hämmerle CH. Soft tissue augmentation of ridge defects in the maxillary anterior area using two different methods: a randomized controlled clinical trial. Clin Oral Implants Res. **2015** Jun; 26(6): 688 – 695.

Akgül AA, Toygar TU. Natural craniofacial changes in the third decade of life: a longitudinal study. Am J Orthod Dentofacial Orthop. **2002** Nov; 122(5): 512 – 522.

Alani A, Maglad A, Nohl F. Br Dent J. The prosthetic management of gingival aesthetics. Br Dent J. **2011** Jan 22; 210(2): 63 – 69.

Albert AM, Ricanek K Jr, Patterson E. A review of the literature on the aging adult skull and face: implications for forensic science research and applications. Forensic Sci Int. **2007** Oct; 172(1): 1 – 9.

Albrektsson T, Zarb G, Worthington P, Eriksson AR. The long-term efficacy of currently used dental implants: a review and proposed criteria of success. Int J Oral Maxillofac Implants. **1986** Summer; 1(1): 11 – 25.

Albrektsson T, Dahlin C, Jemt T, Sennerby L, Turri A, Wennerberg A. Is Marginal Bone Loss around Oral Implants the Result of a Provoked Foreign Body Reaction? Clin Implant Dent Relat Res. **2014**; 16: 155 – 165.

AlGhamdi AS. Successful treatment of early implant failure: a case series. Clin Implant Dent Relat Res. **2012** Jun; 14(3): 380 – 387.

Alharbi HM, Babay N, Alzoman H, Basudan S, Anil S, Jansen JA. Bone morphology changes around two types of bone-level implants installed in fresh extraction sockets—a histomorphometric study in Beagle dogs. Clin Oral Implants Res. **2015** Sep; 26(9): 1106 – 1112.

Al-Nawas B, Brägger U, Meijer HJ, Naert I, Persson R, Perucchi A, Quirynen M, Raghoebar GM, Reichert TE, Romeo E, Santing HJ, Schimmel M, Storelli S, ten Bruggenkate C, Vandekerckhove B, Wagner W, Wismeijer D, Müller F. A double-blind randomized controlled trial (RCT) of Titanium-13Zirconium versus Titanium Grade IV small-diameter bone level implants in edentulous mandibles—results from a 1-year observation period. Clin Implant Dent Relat Res. **2012** Dec; 14(6): 896 – 904.

Altuna P, Lucas-Taulé E, Gargallo-Albiol J, Figueras-Álvarez O, Hernández-Alfaro F, Nart J. Clinical evidence on titanium-zirconium dental implants: a systematic review and meta-analysis. Int J Oral Maxillofac Surg. **2016** Jul; 45(7): 842 – 850.

American Dental Association. 2007 Survey of Current Issues in Dentistry (SCID). **2008.**

Andersson L, Emami-Kristiansen Z, Högström J. Single-tooth implant treatment in the anterior region of the maxilla for treatment of tooth loss after trauma: a retrospective clinical and interview study. Dent Traumatol. **2003** Jun; 19(3): 126 – 131.

Andersson B, Bergenblock S, Fürst B, Jemt T. Long-term function of single-implant restorations: a 17- to 19-year follow-up study on implant infraposition related to the shape of the face and patients' satisfaction. Clin Implant Dent Relat Res. **2013** Aug; 15(4): 471 – 480.

Andreiotelli M, Wenz HJ, Kohal RJ. Are ceramic implants a viable alternative to titanium implants? A systematic literature review. Clin Oral Implants Res. **2009** Sep; 20 (Suppl 4): 32 – 47.

Anitua E, Orive G. Short implants in maxillae and mandibles: a retrospective study with 1 to 8 years of follow-up. J Periodontol. **2010** Jun; 81(6): 819 – 826.

Anitua E, Orive G. A new approach for atraumatic implant explantation and immediate implant installation. Oral Surg Oral Med Oral Pathol Oral Radiol. **2012** Mar; 113(3): e19 – e25.

Annibali S, Bignozzi I, Cristalli MP, Graziani F, La Monaca G, Polimeni A. Peri-implant marginal bone level: a systematic review and meta-analysis of studies comparing platform switching versus conventionally restored implants. J Clin Periodontol. **2012** Nov; 39(11): 1097 – 1113.

Annibali S, Bignozzi I, Cristalli MP, Graziani F, La Monaca G, Polimeni A. Peri-implant marginal bone level: a systematic review and meta-analysis of studies comparing platform switching versus conventionally restored implants. J Clin Periodontol. **2012** Nov; 39(11): 1097 – 1113. (**a**)

Annibali S, Cristalli MP, Dell'Aquila D, Bignozzi I, La Monaca G, Pilloni A. Short dental implants: a systematic review. J Dent Res. **2012** Jan; 91(1): 25 – 32. (**b**)

Antoun H, Sitbon JM, Martinez H, Missika P. A prospective randomized study comparing two techniques of bone augmentation: onlay graft alone or associated with a membrane. Clin Oral Implants Res. **2001** Dec; 12(6): 632 – 639.

Araújo MG, Sonohara M, Hayacibara R, Cardaropoli G, Lindhe J. Lateral ridge augmentation by the use of grafts comprised of autologous bone or a biomaterial. An experiment in the dog. J Clin Periodontol. **2002** Dec; 29(12): 1122 – 1131.

Araújo MG, Sukekava F, Wennström JL, Lindhe J. Ridge alterations following implant placement in fresh extraction sockets: an experimental study in the dog. J Clin Periodontol. **2005** Jun; 32(6): 645 – 652. (**a**)

Araújo MG, Lindhe J. Dimensional ridge alterations following tooth extraction. An experimental study in the dog. J Clin Periodontol. **2005** Feb; 32(2): 212 – 218. (**b**)

Araújo MG, Lindhe J. Ridge alterations following tooth extraction with and without flap elevation: an experimental study in the dog. Clin Oral Implants Res. **2009** Jun; 20(6): 545 – 549. (**a**)

Araújo MG, Lindhe J. Ridge preservation with the use of Bio-Oss collagen: A 6-month study in the dog. Clin Oral Implants Res. **2009** May; 20(5): 433 – 440. (**b**)

Araújo MG, da Silva JC, de Mendonca AF, Lindhe J. Ridge alterations following grafting of fresh extraction sockets in man. A randomized clinical trial. Clin Oral Implants Res. **2015** Apr; 26(4): 417 – 412. (**a**)

Araújo MG, Silva CO, Misawa M, Sukekava F. Alveolar socket healing: what can we learn? Periodontol 2000. **2015** Jun; 68(1): 122 – 134. (**b**)

Ashman A. An immediate tooth root replacement: an implant cylinder and synthetic bone combination. J Oral Implantol. **1990**; 16(1): 28 – 38.

Ata-Ali J, Ata-Ali F, Peñarrocha-Oltra D, Galindo-Moreno P. What is the impact of bisphosphonate therapy upon dental implant survival? A systematic review and meta-analysis. Clin Oral Implants Res. **2016** Feb; 27(2): e38 – 46.

Atieh MA, Ibrahim HM, Atieh AH. Platform switching for marginal bone preservation around dental implants: a systematic review and meta-analysis. J Periodontol. **2010** Oct; 81(10): 1350 – 1366.

Attard NJ, Zarb GA. Immediate and early implant loading protocols: a literature review of clinical studies. J Prosthet Dent. **2005** Sep; 94(3): 242 – 258.

Augthun M, Yildirim M, Spiekermann H, Biesterfeld S. Healing of bone defects in combination with immediate implants using the membrane technique. Int J Oral Maxillofac Implants. **1995** Jul–Aug; 10(4): 421–428.

Avila-Ortiz G, Elangovan S, Kramer KW, Blanchette D, Dawson DV. Effect of alveolar ridge preservation after tooth extraction: a systematic review and meta-analysis. J Dent Res. **2014** Oct; 93(10): 950–958.

Barter S, Stone P, Brägger U. A pilot study to evaluate the success and survival rate of titanium-zirconium implants in partially edentulous patients: results after 24 months of follow-up. Clin Oral Implants Res. **2012** Jul; 23(7): 873–881.

Barzilay I, Irene T. Gingival prostheses—a review. J Can Dent Assoc. **2003** Feb; 69(2): 74–78.

Batista EL Jr., Batista FC, Novaes AB Jr. Management of soft tissue ridge deformities with acellular dermal matrix. Clinical approach and outcome after 6 months of treatment. J Periodontol. **2001** Feb; 72(2): 265–273.

Becker W, Goldstein M, Becker BE, Sennerby L. Minimally invasive flapless implant surgery: a prospective multicenter study. Clin Implant Dent Relat Res. **2005**; 7 (Suppl 1): S21–S27.

Belser UC. Ästhetik-Checkliste für den festsitzenden Zahnersatz. In: Schärer P, Rinn L, Kopp FR (eds). Ästhetische Richtlinien für die rekonstruktive Zahnheilkunde. Berlin: Quintessenz, **1980**. 187–204.

Belser UC, Buser D, Hess D, Schmid B, Bernard JP, Lang NP. Aesthetic implant restorations in partially edentulous patients—a critical appraisal. Periodontol 2000. **1998** Jun; 17: 132–150.

Belser UC, Buser D, Higginbottom F. Consensus statements and recommended clinical procedures regarding esthetics in implant dentistry. Int J Oral Maxillofac Implants. **2004**; 19 (Suppl): 73–74.

Belser UC, Grütter L, Vailati F, Bornstein MM, Weber HP, Buser D. Outcome evaluation of early placed maxillary anterior single-tooth implants using objective esthetic criteria: a cross-sectional, retrospective study in 45 patients with a 2- to 4-year follow-up using pink and white esthetic scores. J Periodontol. **2009** Jan; 80(1): 140–151.

Benic GI, Gallucci GO, Mokti M, Hämmerle CH, Weber HP, Jung RE. Titanium-zirconium narrow-diameter versus titanium regular-diameter implants for anterior and premolar single crowns: 1-year results of a randomized controlled clinical study. J Clin Periodontol. **2013** Nov; 40(11): 1052–1061.

Berberi A, Tehini G, Rifai K, Bou Nasser Eddine F, Badran B, Akl H. Leakage evaluation of original and compatible implant-abutment connections: In vitro study using Rhodamine B. J Dent Biomech. **2014** Aug 11; 5: 1758736014547143.

Berglundh T, Lindhe J. Dimension of the periimplant mucosa. Biological width revisited. J Clin Periodontol. **1996** Oct; 23(10): 971–973.

Berglundh T, Lindhe J. Healing around implants placed in bone defects treated with Bio-Oss. An experimental study in the dog. Clin Oral Implants Res. **1997** Apr; 8(2): 117–124.

Berglundh T, Giannobile WV. Investigational clinical research in implant dentistry: beyond observational and descriptive studies. J Dent Res. **2013** Dec; 92 (12 Suppl): 107S–108S.

Bernard JP, Schatz JP, Christou P, Belser U, Kiliaridis S. Long-term vertical changes of the anterior maxillary teeth adjacent to single implants in young and mature adults. A retrospective study. J Clin Periodontol. **2004** Nov; 31(11): 1024–1028.

Bishara SE, Treder JE, Jakobsen JR. Facial and dental changes in adulthood. Am J Orthod Dentofacial Orthop. **1994** Aug; 106(2): 175–186.

Bonewald LF. The amazing osteocyte. J Bone Miner Res. **2011** Feb; 26(2): 229–238.

Boogaarts JD, Grotenhuis JA, Bartels RH, Beems T. Use of a novel absorbable hydrogel for augmentation of dural repair: results of a preliminary clinical study. Neurosurgery. **2005** Jul; 57 (1 Suppl): 146–151; discussion 146–151.

Bormann KH, Gellrich NC, Kniha H, Dard M, Wieland M, Gahlert M. Biomechanical evaluation of a microstructured zirconia implant by a removal torque comparison with a standard Ti-SLA implant. Clin Oral Implants Res. **2012** Oct; 23(10): 1210–1216.

Bornstein MM, Hart CN, Halbritter SA, Morton D, Buser D. Early loading of nonsubmerged titanium implants with a chemically modified sand-blasted and acid-etched surface: 6-month results of a prospective case series study in the posterior mandible focusing on peri-implant crestal bone changes and implant stability quotient (ISQ) values. Clin Implant Dent Relat Res. **2009** Dec; 11(4): 338–347. (**a**)

Bornstein MM, Heynen G, Bosshardt DD, Buser D. Effect of two bioabsorbable barrier membranes on bone regeneration of standardized defects in calvarial bone: a comparative histomorphometric study in pigs. J Periodontol. **2009** Aug; 80(8): 1289–1299. (**b**)

Bornstein MM, von Arx T, Bosshardt DD: Properties of barrier membranes. In: Buser D (ed). 20 years of guided bone regeneration. Chicago: Quintessence, **2009**: 47–69. (**c**)

Bornstein MM, Wittneben JG, Brägger U, Buser D. Early loading at 21 days of non-submerged titanium implants with a chemically modified sandblasted and acid-etched surface: 3-year results of a prospective study in the posterior mandible. J Periodontol. **2010** Jun; 81(6): 809–818.

Bornstein MM, Scarfe WC, Vaughn VM, Jacobs R. Cone beam computed tomography in implant dentistry: a systematic review focusing on guidelines, indications, and radiation dose risks. Int J Oral Maxillofac Implants. **2014**; 29 (Suppl): 55–77. (**a**)

Bornstein MM, Al-Nawas B, Kuchler U, Tahmaseb A. Consensus statements and recommended clinical procedures regarding contemporary surgical and radiographic techniques in implant dentistry. Int J Oral Maxillofac Implants. **2014**; 29 (Suppl): 78–82. (**b**)

Bosshardt DD. Biological mediators and periodontal regeneration: a review of enamel matrix proteins at the cellular and molecular levels. J Clin Periodontol. **2008** Sep; 35 (8 Suppl): 87–105.

Botha PJ, Gluckman HL. The gingival prosthesis—a literature review. SADJ. **1999** Jul; 54(7): 288–290.

Botticelli D, Persson LG, Lindhe J, Berglundh T. Bone tissue formation adjacent to implants placed in fresh extraction sockets: an experimental study in dogs. Clin Oral Implants Res. **2006** Aug; 17(4): 351–358.

Bottino MC, Thomas V, Schmidt G, Vohra YK, Chu TM, Kowolik MJ, Janowski GM. Recent advances in the development of GTR/GBR membranes for periodontal regeneration--a materials perspective. Dent Mater **2012**; 28: 703–721.

Bouri A, Jr., Bissada N, Al-Zahrani MS, Faddoul F, Nouneh I. Width of keratinized gingiva and the health status of the supporting tissues around dental implants. Int J Oral Maxillofac Implants. **2008** Mar–Apr; 23(2): 323–326.

Brägger U, Hämmerle CH, Lang NP. Immediate transmucosal implants using the principle of guided tissue regeneration (II). A cross-sectional study comparing the clinical outcome 1 year after immediate to standard implant placement. Clin Oral Implants Res. **1996** Sep; 7(3): 268–276.

Brånemark PI, Adell R, Breine U, Hansson BO, Lindström J, Ohlsson A. Intra-osseous anchorage of dental prostheses. I. Experimental studies. Scand J Plast Reconstr Surg. **1969**; 3(2): 81–100.

Bratu EA, Tandlich M, Shapira L. A rough surface implant neck with microthreads reduces the amount of marginal bone loss: a prospective clinical study. Clin Oral Implants Res. **2009** Aug; 20(8): 827–832.

Braut V, Bornstein MM, Belser U, Buser D. Thickness of the anterior maxillary facial bone wall-a retrospective radiographic study using cone beam computed tomography. Int J Periodontics Restorative Dent. **2011** Apr; 31(2): 125–131.

Broggini N, McManus LM, Hermann JS, Medina R, Schenk RK, Buser D, Cochran DL. Peri-implant inflammation defined by the implant-abutment interface. J Dent Res. **2006** May; 85(5): 473–478.

Brown SD, Payne AG. Immediately restored single implants in the aesthetic zone of the maxilla using a novel design: 1-year report. Clin Oral Implants Res. **2011** Apr; 22: 445–454.

Bunyaratavej P, Wang HL. Collagen membranes: a review. J Periodontol. **2001** Feb; 72(2): 215–229.

Burchardt H. The biology of bone graft repair. Clin Orthop Relat Res. **1983**: 28–42.

Burkhardt R, Joss A, Lang NP. Soft tissue dehiscence coverage around endosseous implants: a prospective cohort study. Clin Oral Implants Res. **2008** May; 19(4): 451–457.

Busenlechner D, Tangl S, Arnhart C, Redl H, Schuh C, Watzek G, Gruber R. Resorption of deproteinized bovine bone mineral in a porcine calvaria augmentation model. Clin Oral Implants Res. **2012** Jan; 23(1): 95–99.

Buser D, Weber HP, Lang NP. Tissue integration of non-submerged implants. 1-year results of a prospective study with 100 ITI hollow-cylinder and hollow-screw implants. Clin Oral Implants Res. **1990** Dec; 1(1): 33–40.

Buser, D, Dula K, Belser U, Hirt HP, Berthold H. Localized ridge augmentation using guided bone regeneration. 1. Surgical procedure in the maxilla. Int J Periodontics Restorative Dent. **1993**; 13(1); 29–45.

Buser D, Dula K, Hirt HP, Schenk RK. Lateral ridge augmentation using autografts and barrier membranes: a clinical study with 40 partially edentulous patients. J Oral Maxillofac Surg. **1996** Apr; 54(4): 420–432; discussion 432–423.

Buser D, Mericske-Stern R, Bernard JP, Behneke A, Behneke N, Hirt HP, Belser UC, Lang NP. Long-term evaluation of non-submerged ITI implants. Part 1: 8-year life table analysis of a prospective multi-center study with 2359 implants. Clin Oral Implants Res. **1997** Jun; 8(3): 161–172.

Buser D, Nydegger T, Hirt HP, Cochran DL, Nolte LP. Removal torque values of titanium implants in the maxilla of miniature pigs. Int J Oral Maxillofac Implants. **1998** Sep–Oct; 13(5): 611–619. (**a**)

Buser D, Hoffmann B, Bernard JP, Lussi A, Mettler D, Schenk RK. Evaluation of filling materials in membrane--protected bone defects. A comparative histomorphometric study in the mandible of miniature pigs. Clin Oral Implants Res. **1998** Jun; 9(3): 137–150. (**b**)

Buser D, von Arx T, ten Bruggenkate C, Weingart D. Basic surgical principles with ITI implants. Clin Oral Implants Res. **2000**; 11 (Suppl 1): 59–68.

Buser D, Martin W, Belser UC. Optimizing esthetics for implant restorations in the anterior maxilla: anatomic and surgical considerations. Int J Oral Maxillofac Implants. **2004**; 19 (Suppl): 43–61. (**a**)

Buser D, Broggini N, Wieland M, Schenk RK, Denzer AJ, Cochran DL, Hoffmann B, Lussi A, Steinemann SG. Enhanced bone apposition to a chemically modified SLA titanium surface. J Dent Res. **2004** Jul; 83(7): 529–533. (**b**)

Buser D, Bornstein MM, Weber HP, Grütter L, Schmid B, Belser UC. Early implant placement with simultaneous guided bone regeneration following single-tooth extraction in the esthetic zone: a cross-sectional, retrospective study in 45 subjects with a 2- to 4-year follow-up. J Periodontol. **2008** Sep; 79(9): 1773–1781.

Buser D, Chen ST, Weber HP, Belser UC. Early implant placement following single-tooth extraction in the esthetic zone: biologic rationale and surgical procedures. Int J Periodontics Restorative Dent. **2008** Oct; 28(5): 441–451.

Buser D, Halbritter S, Hart C, Bornstein MM, Grütter L, Chappuis V, Belser UC. Early implant placement with simultaneous guided bone regeneration following single-tooth extraction in the esthetic zone: 12-month results of a prospective study with 20 consecutive patients. J Periodontol. **2009** Jan; 80(1): 152–162.

Buser D, Wittneben J, Bornstein MM, Grütter L, Chappuis V, Belser UC. Stability of contour augmentation and esthetic outcomes of implant-supported single crowns in the esthetic zone: 3-year results of a prospective study with early implant placement postextraction. J Periodontol. **2011** Mar; 82(3): 342–349.

Buser D, Janner SF, Wittneben JG, Brägger U, Ramseier CA, Salvi GE. 10-year survival and success rates of 511 titanium implants with a sandblasted and acid-etched surface: a retrospective study in 303 partially edentulous patients. Clin Implant Dent Relat Res. **2012** Dec; 14(8): 839–851.

Buser D, Chappuis V, Bornstein MM, Wittneben JG, Frei M, Belser UC. Long-term stability of contour augmentation with early implant placement following single tooth extraction in the esthetic zone: a prospective, cross-sectional study in 41 patients with a 5- to 9-year follow-up. J Periodontol. **2013** Nov; 84(11): 1517–1527. (**a**)

Buser D, Chappuis V, Kuchler U, Bornstein MM, Wittneben JG, Buser R, Cavusoglu Y, Belser UC. Long-term stability of early implant placement with contour augmentation. J Dent Res. **2013** Dec; 92 (12 Suppl): 176S–182S. (**b**)

Buser D, Chappuis V, Belser UC, Chen S: Implant placement post extraction in esthetic single tooth sites: when immediate, when early, when late? Periodontol 2000. **2017** Feb; 73(1): 84 – 102.

Butkevica A, Nathanson D, Pober R, Strating H. Measurements of repeated tightening and loosening torque of seven different implant/abutment connection designs and their modifications: an in vitro study. J Prosthodont. **2015** Mar 22. [Epub ahead of print.] .

Byrne PJ, Irwin C, Mullally B, Allen W, Ziada H. Periodontics: 8. Periodontal problems associated with compromised anterior teeth. Dent Update. **2008** Jan – Feb; 35(1): 21 – 22, 24 – 26, 28.

Caballé-Serrano J, Bosshardt DD, Buser D, Gruber R. Proteomic analysis of porcine bone-conditioned medium. Int J Oral Maxillofac Implants. **2014** Sep – Oct; 29(5): 1208 – 1215d.

Cairo F, Pagliaro U, Nieri M. Treatment of gingival recession with coronally advanced flap procedures: a systematic review. J Clin Periodontol. **2008** Sep; 35 (8 Suppl): 136 – 162.

Calcaterra R, Di Girolamo M, Mirisola C, Baggi L. Effects of repeated screw tightening on implant abutment interfaces in terms of bacterial and yeast leakage in vitro: one-time abutment versus the multiscrewing technique. Int J Periodontics Restorative Dent. **2016** Mar – Apr; 36(2): 275 – 280.

Caneva M, Salata LA, de Souza SS, Bressan E, Botticelli D, Lang NP. Hard tissue formation adjacent to implants of various size and configuration immediately placed into extraction sockets: an experimental study in dogs. Clin Oral Implants Res. **2010** Sep; 21(9): 885 – 890.

Capa N. An alternative treatment approach to gingival recession: gingiva-colored partial porcelain veneers: a clinical report. J Prosthet Dent. **2007** Aug; 98(2): 82 – 84.

Carbonell JM, Martin IS, Santos A, Pujol A, Sanz-Moliner JD, Nart J. High-density polytetrafluoroethylene membranes in guided bone and tissue regeneration procedures: a literature review. Int J Oral Maxillofac Surg. **2014** Jan; 43(1): 75 – 84.

Cardaropoli G, Araújo M, Lindhe J. Dynamics of bone tissue formation in tooth extraction sites. An experimental study in dogs. J Clin Periodontol. **2003** Sep; 30(9): 809 – 818.

Cardaropoli D, Re S, Corrente G. The Papilla Presence Index (PPI): a new system to assess interproximal papillary levels. Int J Periodontics Restorative Dent. **2004** Oct; 24(5): 488 – 492.

Carr AB, Brunski JB, Hurley E. Effects of fabrication, finishing, and polishing procedures on preload in prostheses using conventional 'gold' and plastic cylinders. Int J Oral Maxillofac Implants. **1996** Sep – Oct; 11(5): 589 – 598.

Cascione D, Nowzari H, Kim TH. Simulated tissue in modern implant dentistry. Spectrum Dialogue. **2008**: 7: 64 – 76.

Cavalcanti AG, Fonseca FT, Zago CD, Brito Junior RB, França FM. Efficacy of gutta-percha and polytetrafluoroethylene tape to microbiologically seal the screw access channel of different prosthetic implant abutments. Clin Implant Dent Relat Res. **2016** Aug; 18(4): 778 – 787.

Chambrone L, Sukekava F, Araújo MG, Pustiglioni FE, Chambrone LA, Lima LA. Root coverage procedures for the treatment of localised recession-type defects. Cochrane Database Syst Rev. **2009** Apr 15: (2) CD007161.

Chappuis V, Gamer L, Cox K, Lowery JW, Bosshardt DD, Rosen V. Periosteal BMP2 activity drives bone graft healing. Bone. **2012** Oct; 51(4): 800 – 809.

Chappuis V, Buser R, Brägger U, Bornstein MM, Salvi GE, Buser D. Long-term outcomes of dental implants with a titanium plasma-sprayed surface: a 20-year prospective case series study in partially edentulous patients. Clin Implant Dent Relat Res. **2013** Dec; 15(6): 780 – 790. (**a**)

Chappuis V, Engel O, Reyes M, Shahim K, Nolte LP, Buser D. Ridge alterations post-extraction in the esthetic zone: a 3D analysis with CBCT. J Dent Res. **2013** Dec; 92 (12 Suppl): 195S-201S. (**b**)

Chappuis V, Engel O, Shahim K, Reyes M, Katsaros C, Buser D. Soft-tissue alterations in esthetic postextraction sites: a 3-dimensional analysis. J Dent Res. **2015** Sep; 94 (9 Suppl): 187S-193S. (**a**)

Chappuis V, Bornstein MM, Buser D, Belser U. Influence of implant neck design on facial bone crest dimensions in the esthetic zone analyzed by cone beam CT: a comparative study with a 5-to-9-year follow-up. Clin Oral Implants Res. **2016** Sep; 27(9): 1055–1064.

Chappuis V, Cavusoglu Y, Gruber R, Kuchler U, Buser D, Bosshardt DD. Osseointegration of zirconia in the presence of multinucleated giant cells. Clin Implant Dent Relat Res. **2016** Aug; 18(4): 686–698. (**b**)

Chappuis V, Cavusoglu Y, Buser D, von Arx T. Lateral ridge augmentation using autogenous block grafts and guided bone regeneration: a 10-year prospective case series study. Clin Implant Dent Relat Res. **2017** Feb; 19(1): 85–96.

Charalampakis G, Rabe P, Leonhardt A, Dahlen G. A follow-up study of peri-implantitis cases after treatment. J Clin Periodontol. **2011** Sep; 38(9): 864–871.

Chen ST, Buser D. Clinical and esthetic outcomes of implants placed in postextraction sites. Int J Oral Maxillofac Implants. **2009**; 24 (Suppl): 186–217.

Chen ST, Beagle J, Jensen SS, Chiapasco M, Darby I. Consensus statements and recommended clinical procedures regarding surgical techniques. Int J Oral Maxillofac Implants. **2009**; 24 (Suppl): 272–278. (**a**)

Chen ST, Darby IB, Reynolds EC, Clement JG. Immediate implant placement postextraction without flap elevation. J Periodontol. **2009** Jan; 80(1): 163–172. (**b**)

Chen FM, Zhang M, Wu ZF. Toward delivery of multiple growth factors in tissue engineering. Biomaterials. **2010** Aug; 31(24): 6279–6308.

Chen FM, Wu LA, Zhang M, Zhang R, Sun HH. Homing of endogenous stem/progenitor cells for in situ tissue regeneration: Promises, strategies, and translational perspectives. Biomaterials. **2011** Apr; 32(12): 3189–3209.

Chen ST, Buser D. Esthetic outcomes following immediate and early implant placement in the anterior maxilla—a systematic review. Int J Oral Maxillofac Implants. **2014**; 29 (Suppl): 186–215.

Chevalier J. What future for zirconia as a biomaterial? Biomaterials. **2006** Feb; 27(4): 535–543.

Chiapasco M, Zaniboni M, Boisco M. Augmentation procedures for the rehabilitation of deficient edentulous ridges with oral implants. Clin Oral Implants Res. **2006** Oct; 17 (Suppl 2):136–159.

Chiapasco M, Casentini P, Zaniboni M. Bone augmentation procedures in implant dentistry. Int J Oral Maxillofac Implants. **2009**; 24 (Suppl): 237–259. (**a**)

Chiapasco M, Zaniboni M. Clinical outcomes of GBR procedures to correct peri-implant dehiscences and fenestrations: a systematic review. Clin Oral Implants Res. **2009** Sep; 20 (Suppl 4): 113–123. (**b**)

Chiapasco M, Casentini P, Zaniboni M, Corsi E, Anello T. Titanium-zirconium alloy narrow-diameter implants (Straumann Roxolid® for the rehabilitation of horizontally deficient edentulous ridges: prospective study on 18 consecutive patients. Clin Oral Implants Res. **2012** Oct; 23(10): 1136–1141.

Chiapasco M, Colletti G, Coggiola A, Di Martino G, Anello T, Romeo E. Clinical outcome of the use of fresh frozen allogeneic bone grafts for the reconstruction of severely resorbed alveolar ridges: preliminary results of a prospective study. Int J Oral Maxillofac Implants. **2015** Mar–Apr; 30(2): 450–460.

Chiapasco M, Colletti G, Coggiola A, Di Martino G, Anello T, Romeo E. Clinical outcome of the use of fresh frozen allogeneic bone grafts for the reconstruction of severely resorbed alveolar ridges: preliminary results of a prospective study. Int J Oral Maxillofac Implants. **2015** Mar–Apr; 30(2): 450–460. (**a**)

Chiapasco M, Di Martino G, Anello T, Zaniboni M, Romeo E. Fresh frozen versus autogenous iliac bone for the rehabilitation of the extremely atrophic maxilla with onlay grafts and endosseous implants: preliminary results of a prospective comparative study. Clin Implant Dent Relat Res. **2015** Jan; 17 (Suppl 1): e251–266. (**b**)

Chiriac G, Herten M, Schwarz F, Rothamel D, Becker J. Autogenous bone chips: influence of a new piezo-electric device (Piezosurgery) on chip morphology, cell viability and differentiation. J Clin Periodontol. **2005** Sep; 32(9): 994–999.

Cho SC, Shetty S, Froum S, Elian N, Tarnow D. Fixed and removable provisional options for patients undergoing implant treatment. Compend Contin Educ Dent. **2005** Nov; 28(11): 604–608.

Choquet V, Hermans M, Adriaenssens P, Daelemans P, Tarnow DP, Malevez C. Clinical and radiographic evaluation of the papilla level adjacent to single-tooth dental implants. A retrospective study in the maxillary anterior region. J Periodontol **2001**; 72: 1364–1371.

Chrcanovic BR, Albrektsson T, Wennerberg A. Reasons for failures of oral implants. J Oral Rehabil. **2014** Jun; 41(6): 443–476.

Chrcanovic BR, Martins MD, Wennerberg A. Immediate placement of implants into infected sites: a systematic review. Clin Implant Dent Relat Res. **2015** Jan; 17 (Suppl 1): e1-e16.

Christensen GJ. Ridge preservation: why not? J Am Dent Assoc. **1996** May; 127(5): 669–670.

Chu SJ, Tarnow DP. Managing esthetic challenges with anterior implants. Part 1: Midfacial recession defects from etiology to resolution. Compend Contin Educ Dent. **2013** Oct; 34 Spec No 7: 26–31.

Chung DM, Oh TJ, Shotwell JL, Misch CE, Wang HL. Significance of keratinized mucosa in maintenance of dental implants with different surfaces. J Periodontol. **2006** Aug; 77(8): 1410–1420.

Cionca N, Müller N, Mombelli A. Two-piece zirconia implants supporting all-ceramic crowns: a prospective clinical study. Clin Oral Implants Res. **2015** Apr. 26(4): 413–418.

Coachman C, Salama M, Garber D, Calamita M, Salama H, Cabral G. Prosthetic gingival reconstruction in a fixed partial restoration. Part 1: introduction to artificial gingiva as an alternative therapy. Int J Periodontics Restorative Dent. **2009** Oct; 29(5): 471–477.

Coachman C, Salama M, Garber D, Calamita M, Salama H, Cabral G. Prosthetic gingival reconstruction in fixed partial restorations. Part 3: laboratory procedures and maintenance. Int J Periodontics Restorative Dent. **2010** Feb; 30(1): 19–29.

Cochran DL, Morton D, Weber HP. Consensus statements and recommended clinical procedrues regarding loading protocols for endosseous dental implants. Int J Oral Maxillofac Implants. **2004**; 19 (Suppl): 109–113.

Cochran DL, Jackson JM, Bernard JP, ten Bruggenkate CM, Buser D, Taylor TD, Weingart D, Schoolfield JD, Jones AA, Oates TW. A 5-year prospective multicenter study of early-loaded titanium implants with a sandblasted and acid-etched surface. Inf J Oral Maxillofac Implants. **2011** Nov–Dec; 26(6): 1324–1332.

Cochran DL, Mau LP, Higginbottom FL, Wilson TG, Bosshardt DD, Schoolfield J, et al. Soft and hard tissue histologic dimensions around dental implants in the canine restored with smaller-diameter abutments: a paradigm shift in peri-implant biology. Int J Oral Maxillofac Implants. **2013** Mar; 28(2): 494–502.

Colnot C. Skeletal cell fate decisions within periosteum and bone marrow during bone regeneration. J Bone Miner Res. **2009** Feb; 24(2): 274–282.

Cooper LF. Objective criteria: guiding and evaluating dental implant esthetics. J Esthet Restor Dent. **2008**; 20(3): 195–205.

Cordaro L, Amadé DS, Cordaro M. Clinical results of alveolar ridge augmentation with mandibular block bone grafts in partially edentulous patients prior to implant placement. Clin Oral Implants Res. **2002** Feb; 13(1): 103–111.

Cordaro L, Torsello F, Morcavallo S, di Torresanto VM. Effect of bovine bone and collagen membranes on healing of mandibular bone blocks: a prospective randomized controlled study. Clin Oral Implants Res. **2011** Oct; 22(10): 1145–1150.

Cordaro L, Torsello F, Chen S, Ganeles J, Brägger U, Hämmerle C. Implant-supported single tooth restoration in the aesthetic zone: transmucosal and submerged healing provide similar outcome when simultaneous bone augmentation is needed. Clin Oral Implants Res. **2013** Oct; 24(10): 1130–1136.

Cordaro L, Boghi F, Mirisola di Torresanto V, Torsello F. Reconstruction of the moderately atrophic edentulous maxilla with mandibular bone grafts. Clin Oral Implants Res. **2013** Nov; 24(11): 1214–1221.

Cordaro L, Terheyden H. Ridge augmentation procedures in implant patients: a staged approach. Berlin: Quintessence, **2014**.

Cortellini P, Tonetti MS. Microsurgical approach to periodontal regeneration. Initial evaluation in a case cohort. J Periodontol. **2001** Apr; 72(4): 559–569.

Costello FW. Real teeth wear pink. Dent Today. **1995** Apr; 14(4): 52 – 55.

Cosyn J, Hooghe N, De Bruyn H. A systematic review on the frequency of advanced recession following single immediate implant treatment. J Clin Periodontol. **2012** Jun; 39(6): 582 – 589.

Croll BM. Emergence profiles in natural tooth contour. Part II: Clinical considerations. J Prosthet Dent. **1990** Apr; 63(4): 374 – 379.

Cumbo C, Marigo L, Somma F, La Torre G, Minciacchi I, D'Addona A. Implant platform switching concept: a literature review. Eur Rev Med Pharmacol Sci. **2013** Feb; 17(3): 392 – 397.

Cura C, SaraçoÐlu A, Cötert HS. J Prosthet Dent. Alternative method for connecting a removable gingival extension and fixed partial denture: a clinical report. **2002** Jul; 88(1): 1 – 3.

da Cunha HA, Filho HN, Batista JG, Matsumoto MA. Segmental osteotomy for the correction of a malpositioned single implant: an 8-year follow-up. Quintessence Int. **2011** Nov – Dec; 42(1): 817 – 822.

Dahlin C, Gottlow J, Linde A, Nyman S. Healing of maxillary and mandibular bone defects using a membrane technique. An experimental study in monkeys. Scand J Plast Reconstr Surg Hand Surg. **1990**; 24(1): 13 – 19.

Darby I, Chen ST, Buser D. Ridge preservation techniques for implant therapy. Int J Oral Maxillofac Implants. **2009**; 24 (Suppl): 260 – 271.

Dasmah A, Thor A, Ekestubbe A, Sennerby L, Rasmusson L. Particulate vs. block bone grafts: three-dimensional changes in graft volume after reconstruction of the atrophic maxilla, a 2-year radiographic follow-up. J Craniomaxillofac Surg. **2012** Dec; 40(8): 654 – 659.

Dawson A, Chen S (eds). The SAC Classification in implant dentistry. Chicago: Quintessence, **2009**.

De Leonardis D, Garg AK, Pecora GE. Osseointegration of rough acid-etched titanium implants: 5-year follow-up of 100 minimatic implants. Int J Oral Maxillofac Implants. **1999** May – Jun; 14(3): 384 – 391.

De Santis E, Lang NP, Scala A, Vigano P, Salata LA, Botticelli D. Healing outcomes at implants installed in grafted sites: an experimental study in dogs. Clin Oral Implants Res. **2012** Mar; 23(3): 340 – 350.

Degidi M, Nardi D, Piattelli A. Peri-implant tissue and radiographic bone levels in the immediately restored single-tooth implant: a retrospective analysis. J Periodontol. **2008** Feb; 79(2): 252 – 259. (**a**)

Degidi M, Novaes AB Jr, Nardi D, Piattelli A. Outcome analysis of immediately placed, immediately restored implants in the esthetic area: the clinical relevance of different interimplant distances. J Periodontol. **2008** Jun; 79(6): 1056 – 1061. (**b**)

den Hartog L, Meijer HJ, Stegenga B, Tymstra N, Vissink A, Raghoebar GM. Single implants with different neck designs in the aesthetic zone: a randomized clinical trial. Clin Oral Implants Res. **2011** Nov; 22(11): 1289 – 1297.

den Hartog L, Raghoebar GM, Slater JJ, Stellingsma K, Vissink A, Meijer HJ. Single-tooth implants with different neck designs: a randomized clinical trial evaluating the aesthetic outcome. Clin Implant Dent Relat Res. **2013** Jun; 15(3): 311 – 321.

Denry I, Kelly JR. State of the art of zirconia for dental applications. Dent Mater. **2008** Mar; 24(3): 299 – 307.

Depprich R, Zipprich H, Ommerborn M, Naujoks C, Wiesmann HP, Kiattavorncharoen S, Lauer HC, Meyer U, Kubler NR, Handschel J. Osseointegration of zirconia implants compared with titanium: an in vivo study. Head Face Med. **2008** Dec; 4: 30.

Depprich R, Naujoks C, Ommerborn M, Schwarz F, Kubler NR, Handschel J. Current findings regarding zirconia implants. Clin Implant Dent Relat Res. **2014** Feb; 16(1): 124 – 137.

Dhir S, Mahesh L, Kurtzman GM, Vandana KL. Peri-implant and periodontal tissues: a review of differences and similarities. Compend Contin Educ Dent. **2013** Jul – Aug; 34(7): e69 – e75.

Di Giacomo GA, Cury PR, de Araujo NS, Sendyk WR, Sendyk CL. Clinical application of stereolithographic surgical guides for implant placement: preliminary results. J Periodontol. **2005** Apr; 76(4): 503 – 507.

Donos N, Kostopoulos L, Karring T. Alveolar ridge augmentation using a resorbable copolymer membrane and autogenous bone grafts. An experimental study in the rat. Clin Oral Implants Res. **2002** Apr; 13(2): 203–213.

Duncan JD, Swift EJ Jr. Use of tissue-tinted porcelain to restore soft-tissue defects. J Prosthodont. **1994** Jun; 3(2): 59–61.

Egar T, Müller HP, Heincke A. Ultrasonic determination of gingival thickness. Subject variation and influence of tooth type and clinical features. J Clin Periodontol. **1996** Sep; 23(9): 839–845.

Ehrler DM, Vaccaro AR. The use of allograft bone in lumbar spine surgery. Clin Orthop Relat Res. **2000** Feb; (371): 38–45.

Elian N, Ehrlich B, Jalbout ZN, Classi AJ, Cho SC, Kamer AR, Froum S, Tarnow DP. Advanced concepts in implant dentistry: creating the "aesthetic site foundation." Dent Clin North Am. **2007** Apr; 51(2): 547–563, xi-xii. (**a**)

Elian N, Cho SC, Froum S, Smith RB, Tarnow DP. A simplified socket classification and repair technique. Pract Proced Aesthet Dent. **2007** Mar; 19(2): 99–104. (**b**)

Elian N, Tabourian G, Jalbout ZN, Classi A, Cho SC, Froum S, Tarnow DP. Accurate transfer of peri-implant soft tissue emergence profile from the provisional crown to the final prosthesis using an emergence profile cast. J Esthet Restor Dent. **2007**; 19{6): 306–314. (**c**)

Elian N, Bloom M, Trushkowsky RD, Dard MM, Tarnow D. Effect of 3- and 4-mm interimplant distances on the height of interimplant bone crest: a histomorphometric evaluation measured on bone level dental implants in minipig. Implant Dent. **2014** Oct; 23(5): 522–528.

Engfors I, Ortorp A, Jemt T. Fixed implant-supported prostheses in elderly patients: a 5-year retrospective study of 133 edentulous patients older than 79 years. Clin Implant Dent Relat Res. **2004**; 6(4): 190–198.

Ericsson I, Lindhe J. Probing depth at implants and teeth. An experimental study in the dog. J Clin Periodontol. **1993** Oct; 20(9): 623–627.

Erisken C, Kalyon DM, Wang H. Functionally graded electrospun polycaprolactone and beta-tricalcium phosphate nanocomposites for tissue engineering applications. Biomaterials. **2008** Oct; 29(30): 4065–4073.

Ersoy AE, Turkyilmaz I, Ozan O, McGlumphy EA. Reliability of implant placement with stereolithographic surgical guides generated from computed tomography: clinical data from 94 implants. J Periodontol. **2008** Aug; 79(8): 1339–1345.

Esposito M, Ekestubbe A, Gröndahl K. Radiological evaluation of marginal bone loss at tooth surfaces facing single Brånemark implants. Clin Oral Implants Res. **1993** Sep; 4(3): 151–157.

Esposito M, Grusovin MG, Chew YS, Worthington HV, Coulthard P. One-stage versus two-stage implant placement. A Cochrane systematic review of randomised controlled clinical trials. Eur J Implantol. **2009** Summer; 2(2): 91–99.

Evans CD, Chen ST. Esthetic outcomes of immediate implant placements. Clin Oral Implants Res. **2008** Jan; 19(1): 73–80.

Evian CI, Cutler SA. Direct replacement of failed CP titanium implants with larger-diameter, HA-coated Ti-6Al-4V implants: report of five cases. Int J Oral Maxillofac Implants. **1995** Nov–Dec; 10(6): 736–743.

Fava J, Lin M, Zahran M, Jokstad A. Single implant-supported crowns in the aesthetic zone: patient satisfaction with aesthetic appearance compared with appraisals by laypeople and dentists. Clin Oral Implants Res. **2015** Oct; 26(10): 1113–1120.

Favero G, Botticelli D, Favero G, Garcia B, Mainetti T, Lang NP. Alveolar bony crest preservation at implants installed immediately after tooth extraction: an experimental study in the dog. Clin Oral Implants Res. **2013** Jan; 24(1): 7–12.

Felton DA, Kanoy BE, Bayne SC, Wirthman GP. Effect of in vivo crown margin discrepancies on periodontal health. J Prosthet Dent. **1991** Mar; 65(3): 357–364.

Fenner N, Hämmerle CH, Sailer I, Jung RE. Long-term clinical, technical, and esthetic outcomes of all-ceramic vs. titanium abutments on implant supporting single-tooth reconstructions after at least 5 years. Clin Oral Implants Res. **2016** Jun; 27(6): 716–723.

Ferguson SJ, Broggini N, Wieland M, de Wild M, Rupp F, Geis-Gerstorfer J, Cochran DL, Buser D. Biomechanical evaluation of the interfacial strength of a chemically modified sandblasted and acid-etched titanium surface. J Biomed Mater Res A. **2006** Aug; 78(2): 291–297.

Fickl S, Zuhr O, Wachtel H, Bolz W, Hürzeler M. Tissue alterations after tooth extraction with and without surgical trauma: a volumetric study in the beagle dog. J Clin Periodontol. **2008** Apr; 35(4): 356–363.

Filippi A, Pohl Y, von Arx T. Decoronation of an ankylosed tooth for preservation of alveolar bone prior to implant placement. Dent Traumatol. **2001** Apr; 17(2): 93–95.

Foong JK, Judge RB, Palamara JE, Swain MV. Fracture resistance of titanium and zirconia abutments: an in vitro study. J Prosthet Dent. **2013** May; 109(5): 304–312.

Forsberg CM. Facial morphology and ageing: a longitudinal cephalometric investigation of young adults. Eur J Orthod. **1979**; 1(1): 15–23.

Forsberg CM, Eliasson S, Westergren H. Face height and tooth eruption in adults—a 20-year follow-up investigation. Eur J Orthod. **1991** Aug; 13(4): 249–254.

Francetti L, Trombelli L, Lombardo G, Guida L, Cafiero C, Roccuzzo M, Carusi G, Del Fabbro M. Evaluation of efficacy of enamel matrix derivative in the treatment of intrabony defects: a 24-month multicenter study. Int J Periodontics Restorative Dent. **2005** Oct; 25(5): 461–473.

Franz S, Rammelt S, Scharnweber D, Simon JC. Immune responses to implants—a review of the implications for the design of immunomodulatory biomaterials. Biomaterials. **2011** Oct; 32(28): 6692–6709.

Frost NA, Mealey BL, Jones AA, Huynh-Ba G. Periodontal Biotype: Gingival Thickness as It Relates to Probe Visibility and Buccal Plate Thickness. J Periodontol. **2015** Oct; 86(10): 1141–1149.

Froum SJ. Dental implant complications: etiology, prevention, and treatment. Hoboken: Wiley-Blackwell, **2010**.

Fu JH, Yeh CY, Chan HL, Tatarakis N, Leong DJ, Wang HL. Tissue biotype and its relation to the underlying bone morphology. J Periodontol. **2010** Apr; 81(4): 569–574.

Fu JH, Oh TJ, Benavides E, Rudek I, Wang HL. A randomized clinical trial evaluating the efficacy of the sandwich bone augmentation technique in increasing buccal bone thickness during implant placement surgery: I. Clinical and radiographic parameters. Clin Oral Implants Res. **2014** Apr; 25(4): 458–467.

Fuentealba R, Jofré J. Esthetic failure in implant dentistry. Dent Clin North Am. **2015** Jan; 59(1): 227–246.

Fugazzotto PA. Success and failure rates of osseointegrated implants in function in regenerated bone for 6 to 51 months: a preliminary report. Int J Oral Maxillofac Implants. **1997** Jan–Feb; 12(1): 17–24.

Fugazzotto PA. Shorter implants in clinical practice: rationale and treatment results. Int J Oral Maxillofac Implants. **2008** May–Jun; 23(3): 487–496.

Fujihara K, Kotaki M, Ramakrishna S. Guided bone regeneration membrane made of polycaprolactone/calcium carbonate composite nano-fibers. Biomaterials. **2005** Jul; 26(19): 4139–4147.

Fürhauser R, Florescu D, Benesch T, Haas R, Mailath G, Watzek G. Evaluation of soft tissue around single-tooth implant crowns: the pink esthetic score. Clin Oral Implants Res. **2005** Dec; 16(6): 639–644.

Furze D, Byrne A, Donos N, Mardas N. Clinical and esthetic outcomes of single-tooth implants in the anterior maxilla. Quintessence Int. **2012** Feb; 43(2): 127–134.

Furze D, Byrne A, Alam S, Wittneben JG. Esthetic outcome of implant supported crowns with and without peri-implant conditioning using provisional fixed prosthesis: a randomized controlled clinical trial. Clin Implant Dent Relat Res. **2016** Dec; 18(6): 1153–1162.

Gahlert M, Gudehus T, Eichhorn S, Steinhauser E, Kniha H, Erhardt W. Biomechanical and histomorphometric comparison between zirconia implants with varying surface textures and a titanium implant in the maxilla of miniature pigs. Clin Oral Implants Res. **2007** Oct; 18(5): 662–668.

Gahlert M, Röhling S, Sprecher CM, Kniha H, Milz S, Bormann K. In vivo performance of zirconia and titanium implants: a histomorphometric study in mini pig maxillae. Clin Oral Implants Res. **2012** Mar; 23(3): 281–286.

Gahlert M, Burtscher D, Pfundstein G, Grunert I, Kniha H, Röhling S. Dental zirconia implants up to three years in function: a retrospective clinical study and evaluation of prosthetic restorations and failures. Int J Oral Maxillofac Implants. **2013** May–Jun; 28(3): 896–904.

Gahlert M, Kniha H, Weingart D, Schild S, Gellrich NC, Bormann KH. A prospective clinical study to evaluate the performance of zirconium dioxide dental implants in single-tooth gaps. Clin Oral Implants Res. **2016** Dec; 27(12): e176–e184.

Gallucci GO, Belser UC, Bernard JP, Magne P. Modeling and characterization of the CEJ for optimization of esthetic implant design. Int J Periodontics Restorative Dent. **2004** Feb; 24(1): 19–29.

Gallucci GO, Guex P, Vinci D, Belser UC. Achieving natural-looking morphology and surface textures in anterior ceramic fixed rehabilitations. Int J Periodontics Restorative Dent. **2007** Apr; 27(2): 117–125.

Gallucci GO, Grütter L, Nedir R, Bischof M, Belser UC. Esthetic outcomes with porcelain-fused-to-ceramic and all-ceramic single-implant crowns: a randomized clinical trial. Clin Oral Implants Res. **2011** Jan; 22(1): 62–69.

Gapski R, Neugeboren N, Pomeranz AZ, Reissner MW. Endosseous implant failure influenced by crown cementation: A clinical case report. Int J Oral Maxillofac Implants. **2008** Sep–Oct; 23(5): 943–946.

Garber DA, Belser UC. Restoration-driven implant placement with restoration-generated site development. Compend Contin Educ Dent. **1995** Aug; 16(8): 796, 798–802, 804.

Garcia LT, Verrett RG. Metal-ceramic restorations--custom characterization with pink porcelain. Compend Contin Educ Dent. **2004** Apr; 25(4): 242–246.

Gelb DA. Immediate implant surgery: three-year retrospective evaluation of 50 consecutive cases. Int J Oral Maxillofac Implants. **1993**; 8(4): 388–399.

Giannobile WV, Somerman MJ. Growth and amelogenin-like factors in periodontal wound healing. A systematic review. Ann Periodontol. **2003** Dec; 8(1): 193–204.

Giannopoulou C, Bernard JP, Buser D, Carrel A, Belser, UC. Effect of intracrevicular restoration margins on peri-implant health: clinical, biochemical, and microbiologic findings around esthetic implants up to 9 years. Int J Oral Maxillofac Implants. **2003** Mar–Apr; 18(2): 173–181.

Gielkens PF, Schortinghuis J, de Jong JR, Paans AM, Ruben JL, Raghoebar GM, Stegenga B, Bos RR. The influence of barrier membranes on autologous bone grafts. J Dent Res. **2008** Nov; 87(11): 1048–1052.

Gigandet M, Bigolin G, Faoro F, Bürgin W, Brägger U. Implants with original and non-original abutment connections. Clin Implant Dent Relat Res. **2014** Apr; 16(2): 303–311.

Gittens RA, Scheideler L, Rupp F, Hyzy SL, Geis-Gerstorfer J, Schwartz Z, Boyan BD. A review on the wettability of dental implant surfaces. II: Biological and clinical aspects. Acta Biomater. **2014** Jul; 10(7): 2907–2918.

Glauser R, Sailer I, Wohlwend A, Studer S, Schibli M, Schärer P. Experimental zirconia abutments for implant-supported single-tooth restorations in esthetically demanding regions: 4-year results of a prospective clinical study. Int J Prosthodont. **2004** May–Jun; 17: 285–290.

Gobbato L, Paniz G, Mazzocco F, Chierico A, Tsukiyama T, Levi PA Jr, Weisgold AS. Significance of crown shape in the replacement of a central incisor with a single implant-supported crown. Quintessence Int. **2013** May; 44(5): 407–413.

Goldberg VM, Stevenson S. The biology of bone grafts. Semin Arthroplasty. **1993** Apr; 4(2): 58–63.

Goldberg M, Langer R, Jia X. Nanostructured materials for applications in drug delivery and tissue engineering. J Biomater Sci Polym Ed. **2007**; 18(3): 241–268.

Goodacre CJ. Gingival esthetics. J Prosthet Dent. **1990** Jul; 64(1): 1–12.

Gorski JP. Biomineralization of bone: a fresh view of the roles of non-collagenous proteins. Front Biosci (Landmark Ed). **2011** Jun 1; 16: 2598–2621.

Gotfredsen K, Berglundh T, Lindhe J. Anchorage of titanium implants with different surface characteristics: an experimental study in rabbits. Clin Implant Dent Relat Res. **2000**; 2(3): 120–128.

Gottlow J, Dard M, Kjellson F, Obrecht M, Sennerby L. Evaluation of a new titanium-zirconium dental implant: a biomechanical and histological comparative study in the mini pig. Clin Implant Dent Relat Res. **2012** Aug; 14: 538–545.

Graziani F, Gennai S, Cei S, Ducci F, Discepoli N, Carmignani A, Tonetti M. Does enamel matrix derivative application provide additional clinical benefits in residual periodontal pockets associated with suprabony defects? A systematic review and meta-analysis of randomized clinical trials. J Clin Periodontol. **2014** Apr; 41(4): 377–386.

Greene PR. The flexible gingival mask: an aesthetic solution in periodontal practice. Br Dent J. **1998** Jun 13; 184(11): 536–540.

Greenstein G, Greenstein B, Cavallaro J, Elian N, Tarnow D. Flap advancement: practical techniques to attain tension-free primary closure. J Periodontol. **2009** Jan; 80(1): 4–15.

Griffin JD Jr. Excellence in photography: heightening dentist-ceramist communication. Dent Today. **2009** Jul; 28(7): 124–127.

Grossmann Y, Levin L. Success and survival of single dental implants placed in sites of previously failed implants. J Periodontol. **2007** Sep; 78(9): 1670–1674.

Grunder U, Polizzi G, Goené R, Hatano N, Henry P, Jackson WJ, , Kawamura K, Köhler S, Renouard F, Rosenberg R, Triplett G, Werbitt M, Lithner B. A 3-year prospective multicenter follow-up report on the immediate and delayed-immediate placement of implants. Int J Oral Maxillofac Implants. **1999** May–Apr; 14(2): 210–216.

Grunder U. Stability of the mucosal topography around single-tooth implants and adjacent teeth: 1-year results. Int J Periodontics Restorative Dent. **2000** Feb; 20(1): 11–17.

Grunder U, Gracis S, Capelli M. Influence of the 3-D bone-to-implant relationship on esthetics. Int J Periodontics Restorative Dent. **2005** Apr; 25(2): 113–119.

Grunder U. Ideale Schnittführung. In: Grunder U (ed). Implantate in der ästhetischen Zone: Ein Behandlungskonzept step-by step. Berlin: Quintessenz, **2015**. 326–350.

Gruskin E, Doll BA, Futrell FW, Schmitz JP, Hollinger JO. Demineralized bone matrix in bone repair: history and use. Adv Drug Deliv Rev. **2012** Sep; 64(12): 1063–1077.

Grütter L, Belser UC. Implant loading protocols for the partially edentulous esthetic zone. Int J Oral Maxillofac Implants. **2009**; 24 (Suppl): 169–179.

Gurtner GC, Werner S, Barrandon Y, Longaker MT. Wound repair and regeneration. Nature. **2008** May 15; 453(7193): 314–321.

Haack JE, Sakaguchi RL, Sun T, Coffey KP. Elongation and preload stress in dental implant abutment screws. Int J Oral Maxillofac Implants. **1995** Sep–Oct; 10(5): 529–536.

Haag P, Nilner K. Bonding between titanium and dental porcelain: A systematic review. Acta Odontol Scand. **2010** May; 68(3): 154–164.

Haj-Ali R, Walker MP. A provisional fixed partial denture that simulates gingival tissue at the pontic-site defect. J Prosthodont. **2002** Mar; 11(1): 46–48.

Hallman M, Thor A. Bone substitutes and growth factors as an alternative/complement to autogenous bone for grafting in implant dentistry. Periodontol 2000. **2008**; 47: 172–192.

Hamilton A, Judge RB, Palamara JE, Evans C. Evaluation of the fit of CAD/CAM abutments. Int J Prosthodont. **2013** Jul–Aug; 26(4): 370–380.

Hämmerle CH, Jung RE. Bone augmentation by means of barrier membranes. Periodontol 2000. **2003**; 33: 36–53.

Hämmerle CH, Chen ST, Wilson TG Jr. Consensus statements and recommended clinical procedures regarding the placement of implants in extraction sockets. Int J Oral Maxillofac Implants. **2004**; 19 (Suppl): 26–28.

Hämmerle CH, Araújo MG, Simion M. Evidence-based knowledge on the biology and treatment of extraction sockets. Clin Oral Implants Res. **2012** Feb; 23 (Suppl 5): 80–82.

Hämmerle CH, Cordaro L, van Assche N, Benic GI, Bornstein M, Gamper F, Gotfredsen K, Harris D, Hürzeler M, Jacobs R, Kapos T, Kohal RJ, Patzelt SB, Sailer I, Tahmaseb A, Vercruyssen M, Wismeijer D. Digital technologies to support planning, treatment, and fabrication processes and outcome assessments in implant dentistry. Summary and consensus statements. The 4th EAO Consensus Conference 2015. Clin Oral Implants Res. **2015** Sep; 26 (Suppl 11): 97 – 101.

Han CH, Johansson CB, Wennerberg A, Albrektsson T. Quantitative and qualitative investigations of surface enlarged titanium and titanium alloy implants. Clin Oral Implants Res. **1998** Feb; 9(1): 1 – 10.

Hannon SM, Colvin CJ, Zurek DJ. Selective use of gingival-toned ceramics: case reports. Quintessence Int. **1994** Apr; 25(4): 233 – 238.

Harris D, Buser D, Dula K, et al. EAO Guidelines for the use of diagnostic imaging in implant dentistry. Clin Oral Implants Res. **2002**; 13: 566 – 570.

Harris D, Horner K, Gröndahl K, Jacobs R, Helmrot E, Benic GI, Bornstein MM, Dawood A, Quirynen M. EAO guidelines for the use of diagnostic imaging in Implant Dentistry 2011: A consensus workshop organized by the European Association for Osseointegration at the Medical University of Warsaw. Clin Oral Implants Res. **2012** Nov; 23(11): 1243 – 1253.

Heij DG, Opdebeeck H, van Steenberghe D, Kokich VG, Belser U, Quirynen M. Facial development, continuous tooth eruption, and mesial drift as compromising factors for implant placement. Int J Oral Maxillofac Implants. **2006** Nov – Dec; 21(6): 867 – 878.

Heitz-Mayfield LJ, Huynh-Ba G. History of treated periodontitis and smoking as risks for implant therapy. Int J Oral Maxillofac Implants. **2009**; 24 (Suppl): 39 – 68.

Heitz-Mayfield LJ, Mombelli A. The therapy of peri-implantitis: a systematic review. Int J Oral Maxillofac Implants. **2014**; 29 (Suppl): 325 – 345. (**a**)

Heitz-Mayfield LJ, Needleman I, Salvi GE, Pjetursson BE. Consensus statements and clinical recommendations for prevention and management of biologic and technical implant complications. Int J Oral Maxillofac Implants. **2014**; 29 Suppl: 346 – 350. (**b**)

Hermann JS, Buser D. Guided bone regeneration for dental implants. Curr Opin Periodontol. **1996** May – Jun; 3: 168 – 177.

Hermann JS, Cochran DL, Nummikoski PV, Buser D. Crestal bone changes around titanium implants. A radiographic evaluation of unloaded nonsubmerged and submerged implants in the canine mandible. J Periodontol. **1997** Nov: 68(11): 1117 – 1130.

Hermann JS, Buser D, Schenk RK, Cochran DL. Crestal bone changes around titanium implants. A histometric evaluation of unloaded non-submerged and submerged implants in the canine mandible. J Periodontol. **2000** Sep; 71(9): 1412 – 1424.

Hermann JS, Buser D, Schenk RK. Biologic width around one- and two-piece titanium implants. Clin Oral Implants Res. **2001** Dec; 12(6): 559 – 571.

Higginbottom FL, Wilson TG Jr. Three-dimensional templates for placement of root-form dental implants: a technical note. Int J Oral Maxillofac Implants. **1996** Nov – Dec; 11(6): 787 – 793.

Hinds KF. Custom impression coping for an exact registration of the healed tissue in the esthetic implant restoration. Int J Periodontics Restorative Dent. **1997** Dec; 17(6): 584 – 591.

Hinds KF. Intraoral digital impressions to enhance implant esthetics. Compend Contin Educ Dent. **2014** Sep; 35 (3 Suppl): 25 – 33.

Hisbergues M, Vendeville S, Vendeville P. Zirconia: Established facts and perspectives for a biomaterial in dental implantology. J Biomed Mater Res B Appl Biomater. **2009** Feb; 88(2): 519 – 529.

Hjørting-Hansen E. Bone grafting to the jaws with special reference to reconstructive preprosthetic surgery. A historical review. Mund Kiefer Gesichtschir. **2002** Jan; 6(1): 6 – 14.

Ho WF, Chen WK, Wu SC, Hsu HC. Structure, mechanical properties, and grindability of dental Ti-Zr alloys. J Mater Sci Mater Med. **2008** Oct; 19: 3179 – 3186.

Hochman MN, Chu SJ, Tarnow DP. Maxillary anterior papilla display during smiling: a clinical study of the interdental smile line. Int J Periodontics Restorative Dent. **2012** Aug; 32(4): 375 – 383.

Holtzclaw D, Toscano N, Eisenlohr L, Callan D. The safety of bone allografts used in dentistry: a review. J Am Dent Assoc. **2008** Sep; 139(9): 1192 – 1199.

Horowitz R, Holtzclaw D, Rosen PS. A review on alveolar ridge preservation following tooth extraction. J Evid Based Dental Pract. **2012** Sep; 12(3): 149–160.

Huang ZM, Zhang YZ, Kotaki M, Ramakrishna S. A review on polymer nanofibers by electrospinning and their applications in nanocomposites. Compos Sci Technol. **2003** Nov; 63(15): 2223–2253.

Hürzeler MB, Quiñones CR, Schupbach P. Guided bone regeneration around dental implants in the atrophic alveolar ridge using a bioresorbable barrier. An experimental study in the monkey. Clin Oral Implants Res. **1997** Aug; 8(4): 323–331.

Hürzeler MB, Kohal RJ, Naghshbandi J, Mota LF, Conradt J, Hutmacher D, Caffesse RG. Evaluation of a new bioresorbable barrier to facilitate guided bone regeneration around exposed implant threads. An experimental study in the monkey. Int J Oral Maxillofac Surg. **1998** Aug; 27(4): 315–320.

Hürzeler MB, Fickl S, Zuhr O, Wachtel H. Clinical failures and shortfalls of immediate implant procedures. Eur J Esthet Dent. **2006** Aug; 1(2): 128–140.

Hürzeler MB, Zuhr O, Schupbach P, Rebele SF, Emmanouilidis N, Fickl S. The socket-shield technique: a proof-of-principle report. J Clin Periodontol. **2010** Sep; 37(9): 855–862.

Huynh-Ba G, Pjetursson BE, Sanz M, Cecchinato D, Ferrus J, Lindhe J, Lang NP. Analysis of the socket bone wall dimensions in the upper maxilla in relation to immediate implant placement. Clin Oral Implants Res. **2010** Jan; 21(1): 37–42.

Hwang D, Wang HL. Flap thickness as a predictor of root coverage: a systematic review. J Periodontol. **2007** Oct; 77(10): 1625–1634.

Iasella JM, Greenwell H, Miller RL, Hill M, Drisko C, Bohra AA, Scheetz JP. Ridge preservation with freeze-dried bone allograft and a collagen membrane compared to extraction alone for implant site development: a clinical and histologic study in humans. J Periodontol. **2003** Jul; 74(7): 990–999.

Ikarashi Y, Toyoda K, Kobayash E, Doi H, Yoneyama T, Hamanaka H, Tsuchiya T. Improved biocompatibility of titanium-zirconium (Ti-Zr) alloy: tissue reaction and sensitization to Ti-Zr alloy compared with pure Ti and Zr in rat implantation study. Mater Trans. **2005**; 46(10): 2260–2267.

Intini G. The use of platelet-rich plasma in bone reconstruction therapy. Biomaterials. **2009** Oct; 30(28): 4956–4966.

Ioannidis A, Gallucci GO, Jung RE, Borzangy S, Hämmerle CH, Benic GI. Titanium-zirconium narrow-diameter versus titanium regular-diameter implants for anterior and premolar single crowns: 3-year results of a randomized controlled clinical study. J Clin Periodontol. **2015** Nov; 42(11): 1060–1070.

Ishikawa-Nagai S, Da Silva JD, Weber HP, Park SE. Optical phenomenon of peri-implant soft tissue. Part II. Preferred implant neck color to improve soft tissue esthetics. Clin Oral Implants Res. **2007** Oct; 18(5): 575–580.

Jacobs R, Pittayapat P, van Steenberghe D, De Mars G, Gijbels F, Van Der Donck A, Li L, Liang X, Van Assche N, Quirynen M, Naert I. A split-mouth comparative study up to 16 years of two screw-shaped titanium implant systems. J Clin Periodontol. **2010** Dec; 37(12): 1119–1127.

Jacques LB, Coelho AB, Hollweg H, Conti PC. Tissue sculpturing: an alternative method for improving esthetics of anterior fixed prosthodontics. J Prosthet Dent. **1999** May; 81(5): 630–633.

Jaime APG, de Vasconcellos DK, Mesquita AM, Kimpara ET, Bottino MA. Effect of cast rectifiers on the marginal fit of UCLA abutments. Journal of Applied & Oral Science. **2007** Jun; 15(3): 169–174.

Januário AL, Barriviera M, Duarte WR. Soft tissue cone-beam computed tomography: a novel method for the measurement of gingival tissue and the dimensions of the dentogingival unit. J Esthet Restor Dent. **2008**; 20(6): 366–373.

Januário AL, Duarte WR, Barriviera M, Mesti JC, Araújo MG, Lindhe J. Dimension of the facial bone wall in the anterior maxilla: a cone-beam computed tomography study. Clin Oral Implants Res. **2011** Oct; 22(10): 1168–1171.

Jemt T. Regeneration of gingival papillae after single-implant treatment. Int J Periodontics Restorative Dent. **1997** Aug; 17(4): 326–333.

Jemt T, Johansson J. Implant treatment in the edentulous maxillae: a 15-year follow-up study on 76 consecutive patients provided with fixed prostheses. Clin Implant Dent Relat Res. **2006**; 8(2): 61–69.

Jensen SS, Aaboe M, Pinholt EM, Hjorting-Hansen E, Melsen F, Ruyter IE. Tissue reaction and material characteristics of four bone substitutes. Int J Oral Maxillofac Implants. **1996** Jan – Feb; 11(1): 55 – 66.

Jensen J, Joss A, Lang NP. The smile line of different ethnic groups depending on age and gender. Acta Med Dent Helv. **1999;** 4: 38 – 46.

Jensen SS, Broggini N, Weibrich G, Hjørting-Hansen E, Schenk R, Buser D. Bone regeneration in standardized bone defects with autografts or bone substitutes in combination with platelet concentrate: a histologic and histomorphometric study in the mandibles of minipigs. Int J Oral Maxillofac Implants. **2005** Sep – Oct; 20(5): 703 – 12.

Jensen SS, Broggini N, Hjørting-Hansen E, Schenk R, Buser D. Bone healing and graft resorption of autograft, anorganic bovine bone and beta-tricalcium phosphate. A histologic and histomorphometric study in the mandibles of minipigs. Clin Oral Implants Res. **2006** Jun; 17(3): 237 – 243.

Jensen SS, Yeo A, Dard M, Hunziker E, Schenk R, Buser D. Evaluation of a novel biphasic calcium phosphate in standardized bone defects: a histologic and histomorphometric study in the mandibles of minipigs. Clin Oral Implants Res. **2007** Dec; 18(6): 752 – 760.

Jensen SS, Terheyden H. Bone augmentation procedures in localized defects in the alveolar ridge: clinical results with different bone grafts and bone-substitute materials. Int J Oral Maxillofac Implants, **2009;** 24 (Suppl): 218 – 236.

Jensen SS, Bosshardt DD, Gruber R, Buser D. Long-term stability of contour augmentation in the esthetic zone. Histologic and histomorphometric evaluation of 12 human biopsies 14 to 80 months after augmentation. J Periodontol. **2014** Nov: 85(11): 1 – 15.

Jensen SS, Gruber R, Buser D, Bosshardt DD. Osteoclast-like cells on deproteinized bovine bone mineral and biphasic calcium phosphate: light and transmission electron microscopical observations. Clin Oral Implants Res. **2015** Aug; 26(8): 859 – 864.

Jimbo R, Naito Y, Galli S, Berner S, Dard M, Wennerberg A. Biomechanical and histomorphometrical valuation of TiZr alloy implants: an in vivo study in the rabbit. Clin Implant Dent Relat Res. **2015** Oct; 17 (Suppl 2): e670 – e678.

Joda T, Wittneben JG, Brägger U. Digital implant impressions with the Individualized Scanbody Technique for emergence profile support. Clin Oral Implants Res. **2014** Mar; 25(3): 395 – 397.

Joda, T, Bürki A, Bethge S, Brägger U, Zysset O. Stiffness, strength, and failure modes of implant-supported monolithic lithium disilicate crowns: influence of titanium and zirconia abutments. Int J Oral Maxillofac Implants. **2015** Nov – Dec; 30(6): 1272 – 1279.

Johansson CB, Han CH, Wennerberg A, Albrektsson T. A quantitative comparison of machined commercially pure titanium and titanium-aluminum-vanadium implants in rabbit bone. Int J Oral Maxillofac Implants. **1998** May – Jun; 13(3): 315 – 321.

Jones AR, Martin W. Comparing pink and white esthetic scores to layperson perception in the single-tooth implant patient. Int J Oral Maxillofac Implants. **2014** Nov – Dec; 29(6): 1348 – 1353.

Jovanovic SA, Spiekermann H, Richter EJ. Bone regeneration around titanium dental implants in dehisced defect sites: a clinical study. Int J Oral Maxillofac Implants. **1992** Summer; 7(2): 233 – 245.

Jovanovic SA, Nevins M. Bone formation utilizing titanium-reinforced barrier membranes. Int J Periodontics Restorative Dent. **1995** Feb; 15(1): 56 – 69.

Jung RE, Siegenthaler DW, Hämmerle CH. Postextraction tissue management: a soft tissue punch technique. Int J Periodontics Restorative Dent. **2004** Dec; 24(6): 545 – 553. (**a**)

Jung R. Replacement of an upper right central incisor with a regular neck implant restored with an all-ceramic crown, cemented. In: Belser U, Buser D, Hämmerle C, Jung R, Martin W, Morton D, Schmid B. ITI Treatment Guide, Vol. 1. Implant therapy in the esthetic zone: single-tooth replacements. Editors: Belser U, Buser D, Wismeijer D. Berlin: Quintessence, **2006.** (**b**)

Jung RE, Cochran DL, Domken O, Seibl R, Jones AA, Buser D, Hämmerle CH. The effect of matrix bound parathyroid hormone on bone regeneration. Clin Oral Implants Res. **2007** Jun; 18(3): 319 – 325.

Jung RE, Sailer I, Hämmerle CH, Attin T, Schmidlin P. In vitro color changes of soft tissues caused by restorative materials. Int J Periodontics Restorative Dent. **2007** Jun; 27(3): 251 – 257.

Jung RE, Thoma DS, Hämmerle CH. Assessment of the potential of growth factors for localized alveolar ridge augmentation: a systematic review. J Clin Periodontol. **2008** Sep; 35 (8 Suppl): 255–281.

Jung RE, Holderegger C, Sailer I, Khraisat , Suter A, Hämmerle CH. The effect of all-ceramic and porcelain-fused-to-metal restorations on marginal peri-implant soft tissue color: a randomized controlled clinical trial. Int J Periodontics Restorative Dent. **2008** Aug; 28(4): 357–365.

Jung RE, Schneider D, Ganeles J, Wismeijer D, Zwahlen M, Hämmerle CH, Tahmaseb A. Computer technology applications in surgical implant dentistry: a systematic review. Int J Oral Maxillofac Implants. **2009**; 24 (Suppl): 92–109.

Jung RE, Zembic A, Pjetursson BE, Zwahlen M, Thoma DS. Systematic review of the survival rate and the incidence of biological, technical, and aesthetic complications of single crowns on implants reported in longitudinal studies with a mean follow-up of 5 years. Clin Oral Implants Res. **2012** Oct; 23 (Suppl 6): 2–21.

Jung RE, Fenner N, Hämmerle CH, Zitzmann NU. Long-term outcome of implants placed with guided bone regeneration (GBR) using resorbable and non-resorbable membranes after 12–14 years. Clin Oral Implants Res. **2013** Oct; 24(10): 1065–1073. (**H365**)

Jung RE, Philipp A, Annen BM, Signorelli L, Thoma DS, Hämmerle CH, Attin T, Schmidlin P. Radiographic evaluation of different techniques for ridge preservation after tooth extraction: a randomized controlled clinical trial. J Clin Periodontol. **2013** Jan; 40(1): 90–98. (**b**)

Kaitsas R, Paolone MG, Paolone G. Guided orthodontic regeneration: a tool to enhance conventional regenerative techniques in implant surgery. Int Orthod. **2015** Dec; 13(4): 539–554.

Kamalakidis S, Paniz G, Kang KH, Hirayama H. Nonsurgical management of soft tissue deficiencies for anterior single implant-supported restorations: a clinical report. J Prosthet Dent. **2007** Jan; 97(1): 1–5.

Kan JY, Rungcharassaeng K, Umezu K, Kois JC. Dimensions of peri-implant mucosa: an evaluation of maxillary anterior single implants in humans. J Periodontol. **2003** Apr; 74(4): 557–562.

Kan JY, Rungcharassaeng K, Umezu K, Kois JC. Dimensions of peri-implant mucosa: an evaluation of maxillary anterior single implants in humans. J Periodontol. **2003** Apr; 74(4): 557–562. (**a**)

Kan JY, Rungcharassaeng K. Interimplant papilla preservation in the esthetic zone: a report of six consecutive cases. Int J Periodontics Restorative Dent. **2003** Jun; 23(3): 249–259. (**b**)

Kan JY, Rungcharassaeng K, Sclar A, Lozada JL. Effects of the facial osseous defect morphology on gingival dynamics after immediate tooth replacement and guided bone regeneration: 1-year results. J Oral Maxillofac Surg. **2007** Jul; 65 (7 Suppl 1): 13–19.

Kan JY, Rungcharassaeng K, Fillman M, Caruso J. Tissue architecture modification for anterior implant esthetics: an interdisciplinary approach. Eur J Esthet Dent. **2009** Summer; 4(2): 104–117. (**a**)

Kan JY, Rungcharassaeng K, Morimoto T, Lozada J. Facial gingival tissue stability after connective tissue graft with single immediate tooth replacement in the esthetic zone: Consecutive case report. J Oral Maxillofac Surg. **2009**; 67: 40–48. (**b**)

Kan JY, Morimoto T, Rungcharassaeng K, Roe P, Smith DH. Gingival biotype assessment in the esthetic zone: visual versus direct measurement. Int J Periodontics Restorative Dent. **2010** Jun; 30(3): 237–243.

Kan JYK, Roe P, Rungcharassaeng K, Patel RD, Waki T, Lozada JL, Zimmerman G. Classification of sagittal root position in relation to the anterior maxillary osseous housing for immediate implant placement: a cone beam computed tomography study. Int J Oral Maxillofac Implants. **2011** Jul; 26(4): 873–876.

Kapos T, Evans C. CAD/CAM technology for implant abutments, crowns, and superstructures. Int J Oral Maxillofac Implants. **2014**; 29 (Suppl): 117–136.

Karageorgiou V, Kaplan D. Porosity of 3D biomaterial scaffolds and osteogenesis. Biomaterials. **2005** Sep; 26(27): 5474–5491.

Karl M, Krafft T, Kelly JR. Fracture of a narrow-diameter roxolid implant: clinical and fractographic considerations. Int J Oral Maxillofac Implants. **2014** Sep–Oct; 29(5): 1193–1196.

Karoussis IK, Brägger U, Salvi GE, Burgin W, Lang NP. Effect of implant design on survival and success rates of titanium oral implants: a 10-year prospective cohort study of the ITI Dental Implant System. Clin Oral Implants Res. **2004** Feb; 15(1): 8 – 17.

Kassolis JD, Baer ML, Reynolds MA. The segmental osteotomy in the management of malposed implants: a case report and literature review. J Periodontol. **2003** Apr; 74(4): 529 – 536.

Keith JD, Jr., Petrungaro P, Leonetti JA, Elwell CW, Zeren KJ, Caputo C, Nikitakis NG, Schopf C, Warner MM. Clinical and histologic evaluation of a mineralized block allograft: results from the developmental period (2001 – 2004). Int J Periodontics Restorative Dent. **2006** Aug; 26(4): 321 – 327.

Kelly JR, Denry I. Stabilized zirconia as a structural ceramic: An overview. Dent Mater. **2008** Mar; 24(3): 289 – 298.

Kelly JR, Benetti P. Ceramic materials in dentistry: historical evolution and current practice. Aust Dent J. **2011** Jun; 56 (Suppl): 84 – 96.

Khan SN, Bostrom MP, Lane JM. Bone growth factors. Orthop Clin North Am. **2000** Jul; 31(3): 375 – 388.

Khoury F, Hanser T. Mandibular bone block harvesting from the retromolar region: a 10-year prospective clinical study. Int J Oral Maxillofac Implants. **2015** May – Jun; 30(3): 688 – 397.

Kim TH, Cascione D, Knezevic A. Simulated tissue using a unique pontic design: a clinical report. J Prosthet Dent. **2009** Oct; 102(4): 205 – 210. (**a**)

Kim BS, Kim YK, Yun PY, Yi YJ, Lee HJ, Kim SG, Son JS. Evaluation of peri-implant tissue response according to the presence of keratinized mucosa. Oral Surg Oral Med Oral Pathol Oral Radiol Endod. **2009** Mar; 107(3): e24 – 28. (**b**)

Kim TH, Cascione D, Knezevic A, Nowzari H. Restoration using gingiva-colored ceramic and a ridge lap pontic with circumferential pressure: a clinical report. J Prosthet Dent. **2010** Aug; 104(2): 71 – 76.

Klein MO, Schiegnitz E, Al-Nawas B. Systematic review on success of narrow-diameter dental implants. Int J Oral Maxillofac Implants. **2014**; 29 (Suppl): 43 – 54.

Kleinheinz J, Büchter A, Kruse-Lösler B, Weingart D, Joos U. Incision design in implant dentistry based on vascularization of the mucosa. Clin Oral Implants Res. **2005** Oct, 16(5): 518 – 523.

Klinge B, Meyle J. Peri-implant tissue destruction. The Third EAO Consensus Conference. Clin Oral Implants Res. **2012** Oct; 23 (Suppl 6): 108 – 110.

Klokkevold PR. Cone beam computed tomography for the dental implant patient. J Calif Dent Assoc. **2015** Sep; 43(9): 521 – 530.

Klotz MW, Taylor TD, Goldberg AD. Wear at the titanium-zirconia implant-abutment interface: a pilot study. Int J Oral Maxillofac Implants. **2011** Sep – Oct; 26(5): 970 – 975.

Kobayashi E, Matsumoto S, Doi H, Yoneyama T, Hamanaka H. Mechanical properties of the binary titanium-zirconium alloys and their potential for biomedical materials. J Biomed Mater Res. **1995** Aug; 29(8): 943 – 950.

Kohal RJ, Weng D, Bächle M, Strub JR. Loaded custom-made zirconia and titanium implants show similar osseointegration: an animal experiment. J Periodontol. **2004** Sep; 75(9): 1262 – 1268.

Kois JC. Predictable single tooth peri-implant esthetics: five diagnostic keys. Compend Contin Educ Dent. **2001** Mar; 22(3): 199 – 206.

Kokich VO Jr, Kiyak HA, Shapiro PA. Comparing the perception of dentists and lay people to altered dental esthetics. J Esthet Dent. **1999**; 11(6): 311 – 324.

Kolk A, Handschel J, Drescher W, Rothamel D, Kloss F, Blessmann M, Heiland M, Wolff KD, Smeets R. Current trends and future perspectives of bone substitute materials—from space holders to innovative biomaterials. J Craniomaxillofa Surg. **2012** Dec; 40(8): 706 – 718.

Komiyama A, Klinge B, Hultin M. Treatment outcome of immediately loaded implants installed in edentulous jaws following computer-assisted virtual treatment planning and flapless surgery. Clin Oral Implants Res. **2008** Jul; 19(7): 677 – 685.

Koutouzis T, Neiva R, Lipton D, Lundgren T. The effect of interimplant distance on peri-implant bone and soft-tissue dimensional changes: a nonrandomized, prospective, 2-year follow-up study. Int J Oral Maxillofac Implants. **2015** Jul – Aug; 30(4): 900 – 908.

Krennmair G, Piehslinger E, Wagner H. Status of teeth adjacent to single-tooth implants. Int J Prosthodont. **2003** Sep – Oct; 16(5): 524 – 528.

Kuchler U, von Arx T. Horizontal ridge augmentation in conjunction with or prior to implant placement in the anterior maxilla: a systematic review. Int J Oral Maxillofac Implants. **2014**; 29 (Suppl): 14 – 24.

Lang NP, Berglundh T, Working Group 4 of Seventh European Workshop on Periodontology. Periimplant diseases: where are we now?—Consensus of the Seventh European Workshop on Periodontology. J Clin Periodontol. **2011** Mar; 38 (Suppl 11): 178 – 181.

Langer B. Spontaneous in situ gingival augmentation. Int J Periodontics Restorative Dent. **1994** Dec; 14(6): 524 – 535.

Langer L, Langer B, Salem D. Unintentional root fragment retention in proximity to dental implants: a series of six human case reports. Int J Periodontics Restorative Dent. **2015** May – Jun; 35(3): 305 – 313.

Lanyon LE. Osteocytes, strain detection, bone modeling and remodeling. Calcif Tissue Int. **1993**; 53 (Suppl 1): S102 – S106; discussion S106 – S107.

Lazzara RJ. Immediate implant placement into extraction sites: surgical and restorative advantages. Int J Periodontics Restorative Dent. **1989**; 9(5): 332 – 343.

Lazzara RJ, Porter SS. Platform switching: a new concept in implant dentistry for controlling postrestorative crestal bone levels. Int J Periodontics Restorative Dent. **2006** Feb; 26(1): 9 – 17.

Le Guéhennec L, Soueidan A, Layrolle P, Amouriq Y. Surface treatments of titanium dental implants for rapid osseointegration. Dent Mater. **2007** Jul; 23(7): 844 – 854.

Lee K, Silva EA, Mooney DJ. Growth factor delivery-based tissue engineering: general approaches and a review of recent developments. J R Soc Interface. **2011** Feb 6; 8(55): 153 – 170.

LeGeros RZ, Lin S, Rohanizadeh R, Mijares D, LeGeros JP. Biphasic calcium phosphate bioceramics: preparation, properties and applications. J Mater Sci Mater Med. **2003** Mar; 14(3): 201 – 209.

LeGeros RZ. Calcium phosphate-based osteoinductive materials. Chem Rev. **2008** Nov; 108(11): 4742 – 4753.

Lekholm U, Gunne J, Henry P, Higuchi K, Lindén U, Bergström C, van Steenberghe D. Survival of the Brånemark implant in partially edentulous jaws: a 10-year prospective multicenter study. Int J Oral Maxillofac Implants. **1999** Sep – Oct; 14(5): 639 – 645.

Levin L, Schwartz-Arad D. The effect of cigarette smoking on dental implants and related surgery. Implant Dent. **2005** Dec; 14(4): 357 – 361.

Levine RA, Huynh-Ba G, Cochran DL. Soft tissue augmentation procedures for mucogingival defects in esthetic sites. Int J Oral Maxillofac Implants. **2014**; 29 (Suppl): 155 – 185.

Lewis S, Beumer J 3rd, Hornburg W, Moy P. The "UCLA" abutment. Int J Oral Maxillofac Implants. **1998** Fall; 3(3): 183 – 189.

Liao S, Wang W, Uo M, Ohkawa S, Akasaka T, Tamura K, Cui F, Watari F. A three-layered nano-carbonated hydroxyapatite/collagen/PLGA composite membrane for guided tissue regeneration. Biomaterials. **2005** Dec; 26(36): 7564 – 7571.

Lin GH, Chan HL, Wang HL. The significance of keratinized mucosa on implant health: a systematic review. J Periodontol. **2013** Dec; 84(12): 1755 – 1767. (**a**)

Lin WS, Harris BT, Morton D. Use of implant-supported interim restorations to transfer periimplant soft tissue profiles to a milled polyurethane definitive cast. J Prosthet Dent. **2013** May; 109(5): 333 – 337.

Lin WS, Harris B, Zandinejad A, Martin WC, Morton D. Use of prefabricated titanium abutments and customized anatomic lithium disilicate structures for cement-retained implant restorations in the esthetic zone. J Prosthet Dent. **2014** Mar; 111(3): 181 – 185.

Lindeboom JA, Tjiook Y, Kroon FH. Immediate placement of implants in periapical infected sites: a prospective randomized study in 50 patients. Oral Surg Oral Med Oral Pathol Oral Radiol Endod. **2006** Jun; 101(6): 705 – 710.

Lindfors LT, Tervonen EA, Sándor GK, Ylikontiola LP. Guided bone regeneration using a titanium-reinforced ePTFE membrane and particulate autogenous bone: the effect of smoking and membrane exposure. Oral Surg Oral Med Oral Pathol Oral Radiol Endod. **2010** Jun; 109(6): 825 – 830.

Lindhe J, Socransky SS, Nyman S, Westfelt E. Dimensional alteration of the periodontal tissues following therapy. Int J Periodontics Restorative Dent. **1987**; 7(2): 9 – 21.

Lindhe J, Meyle J. Peri-implant diseases: Consensus Report of the Sixth European Workshop on Periodontology. J Clin Periodontol. **2008** Sep; 35 (8 Suppl): 282 – 285.

Lindquist LW, Carlsson GE, Jemt T. A prospective 15-year follow-up study of mandibular fixed prostheses supported by osseointegrated implants. Clinical results and marginal bone loss. Clin Oral Implants Res. **1996** Dec; 7(4): 329 – 336.

Linkevicius T, Apse P. Influence of abutment material on stability of peri-implant tissues: a systematic review. Int J Oral Maxillofac Implants. **2008** May – Jun; 23(3): 449 – 456.

Linkevicius T, Vindasiute E, Puisys A, Peciuliene V. The influence of margin location on the amount of undetected cement excess after delivery of cement-retained implant restorations. Clin Oral Implants Res. **2011** Dec; 22(12): 1379 – 1384.

Linkevicius T, Vindasiute E, Puisys A, Linkeviciene L, Maslova N, Puriene A. The influence of the cementation margin position on the amount of undetected cement. A prospective clinical study. Clin Oral Implants Res. **2013** Jan; 24(1): 71 – 76.

Linkevicius T, Vaitelis J. The effect of zirconia or titanium as abutment material on soft peri-implant tissues: a systematic review and meta-analysis. Clin Oral Implants Res. **2015** Sep; 26 (Suppl 11): 139 – 147.

Lops D, Chiapasco M, Rossi A, Bressan E, Romeo E. Incidence of inter-proximal papilla between a tooth and an adjacent immediate implant placed into a fresh extraction socket: 1-year prospective study. Clin Oral Implants Res. **2008** Nov; 19(11): 1135 – 1140.

Lorenzana ER, Allen EP. The single-incision palatal harvest technique: a strategy for esthetics and patient comfort. Int J Periodontics Restorative Dent. **2000** Jun; 20(3): 297 – 305.

Lozano FE. Overview of dental photography. Lab communication: Part 1. Forum Implantologicum. **2014**; 10(1): 84 – 87.

Lozano FE. Overview of dental photography: white balance explained. Forum Implantologicum. **2015**; 11(2): 122 – 125. (**a**)

Lozano FE, Gonzaga LH. Overview of dental photography. Lab Communication: Part 2. Complex elements of lab communication. Forum Implantologicum. **2015**; 11(1): 40 – 43. (**b**)

Lughi V, Sergo V. Low temperature degradation—aging—of zirconia: a critical review of the relevant aspects in dentistry. Dent Mater. **2010** Aug; 26(8): 807 – 820.

Lutolf MP, Lauer-Fields JL, Schmoekel HG, Metters AT, Weber FE, Fields GB, Hubbell JA. Synthetic matrix metalloproteinase-sensitive hydrogels for the conduction of tissue regeneration: engineering cell-invasion characteristics. Proc Natl Acad Sci U S A. **2003** Apr 29; 100(9): 5413 – 5418.

Lutolf MP, Hubbell JA. Synthetic biomaterials as instructive extracellular microenvironments for morphogenesis in tissue engineering. Nat Biotechnol. **2005** Jan; 23(1): 47 – 55.

Machtei EE. The effect of membrane exposure on the outcome of regenerative procedures in humans: a meta-analysis. J Periodontol. **2001** Apr; 72(4): 512 – 516.

Machtei EE, Mahler D, Oettinger-Barak O, Zuabi O, Horwitz J. Dental implants placed in previously failed sites: survival rate and factors affecting the outcome. Clin Oral Implants Res. **2008** Mar; 19(3): 259 – 264.

Maeda Y, Miura J, Taki I, Sogo M. Biomechanical analysis on platform switching: is there any biomechanical rationale? Clin Oral Implants Res. **2007** Oct; 18(5): 581 – 584.

Magne P, Belser UC (eds). Bonded porcelain restorations in the anterior dentition: a biomimetic approach. Chicago: Quintessence, **2002**.

Maiorana C, Beretta M, Salina S, Santoro F. Reduction of autogenous bone graft resorption by means of Bio-Oss coverage: a prospective study. Int J Periodontics Restorative Dent. **2005** Feb; 25(1): 19–25.

Mankoo T. Maintenance of interdental papillae in the esthetic zone using multiple immediate adjacent implants to restore failing teeth—a report of ten cases at 2 to 7 years follow-up. European Journal of Esthetic Dentistry. **2008** Winter; 3(4): 304–322.

Manzano-Moreno FJ, Herrera-Briones FJ, Linares-Recatala M, Ocaña-Peinado FM, Reyes-Botella C, Valle-cillo-Capilla MF. Bacterial contamination levels of autogenous bone particles collected by 3 different techniques for harvesting intraoral bone grafts. J Oral Maxillofac Surg. **2015** Mar; 73(3): 424–429.

Mao JJ, Giannobile WV, Helms JA, Hollister SJ, Krebsbach PH, Longaker MT, Shi S. Craniofacial tissue engineering by stem cells. J Dent Res. **2006** Nov; 85(11): 966–979.

Mardinger O, Ben Zvi Y, Chaushu G, Nissan J, Manor Y. A retrospective analysis of replacing dental implants in previously failed sites. Oral Surg Oral Med Oral Pathol Oral Radiol. **2012** Sep; 114(3): 290–293.

Markus SJ. Interim esthetic restorations in conjunction with anterior implants. J Prosthet Dent. **1999** Aug; 82(2): 233–236.

Martin W, Morton D, Buser D. Pre-operative analysis and prosthetic treatment planning in esthetic implant dentistry. In: Belser U, Buser D, Hämmerle C, Jung R, Martin W, Morton D, Schmid B. ITI Treatment Guide, Vol. 1. Implant therapy in the esthetic zone: single-tooth replacements. Editors: Belser U, Buser D, Wismeijer D. Berlin: Quintessence, **2006**.

Martin WC, Pollini A, Morton D. The influence of restorative procedures on esthetic outcomes in implant dentistry: a systematic review. Int J Oral Maxillofac Implants. **2014**; 29 (Suppl): 142–154.

Marx RE, Carlson ER, Eichstaedt RM, Schimmele SR, Strauss JE, Georgeff KR. Platelet-rich plasma: Growth factor enhancement for bone grafts. Oral Surg Oral Med Oral Pathol Oral Radiol Endod. **1998** Jun; 85(6): 638–646.

Matarasso S, Iorio Siciliano V, Aglietta M, Andreuccetti G, Salvi GE. Clinical and radiographic outcomes of a combined resective and regenerative approach in the treatment of peri-implantitis: a prospective case series. Clin Oral Implants Res. **2014** Jul; 25(7): 761–767.

Mattheos N, Janda MS. Exotic encounters with dental implants: managing complications with unidentified systems. Aust Dent J. **2012** Jun; 57(2): 236–242.

McAllister BS, Haghighat K. Bone augmentation techniques. J Periodontol. **2007** Mar; 78(3): 377–396.

McClure MJ, Sell SA, Simpson DG, Walpoth BH, Bowlin GL. A three-layered electrospun matrix to mimic native arterial architecture using polycaprolactone, elastin, and collagen: a preliminary study. Acta Biomater. **2010** Jul; 6(7): 2422–2433.

Meijer HJ, Stellingsma K, Meijndert L, Raghoebar GM. A new index for rating aesthetics of implant-supported single crowns and adjacent soft tissues—the Implant Crown Aesthetic Index. Clin Oral Implants Res. **2005** Dec; 16(6): 645–649.

Mendelson MR. Effective laboratory communication… it's a two-way street. Dent Today. **2006** Jul; 25(7): 96–98.

Michaeli E, Weinberg I, Nahlieli O. Dental implants in the diabetic patient: systemic and rehabilitative considerations. Quintessence Int. **2009** Sep; 40(8): 639–645.

Miguel BS, Ghayor C, Ehrbar M, Jung RE, Zwahlen RA, Hortschansky P, Schmoekel HG, Weber FE. N-methyl pyrrolidone as a potent bone morphogenetic protein enhancer for bone tissue regeneration. Tissue Eng Part A. **2009** Oct; 15(10): 2955–2963.

Milella E, Ramires PA, Brescia E, La Sala G, Di Paola L, Bruno V. Physicochemical, mechanical, and biological properties of commercial membranes for GTR. J Biomed Mater Res. **2001**; 58(4): 427–435.

Miron RJ, Hedbom E, Saulacic N, Zhang Y, Sculean A, Bosshardt DD, Buser D. Osteogenic potential of autogenous bone grafts harvested with four different surgical techniques. J Dent Res. **2011** Dec; 90(12): 1428–1433.

Miron RJ, Gruber R, Hedbom E, Saulacic N, Zhang Y, Sculean A, Bosshardt DD, Buser D. Impact of bone harvesting techniques on cell viability and the release of growth factors of autografts. Clin Implant Dent Relat Res. **2013** Aug; 15(4): 481–489.

Mitrani R, Adolfi D, Tacher, S. implant-supported restorations in the esthetic zone: understanding the biology. J Esthet Restor Dent. **2005**; 17(4): 211–223.

Miyakawa O, Watanabe K, Okawa S, Nakano S, Kobayashi M, Shiokawa N. Layered structure of cast titanium surface. Dental Mater J. **1989** Dec; 8(2): 175–185.

Mombelli A, Wick P. Peri-implantitis treated by an antimicrobial and regenerative approach. In: Nrägger U, Heitz-Mayfield LJA. ITI Treatment Guide, Vol. 8. Biological and hardware complications in implant dentistry. Editors: Wismeijer D, Buser D, Chen S. Berlin: Quintessence, **2015**.

Montoya-Salazar V, Castillo-Oyagüe R, Torres-Sánchez C, Lynch CD, Gutiérrez-Pérez JL, Torres-Lagares D. Outcome of single immediate implants placed in post-extraction infected and non-infected sites, restored with cemented crowns: a 3-year prospective study. J Dent. **2014** Jun; 42(6): 645–652.

Moráguez OD, Belser UC. The use of polytetrafluoroethylene tape for the management of screw access channels in implant-supported prostheses. J Prosthet Dent. **2010** Mar; 103(3): 189–191.

Moraschini V, Barboza ES. Effect of autologous platelet concentrates for alveolar socket preservation: a systematic review. Int J Oral Maxillofac Surg. **2015** May; 44(5): 632–641.

Morris HF, Ochi S, Winkler S. Implant survival in patients with type 2 diabetes: placement to 36 months. Ann Periodontol. **2000** Dec; 5(1): 157–165.

Morton D, Bornstein MM, Wittneben JG, Martin WC, Ruskin JD, Hart CN, Buser D. Early loading after 21 days of healing of nonsubmerged titanium implants with a chemically modified sandblasted and acid-etched surface: Two-year results of a prospecive two-center study. Implant Dent Relat Res. **2010** Mar; 12(1): 9–17.

Morton D, Chen ST, Martin WC, Levine RA, Buser D. Consensus statements and recommended clinical procedures regarding optimizing esthetic outcomes in implant dentistry. Int J Oral Maxillofac Implants. **2014**; 29 (Suppl): 216–220.

Moskowitz EM, Sheridan JJ, Celenza F Jr, Tovilo K, Muñoz AM. Essix appliances. Provisional anterior prosthesis for pre and post implant patients. N Y State Dent J. **1997** Apr; 63(4): 32–35.

Moy PK, Medina D, Shetty V, Aghaloo TL. Dental implant failure rates and associated risk factors. Int J Oral Maxillofac Implants. **2005** Jul–Aug; 20(4): 569–577.

Müller HP, Heinecke A, Schaller N, Eger T. Masticatory mucosa in subjects with different periodontal phenotypes. J Clin Periodontol. **2000** Sep; 27(9): 621–626.

Müller F, Al-Nawas B, Storelli S, Quirynen M, Hicklin S, Castro-Laza J, Bassetti R, Schimmel M, Roxolid Study Group. Small-diameter titanium grade IV and titanium-zirconium implants in edentulous mandibles: five-year results from a double-blind, randomized controlled trial. BMC Oral Health. **2015** Oct 12; 15(1): 123.

Nauta A, Gurtner G, Longaker MT. Wound healing and regenerative strategies. Oral Dis. **2011** Sep; 17(6): 541–549.

Nemcovsky CE, Artzi Z. Comparative study of buccal dehiscence defects in immediate, delayed, and late maxillary implant placement with collagen membranes: clinical healing between placement and second-stage surgery. J Periodontol. **2002** Jul; 73(7): 754–761.

Nickenig HJ, Wichmann M, Schlegel KA, Nkenke E, Eitner S. Radiographic evaluation of marginal bone levels adjacent to parallel-screw cylinder machined-neck implants and rough-surfaced microthreaded implants using digitized panoramic radiographs. Clin Oral Implants Res. **2009** Jun; 20(6): 550–554.

Nissan J, Mardinger O, Calderon S, Romanos GE, Chaushu G. Cancellous bone block allografts for the augmentation of the anterior atrophic maxilla. Clin Implant Dent Relat Res. **2011** Jun; 13(2): 104–111.

Nyström E, Nilson H, Gunne J, Lundgren S. A 9 – 14 year follow-up of onlay bone grafting in the atrophic maxilla. Int J Oral Maxillofac Surg. **2009** Feb; 38(2): 111 – 116.

Oates TW, Valderrama P, Bischof M, Nedir R, Jones A, Simpson J, Toutenburg H, Cochran DL. Enhanced implant stability with a chemically modified SLA surface: a randomized pilot study. Int J Oral Maxillofac Implants. **2007** Sep – Oct; 22(5): 755 – 760.

Oliva J, Oliva X, Oliva JD. Five-year success rate of 831 consecutively placed Zirconia dental implants in humans: a comparison of three different rough surfaces. Int J Oral Maxillofac Implants. **2010** Mar – Apr; 25(2): 336 – 344.

Olsson M, Lindhe J. Periodontal characteristics in individuals with varying form of the upper central incisors. J Clin Periodontol **1991** Jan; 18(1): 78 – 82.

Osburn RC. Preservation of the alveolar ridge: a simplified technique for retaining teeth beneath removable appliances. J Indiana State Dent Assoc. **1974** Jan – Feb; 53(1): 8 – 11.

Ozaki W, Buchman SR. Volume maintenance of onlay bone grafts in the craniofacial skeleton: micro-architecture versus embryologic origin. Plast Reconstr Surg. **1998** Aug; 102(2): 291 – 299.

Palacci P, Nowzari H. Soft tissue enhancement around dental implants. Periodontol 2000. **2008**; 47: 113 – 132.

Pallesen L, Schou S, Aaboe M, Hjørting-Hansen E, Nattestad A, Melsen F. Influence of particle size of autogenous bone grafts on the early stages of bone regeneration: a histologic and stereologic study in rabbit calvarium. Int J Oral Maxillofac Implants. **2002** Jul – Aug; 17(4): 498 – 506.

Palmer SH, Gibbons CL, Athanasou NA. The pathology of bone allograft. J Bone Joint Surg Br. **1999** Mar; 81(2): 333 – 335.

Park SE, Da Silva JD, Weber HP, Ishikawa-Nagai S. Optical phenomenon of peri-implant soft tissue. Part I. Spectrophotometric assessment of natural tooth gingiva and peri-implant mucosa. Clin Oral Implants Res. **2007** Oct; 18(5): 569 – 474.

Park SH, Lee KW, Oh TJ, Misch CE, Shotwell J, Wang HL. Effect of absorbable membranes on sandwich bone augmentation. Clin Oral Implants Res. **2008** Jan; 19(1): 32 – 41.

Park JC, Kim CS, Choi SH, Cho KS, Chai JK, Jung UW. Flap extension attained by vertical and periosteal-releasing incisions: a prospective cohort study. Clin Oral Implants Res. **2012** Aug; 23(8): 993 – 998.

Patras M, Martin W. Simplified custom impression post for implant-supported restorations. J Prosthet Dent. **2016** May; 115(5): 556 – 559.

Pauletto N, Lahiffe BJ, Walton JN. Complications associated with excess cement around crowns on osseointegrated implants: a clinical report. Int J Oral Maxillofac Implants. **1999** Nov – Dec; 14(6): 865 – 868.

Payer M, Heschl A, Koller M, Arnetzl G, Lorenzoni M, Jakse N. All-ceramic restoration of zirconia two-piece implants—a randomized controlled clinical trial. Clin Oral Implants Res. **2015** Apr; 26(4): 371 – 376.

Peixoto A, Marques TM, Correia A. Gingival biotype characterization—a study in a Portuguese sample. Int J Esthet Dent. **2015** Winter; 10(4): 534 – 546.

Piattelli A, Scarano A, Russo P, Matarasso S. Evaluation of guided bone regeneration in rabbit tibia using bioresorbable and non-resorbable membranes. Biomaterials. **1996** Apr; 17(8): 791 – 796.

Piattelli M, Favero GA, Scarano A, Orsini G, Piattelli A. Bone reactions to anorganic bovine bone (Bio-Oss) used in sinus augmentation procedures: a histologic long-term report of 20 cases in humans. Int J Oral Maxillofac Implants. **1999** Nov – Dec; 14(6): 835 – 840.

Piattelli A, Vrespa G, Petrone G, Iezzi G, Annibali S, Scarano A. Role of the microgap between implant and abutment: a retrospective histologic evaluation in monkeys. J Periodontol. **2003** Mar; 74(3): 346 – 352.

Pjetursson BE, Tan K, Lang NP, Brägger U, Egger M, Zwahlen M. A systematic review of the survival and complication rates of fixed partial dentures (FPDs) after an observation period of at least 5 years. Clin Oral Implants Res. **2004** Dec; 15(8): 625 – 642.

Pjetursson BE, Asgeirsson AG, Zwahlen M, Sailer I. Improvements in implant dentistry over the last decade: comparison of survival and complication rates in older and newer publications. Int J Oral Maxillofac Implants. **2014**; 29 (Suppl): 308 – 324.

Polack MA. Simple method of fabricating an impression coping to reproduce peri-implant gingiva on the master cast. J Prosthet Dent. **2002** Aug; 88(2): 221 – 223.

Polimeni G, Albandar JM, Wikesjö UM. Prognostic factors for alveolar regeneration: effect of space provision. J Clin Periodontol. **2005** Sep; 32(9): 951 – 954.

Pontoriero R, Wennström J, Lindhe J. The use of barrier membranes and enamel matrix proteins in the treatment of angular bone defects. A prospective controlled clinical study. J Clin Periodontol. **1999** Dec; 26(12): 833 – 840.

Priest GF, Lindke L. Gingival-colored porcelain for implant-supported prostheses in the aesthetic zone. Pract Periodontics Aesthet Dent. **1998** Nov – Dec; 10(9): 1231 – 1240.

Priest G. Virtual-designed and computer-milled implant abutments. J Oral Maxillofac Surg. **2005** Sep; 63(9 Suppl 2): 22 – 32.

Priest GF. The esthetic challenge of adjacent implants. J Oral Maxillofac Surg. **2007** Jul; 65 (7 Suppl 1): 2 – 12.

Proussaefs P, Lozada J. The use of resorbable collagen membrane in conjunction with autogenous bone graft and inorganic bovine mineral for buccal/labial alveolar ridge augmentation: a pilot study. J Prosthet Dent. **2003** Dec; 90(6): 530 – 538.

Qahash M, Susin C, Polimeni G, Hall J, Wikesjö UM. Bone healing dynamics at buccal peri-implant sites. Clin Oral Implants Res. **2008** Feb; 19(2): 166 – 172.

Rathe F, Junker R, Chesnutt BM, Jansen JA. The effect of enamel matrix derivative (Emdogain) on bone formation: a systematic review. Tissue Eng Part B Rev. **2009** Sep; 15(3): 215 – 224.

Reddi AH. Morphogenesis and tissue engineering of bone and cartilage: inductive signals, stem cells, and biomimetic biomaterials. Tissue Eng. **2000** Aug; 6(4): 351 – 359.

Richter WA, Ueno H. Relationship of crown margin placement to gingival inflammation. J Prosthet Dent. **1973** Aug; 30(2): 156 – 161.

Rocchietta I, Simion M, Hoffmann M, Trisciuoglio D, Benigni M, Dahlin C. Vertical bone augmentation with an autogenous block or particles in combination with guided bone regeneration: a clinical and histological preliminary study in humans. Clin Implant Dent Relat Res. **2016** Feb; 18(1): 19 – 29.

Roccuzzo M, Bunino M, Needleman I, Sanz M. Periodontal plastic surgery for treatment of localized gingival recessions: a systematic review. J Clin Periodontol. **2002**; 29 (Suppl 3): 178 – 194; discussion 195 – 196.

Roccuzzo M, Gaudioso L, Bunino M, Dalmasso P. Surgical treatment of buccal soft tissue recessions around single implants: 1-year results from a prospective pilot study. Clin Oral Implants Res. **2014** Jun; 25(6): 641 – 646.

Roe P, Kan JY, Rungcharassaeng K, Caruso JM, Zimmerman G, Mesquida J. Horizontal and vertical dimensional changes of peri-implant facial bone following immediate placement and provisionalization of maxillary anterior single implants: a 1-year cone beam computed tomography study. Int J Oral Maxillofac Implants. **2012** Mar – Apr; 27(2): 393 – 400.

Roffi A, Filardo G, Kon E, Marcacci M. Does PRP enhance bone integration with grafts, graft substitutes, or implants? A systematic review. BMC Musculoskelet Disord. **2013** Nov 21; 14: 330.

Röhling S, Meng B, Cochren D. Sandblasted and acid etched implant surfaces with or without high surface free energy —+H482 experimental and clinical background. In: Wennerberg A, Albrektsson T, Jimbo R: Implant surfaces and their biological and clinical impact. Springer Science, **2014**.

Romanos GE, Javed F. Platform switching minimises crestal bone loss around dental implants: truth or myth? J Oral Rehabil. **2014** Sep; 41(9): 700 – 708.

Roos-Jansåker AM, Renvert H, Lindahl C, Renvert S. Surgical treatment of peri-implantitis using a bone substitute with or without a resorbable membrane: a prospective cohort study. J Clin Periodontol. **2007** Jul; 34(7): 625 – 632.

Rothamel D, Schwarz F, Sager M, Herten M, Sculean A, Becker J. Biodegradation of differently cross-linked collagen membranes: an experimental study in the rat. Clin Oral Implants Res. **2005** Jun; 16(3): 369 – 378.

Rothamel D, Schwarz F, Fienitz T, Smeets R, Dreiseidler T, Ritter L, Happe A, Zöller J. Biocompatibility and biodegradation of a native porcine pericardium membrane: results of in vitro and in vivo examinations. Int J Oral Maxillofac Implants. **2012** Jan – Feb; 27(1): 146 – 154.

Rotstein I, Zalkind M, Mor C, Tarabeah A, Friedman S. In vitro efficacy of sodium perborate preparations used for intracoronal bleaching of discolored non-vital teeth. Endod Dent Traumatology. **1991** Aug; 7(4); 177 – 180.

Rungcharassaeng K, Kan Joseph YK, Yoshino S, Morimoto T, Zimmerman G. Immediate implant placement and provisionalization with and without a vonnective tissue graft: an analysis of facial gingival tissue thickness. Int J Periodontics Restorative Dent. **2012** Dec; 32(6): 657 – 663.

Sadrimanesh R, Siadat H, Sadr-Eshkevari P, Monzavi A, Maurer P, Rashad A. Alveolar bone stress around implants with different abutment angulation: an FE-analysis of anterior maxilla. Implant Dent. **2012** Jun; 21(3): 196 – 201.

Sailer I, Zembic A, Jung RE, Hämmerle CH, Mattiola A. Single-tooth implant reconstructions: esthetic factors influencing the decision between titanium and zirconia abutments in anterior regions. Eur J Esthet Dent. **2007** Autumn; 2(3): 296 – 310.

Sailer I, Philipp A, Zembic A, Pjetursson BE, Hämmerle CH, Zwahlen M. A systematic review of the performance of ceramic and metal implant abutments supporting fixed implant reconstructions. Clin Oral Implants Res. **2009** Sep; 20 (Suppl 4): 4 – 31. (**a**)

Sailer I, Sailer T, Stawarczyk B, Jung RE, Hämmerle CH. In vitro study of the influence of the type of connection on the fracture load of zirconia abutments with internal and external implant-abutment connections. Int J Oral Maxillofac Implants. **2009** Sep – Oct; 24(2): 850 – 858. (**b**)

Sailer I, Mühlemann S, Zwahlen M, Hämmerle CH, Schneider D. Cemented and screw-retained implant reconstructions: a systematic review of the survival and complication rates. Clin Oral Implants Res. **2012** Oct; 23 (Suppl 6): 163 – 201.

Sailer I, Fehmer V, Ioannidis A, Hämmerle CH, Thoma DS. Threshold value for the perception of color changes of human gingiva. Int J Periodontics Restorative Dent. **2014** Nov – Dec; 34(6): 757 – 762.

Sailer I, Makarov NA, Thoma DS, Zwahlen M, Pjetursson BE. All-ceramic or metal-ceramic tooth-supported fixed dental prostheses (FDPs)? A systematic review of the survival and complication rates. Part I: Single crowns (SCs). Dent Mater. **2014** Jun; 31(6): 603 – 623.

Salama H, Salama M, Kelly J. The orthodontic-periodontal connection in implant site development. Pract Periodontics Aesthet Dent. **1996** Nov – Dec; 8(9): 923 – 932.

Salama M, Coachman C, Garber D, Calamita M, Salama H, Cabral G. Prosthetic gingival reconstruction in the fixed partial restoration. Part 2: diagnosis and treatment planning. Int J Periodontics Restorative Dent. **2009** Dec; 29(6): 573 – 581.

Salvi GE, Brägger U. Mechanical and technical risks in implant therapy. Int J Oral Maxillofac Implants. **2009**; 24 Suppl: 69 – 85.

Salvi GE, Zitzmann NU. The effects of anti-infective preventive measures on the occurrence of biologic implant complications and implant loss: a systematic review. Int J Oral Maxillofac Implants. **2014**; 29 (Suppl): 292 – 307.

Sanavi F, Weisgold AS, Rose LF. Biologic width and its relation to periodontal biotypes. J Esthet Dent. **1998**; 10(3): 157 – 163.

Santling HJ, Raghoebar GM, Vissink A, den Fartog L, Meijer HJ. Performance of the Straumann Bone Level Implant System for anterior single-tooth replacement in augmented and nonaugmented sites: a prospective cohort study with 60 consecutive patients. Clin Oral Implants Res. **2013** Aug; 24(8): 941 – 948.

Santosa RE, Martin W, Morton D. Effects of a cementing technique in addition to luting agent on the uniaxial retention force of a single-tooth implant-supported restoration: an in vitro study. Int J Oral Maxillofac Implants. **2010** Nov – Dec; 25(6): 1145 – 1152.

Sanz M, Lorenzo R, Aranda JJ, Martin C, Orsini M. Clinical evaluation of a new collagen matrix (Mucograft prototype) to enhance the width of keratinized tissue in patients with fixed prosthetic restorations: a randomized prospective clinical trial. J Clin Peridontol. **2009** Oct; 36(10): 868 – 876.

Sanz I, Garcia-Gargallo M, Herrera D, Martin C, Figuero E, Sanz M. Surgical protocols for early implant placement in post-extraction sockets: a systematic review. Clin Oral Implants Res. **2012** Feb; 23 (Suppl 5): 67–79.

Sanz-Sánchez I, Ortiz-Vigón A, Sanz-Martín I, Figuero E, Sanz M. Effectiveness of lateral bone augmentation on the alveolar crest dimension: a systematic review and meta-analysis. J Dent Res. **2015** Sep; 94 (9 Suppl): 128S–142S.

Saulacic N, Bosshardt DD, Bornstein MM, Berner S, Buser D. Bone apposition to a titanium-zirconium alloy implant, as compared to two other titanium-containing implants. Eur Cell Mater. **2012** Apr 10; 23: 273–286; discussion 286–288.

Saulacic N, Erdösi R, Bosshardt DD, Gruber R, Buser D. Acid and alkaline etching of sandblasted zirconia implants: a histomorphometric study in miniature pigs. Clin Implant Dent Relat Res. **2014** Jun; 16(3): 312–322.

Sbordone L, Toti P, Menchini-Fabris GB, Sbordone C, Piombino P, Guidetti F. Volume changes of autogenous bone grafts after alveolar ridge augmentation of atrophic maxillae and mandibles. Int J Oral Maxillofac Surg. **2009** Oct; 38(19): 1059–1065.

Scarano A, Piattelli M, Caputi S, Favero GA, Piattelli A. Bacterial adhesion on commercially pure titanium and zirconium oxide disks: an in vivo human study. J Periodontol. **2004** Feb; 75(2): 292–206.

Schenk RK, Buser D, Hardwick WR, Dahlin C. Healing pattern of bone regeneration in membrane-protected defects: a histologic study in the canine mandible. Int J Oral Maxillofac Implants. **1994** Jan–Feb; 9(1): 13–29.

Schimmel M, Srinivasan M, Herrmann F.R., Müller F. Loading protocols for implant-supported overdentures in the edentulous jaw: a systematic review and meta-analysis. Int J Oral Maxillofac Implants. **2014**; 29 (Suppl): 271–286.

Schlegel AK, Möhler H, Busch F, Mehl A. Preclinical and clinical studies of a collagen membrane (Bio-Gide). Biomaterials. **1997** Apr; 18(7): 535–538.

Schliephake H. Bone growth factors in maxillofacial skeletal reconstruction. Int J Oral Maxillofac Surg. **2002** Oct; 31(5): 469–484.

Schneider D, Grunder U, Ender A, Hämmerle CH, Jung RE. Volume gain and stability of peri-implant tissue following bone and soft tissue augmentation: 1-year results from a prospective cohort study. Clin Oral Implants Res. **2011** Jan; 22(1): 28–37.

Schneider D, Weber FE, Grunder U, Andreoni C, Burkhardt R, Jung RE. A randomized controlled clinical multicenter trial comparing the clinical and histological performance of a new, modified polylactide-co-glycolide acid membrane to an expanded polytetrafluorethylene membrane in guided bone regeneration procedures. Clin Oral Implants Res. **2014** Feb; 25(2): 150–158.

Schoenbaum TR, Han TJ. Direct custom implant impression copings for the preservation of the pontic receptor site architecture. J Prosthet Dent. **2012** Mar; 107(3): 203–206.

Schroeder A, Pohler O, Sutter F. [Tissue reaction to an implant of a titanium hollow cylinder with a titanium surface spray layer]. SSO Schweiz Monatsschr Zahnheilkd. **1976**; 86: 713–727.

Schroeder A, Sutter F, Krekeler G. Oral implantology: basics, ITI hollow cylinder system. New York: Thieme, **1991**.

Schropp L, Isidor F. Papilla dimension and soft tissue level after early vs. delayed placement of single-tooth implants: 10-year results from a randomized controlled clinical trial. Clin Oral Implants Res. **2015** Mar; 26(3): 278–286.

Schrott AR, Jimenez M, Hwang JW, Fiorellini J, Weber HP. Five-year evaluation of the influence of keratinized mucosa on peri-implant soft-tissue health and stability around implants supporting full-arch mandibular fixed prostheses. Clin Oral Implants Res. **2009** Oct; 20(10): 1170–1177.

Schulte W, Kleineikenscheidt H, Lindner K, Schareyka R. [The Tübingen immediate implant in clinical studies.] Dtsch Zahnärztl Z. **1978**; 33(5): 348–359.

Schwartz-Arad D, Levin L, Sigal L. Surgical success of intraoral autogenous block onlay bone grafting for alveolar ridge augmentation. Implant Dent. **2005** Jun; 14(2): 131–138.

Schwartz-Arad D, Bichacho N. Effect of age on single implant submersion rate in the central maxillary incisor region: a long-term retrospective study. Clin Implant Dent Relat Res. **2015** Jun; 17(3): 509–514.

Schwarz F, Ferrari D, Herten M, Mihatovic I, Wieland M, Sager M, Becker J. Effects of surface hydrophilicity and microtopography on early stages of soft and hard tissue integration at non-submerged titanium implants: an immunohistochemical study in dogs. J Periodontol. **2007** Nov; 78(11): 2171–2184.

Schwarz F, Rothamel D, Herten M, Ferrari D, Sager M, Becker J. Lateral ridge augmentation using particulated or block bone substitutes biocoated with rhGDF-5 and rhBMP-2: an immunohistochemical study in dogs. Clin Oral Implants Res. **2008** Jul; 19(7): 642–652.

Schwarz F, Sahm N, Schwarz K, Becker J. Impact of defect configuration on the clinical outcome following surgical regenerative therapy of peri-implantitis. J Clin Periodontol. **2010** May; 37(5): 449–455.

Sclar AG. Guidelines for flapless surgery. J Oral Maxillofac Surg. **2007** Jul; 65 (7 Suppl 1): 20–32.

Sculean A, Donos N, Blaes A, Lauermann M, Reich E, Brecx M. Comparison of enamel matrix proteins and bioabsorbable membranes in the treatment of intrabony periodontal defects. A split-mouth study. J Periodontol. **1999** Mar; 70(3): 255–262.

Sculean A, Gruber R, Bosshardt DD. Soft tissue wound healing around teeth and dental implants. J Clin Periodontol. **2014** Apr; 41 (Suppl 15): S6–S22.

Shegarfi H, Reikeras O. Review article: bone transplantation and immune response. J Orthop Surg (Hong Kong). **2009** Aug; 17(2): 206–211.

Shin YK, Han CH, Heo SJ, Kim S, Chun HJ. Radiographic evaluation of marginal bone level around implants with different neck designs after 1 year. Int J Oral Maxillofac Implants. **2006** Sep–Oct; 21(5): 789–794.

Shor A, Schuler R, Goto Y. Indirect implant-supported fixed provisional restoration in the esthetic zone: fabrication technique and treatment workflow. J Esthet Restor Dent. **2008**; 20(2): 82–95.

Siddiqi A, Kieser JA, De Silva RK, Thomson WM, Duncan WJ. Soft and hard tissue response to zirconia versus titanium one-piece implants placed in alveolar and palatal sites: a randomized control trial. Clin Implant Dent Relat Res. **2015** Jun; (17(3): 483–496.

Sigurdsson TJ, Nygaard L, Tatakis DN, Fu E, Turek TJ, Jin L, Wozney JM, Wikesjö UM. Periodontal repair in dogs: evaluation of rhBMP-2 carriers. Int J Periodontics Restorative Dent. **1996** Dec; 16(6): 524–537.

Silva TM, Salvia AC, Carvalho RF, Pagani C, Rocha DM, Silva EG. Polishing for glass ceramics: which protocol? J Prosthodont Res. **2014** Jul; 58(3): 160–170.

Simion M, Baldoni M, Rossi P, Zaffe D. A comparative study of the effectiveness of e-PTFE membranes with and without early exposure during the healing period. Int J Periodontics Restorative Dent. **1994** Apr; 14(2): 166–180. (**a**)

Simion M, Trisi P, Piattelli A. Vertical ridge augmentation using a membrane technique associated with osseointegrated implants. Int J Periodontics Restorative Dent. **1994** Dec; 14(6): 496–511. (**b**)

Simion M, Misitano U, Gionso L, Salvato A. Treatment of dehiscences and fenestrations around dental implants using resorbable and nonresorbable membranes associated with bone autografts: a comparative clinical study. Int J Oral Maxillofac Implants. **1997** Mar–Apr; 12(2): 159–167.

Simion M, Jovanovic SA, Trisi P, Scarano A, Piattelli A. Vertical ridge augmentation around dental implants using a membrane technique and autogenous bone or allografts in humans. Int J Periodontics Restorative Dent. **1998** Feb; 18(1): 8–23.

Simion M, Fontana F, Rasperini G, Maiorana C. Long-term evaluation of osseointegrated implants placed in sites augmented with sinus floor elevation associated with vertical ridge augmentation: a retrospective study of 38 consecutive implants with 1- to 7-year follow-up. Int J Periodontics Restorative Dent. **2004** Jun; 24(3): 208–221.

Simion M, Fontana F, Rasperini G, Maiorana C. Vertical ridge augmentation by expanded-polytetrafluoroethylene membrane and a combination of intraoral autogenous bone graft and deproteinized anorganic bovine bone (Bio-Oss). Clin Oral Implants Res. **2007** Oct; 18(5): 620–629.

Simion M, Rocchietta I, Fontana F, Dellavia C. Evaluation of a resorbable collagen matrix infused with rh-PDGF-BB in peri-implant soft tissue augmentation: a preliminary report with 3.5 years of observation. Int J Periodontics Restorative Dent. **2012** Jun; 32(3): 273–282.

Smith DE, Zarb GA. Criteria for success of osseointegrated endosseous implants. J Prosthet Dent. **1989** Nov; 62(5): 567–572.

Sohrabi K, Mushantat A, Esfandiari S, Feine J. How successful are small-diameter implants? A literature review. Clin Oral Implants Res. **2012** May; 23(5): 515–525.

Spear FM, Kokich VG. A multidisciplinary approach to esthetic dentistry. Dent Clin North Am. **2007** Apr; 51(2): 487–505.

Speroni S, Cicciu M, Maridati P, Grossi GB, Maiorana C. Clinical investigation of mucosal thickness stability after soft tissue grafting around implants: a 3-year retrospective study. Indian J Dent Res. **2010** Oct–Dec; 21(4): 474–479.

Spin-Neto R, Stavropoulos A, Coletti FL, Pereira LA, Marcantonio E Jr, Wenzel A. Remodeling of cortical and corticocancellous fresh-frozen allogeneic block bone grafts—a radiographic and histomorphometric comparison to autologous bone grafts. Clin Oral Implants Res. **2015** Jul; 26(7): 747–752.

Spray JR, Black CG, Morris HF, Ochi S. The influence of bone thickness on facial marginal bone response: stage 1 placement through stage 2 uncovering. Ann Periodontol. **2000** Dec; 5(1): 119–128.

Springer IN, Terheyden H, Geiss S, Harle F, Hedderich J, Açil Y. Particulated bone grafts—effectiveness of bone cell supply. Clin Oral Implants Res. **2004** Apr; 15(2): 205–212.

Spyropoulou PE, Razzoog M, Sierraalta M. Restoring implants in the esthetic zone after sculpting and capturing the periimplant tissues in rest position: a clinical report. J Prosthet Dent. **2009** Dec; 102(6): 345–347.

Srinivasan M, Vazquez L, Rieder P, Moraguez O, Bernard JP, Belser UC. Survival rates of short (6 mm) micro-rough surface implants: a review of literature and meta-analysis. Clin Oral Implants Res. **2014** May; 25(5): 539–545.

Stacchi C, Costantinides F, Biasotto M, Di Lenarda R. Relocation of a malpositioned maxillary implant with piezoelectric osteotomies: a case report. Int J Periodontics Restorative Dent. **2008** Oct; 28(5): 489–495.

Stellini E, Comuzzi L, Mazzocco F, Parente N, Gobbato L. Relationships between different tooth shapes and patient's periodontal phenotype. J Periodontal Res. **2013** Oct; 48(5): 657–662.

Stenport VF, Johansson CB. Evaluations of bone tissue integration to pure and alloyed titanium implants. Clin Implant Dent Relat Res. **2008** Sep; 10(3): 191–199.

Stimmelmayr M, Edelhoff F, Guth FJ, Erdelt K, Happe A, Beuer F. Wear at the titanium-titanium and the titanium-zirconia implant-abutment interface: a comparative in vitro study. Dent Mater. **2012** Dec; 28(12): 1215–1220.

Strietzel FP, Khongkhunthian P, Khattiya R, Patchanee P, Reichart PA. Healing pattern of bone defects covered by different membrane types--a histologic study in the porcine mandible. J Biomed Mater Res B Appl Biomater. **2006** Jul(1); 78: 35–46.

Strietzel FP, Neumann K, Hertel M. Impact of platform switching on marginal peri-implant bone-level changes. A systematic review and meta-analysis. Clin Oral Implants Res. **2015** Mar; 26(3): 342–358**.**

Strub JR, Rekow ED, Witkowski S. Computer-aided design and fabrication of dental restorations: current systems and future possibilities. J Am Dent Assoc. **2006** Sep; 137(9): 1289–1296.

Sui X, Wei H, Wang D, Han Y, Deng J, Wang Y, Wang J, Yang J. Experimental research on the relationship between fit accuracy and fracture resistance of zirconia abutments. J Dent. **2014** Oct; 42(10): 1353–1359.

Svanborg LM, Andersson M, Wennerberg A. Surface characterization of commercial oral implants on the nanometer level. J Biomed Mater Res B Appl Biomater. **2010** Feb; 92(2): 462–469.

Tahmaseb A, Wismeijer D, Coucke W, Derksen W. Computer technology application in durgical implant dentistry: a systematic review. Int J Oral Maxillofac Implants. **2014**; 29 (Suppl): 25–42.

Takei HH. The interdental space. Dent Clin North Am. **1980** Apr; 24(2): 169–176.

Tarnow DP, Cho SC, Wallace SS. The effect of inter-implant distance on the height of inter-implant bone crest. J Periodontol. **2000** Apr; 71(4): 546–549.

Tarnow D, Elian N, Fletcher P, Froum S, Magner A, Cho SC, Salama M, Salama H, Garber DA. Vertical distance from the crest of bone to the height of the interproximal papilla between adjacent implants. J Periodontol. **2003** Dec; 74(12): 1785 – 1788.

Tatakis DN, Chambrone L, Allen EP, Langer B, McGuire MK, Richardson CR, Zabalegui I, Zadeh HH. Periodontal soft tissue root coverage procedures: a consensus report from the AAP Regeneration Workshop. J Periodontol. **2015** Feb; 86 (2 Suppl): S52 – S55.

Tettamanti S, Millen C, Gavric J, Buser D, Belser UC, Brägger U, Wittneben JG. Esthetic evaluation of implant crowns and peri-implant soft tissue in the anterior maxilla: comparison and reproducibility of three different indices. Clin Implant Dent Relat Res. **2016** Jun; 18(3): 517 – 526.

Teughels W, Van Assche N, Sliepen I, Quirynen M. Effect of material characteristics and/or surface topography on biofilm development. Clin Oral Implants Res. **2006** Oct; 17 (Suppl 2): 68 – 81.

Theoharidou, A, Petridis HP, Tzannas K, Garefis P. Abutment screw loosening in single-implant restorations: A systematic review. Int J Oral Maxillofac Implants. **2008** Jul – Aug; 23(4): 681 – 690.

Thoma DS, Benić GI, Zwahlen M, Hämmerle CH, Jung RE. A systematic review assessing soft tissue augmentation techniques. Clin Oral Implants Res. **2009** Sep; 20 (Suppl 4): 146 – 165.

Thoma DS, Jones AA, Dard M, Grize L, Obrecht M, Cochran DL. Tissue integration of a new titanium-zirconium dental implant: a comparative histologic and radiographic study in the canine. J Periodontol. **2011** Oct; 82: 1453 – 1461.

Thoma DS, Dard MM, Halg GA, Ramel CF, Hammerle CH, Jung RE. Evaluation of a biodegradable synthetic hydrogel used as a guided bone regeneration membrane: an experimental study in dogs. Clin Oral Implants Res. **2012** Feb; 23(2): 160 – 168. (**a**)

Thoma DS, Sancho-Puchades M, Ettlin DA, Hämmerle CH, Jung RE. Impact of a collagen matrix on early healing, aesthetics and patient morbidity in oral mucosal wounds—a randomized study in humans. J Clin Periodontol. **2012** Feb; 39(2); 157 – 165. (**b**)

Thoma DS, Buranawat B, Hämmerle CH, Held U, Jung RE. Efficacy of soft tissue augmentation around dental implants and in partially edentulous areas: a systematic review. J Clin Periodontol. **2014** Apr; 41 (Suppl 15): S77 – S91. (**a**)

Thoma DS, Mühlemann S, Jung RE. Critical soft-tissue dimensions with dental implants and treatment concepts. Periodontol 2000. **2014** Oct; 66(1): 106 – 118. (**b**)

Thoma DS, Kruse A, Ghayor C, Jung RE, Weber FE. Bone augmentation using a synthetic hydroxyapatite/silica oxide-based and a xenogenic hydroxyapatite-based bone substitute materials with and without recombinant human bone morphogenetic protein-2. Clin Oral Implants Res. **2015** May; 26(5): 592 – 598.

Thoma DS, Ioannidis A, Cathomen E, Hämmerle CH, Hüsler J, Jung RE. Discoloration of the peri-implant mucosa caused by zirconia and titanium implants. Int J Periodontics Restorative Dent. **2016** Jan – Feb; 36(1): 39 – 45. (**a**)

Thoma DS, Zeltner M, Hilbe M, Hämmerle CH, Hüsler J, Jung RE. Randomized controlled clinical study evaluating effectiveness and safety of a volume-stable collagen matrix compared to autogenous connective tissue grafts for soft tissue augmentation at implant sites. J Clin Periodontol. **2016** Oct; 43(10): 874 – 875. (**b**)

Thoma DS, Brandenberg F, Fehmer V, Knechtle N, Hämmerle CH, Sailer I. The esthetic effect of veneered zirconia abutments for single-tooth implant reconstructions: a randomized controlled clinical trial. Clin Implant Dent Relat Res. **2016** Dec; 18(6): 1210 – 1217. (**c**)

Thomas V, Zhang X, Vohra YK. A biomimetic tubular scaffold with spatially designed nanofibers of protein/PDS bio-blends. Biotechnol Bioeng. **2008** Dec 1; 104(5): 1025 – 1033.

Thulasidas S, Givan DA, Lemons JE, O'Neal SJ, Ramp LC, Liu PR. Influence of implant angulation on the fracture resistance of zirconia abutments. J Prosthodont. **2015** Feb; 24(2): 127 – 135.

Tjan AH, Miller GD, The JG. Some esthetic factors in a smile. J Prosthet Dent. **1984** Jan; 51(1): 24 – 28.

Tonetti MS, Lang NP, Cortellini P, Suvan JE, Adriaens P, Dubravec D, Fonzar A, Fourmousis I, Mayfield L, Rossi R, Silvestri M, Tiedemann C, Topoll H, Vangsted T, Wallkamm B. Enamel matrix proteins in the regenerative therapy of deep intrabony defects. J Clin Periodontol. **2002** Apr; 29(4): 317 – 325.

Traore A, Yombi JC, Tribak K, Cornu O. Risk of virus transmission through femoral head allografts: a Belgian appraisal. J Clin Orthop Trauma. **2013** Sep; 4(3): 119 – 122.

Tsuji K, Bandyopadhyay A, Harfe BD, Cox K, Kakar S, Gerstenfeld L, Einhorn T, Tabin CJ, Rosen V. BMP2 activity, although dispensable for bone formation, is required for the initiation of fracture healing. Nat Genet. **2006** Dec; 38(12): 1424 – 1429.

Urban IA, Lozada JL, Jovanovic SA, Nagursky H, Nagy K. Vertical ridge augmentation with titanium-reinforced, dense-PTFE membranes and a combination of particulated autogenous bone and anorganic bovine bone-derived mineral: a prospective case series in 19 patients. Int J Oral Maxillofac Implants. **2014** Jan – Feb; 29(1): 185 – 193.

Urban IA, Monje A, Wang HL. Vertical ridge augmentation and soft tissue reconstruction of the anterior atrophic maxillae: a case series. Int J Periodontics Restorative Dent. **2015** Sep – Oct; 35(5): 613 – 623.

Urban IA, Lozada JL, Nagy K, Sanz M. Treatment of severe mucogingival defects with a combination of strip gingival grafts and a xenogenic collagen matrix: a prospective case series study. Int J Periodontics Restorative Dent. **2015** May – Jun; 35(3): 345 – 353.

Urist MR. Bone: formation by autoinduction. Science. **1965** Nov 12; 150(3698): 893 – 899.

Urist MR, Silverman BF, Büring K, Dubuc FL, Rosenberg JM. The bone induction principle. Clin Orthop Relat Res. **1967** Jul – Aug; 53: 243 – 283.

Vailati F, Belser U. Implant-supported fixed prostheses with integrated artificial gingiva for the esthetic zone: the Pink Power Concept. Forum Implantologicum. **2011**; 7(2): 108 – 123.

Van Assche N, Michels S, Naert I, Quirynen M. Randomized controlled trial to compare two bone substitutes in the treatment of bony dehiscences. Clin Implant Dent Relat Res. **2013** Aug; 15(4): 558 – 568.

van Brakel R, Noordmans HJ, Frenken J, de Roode R, de Wit GC, Cune MS. The effect of zirconia and titanium implant abutments on light reflection of the supporting soft tissues. Clin Oral Implants Res. **2011** Oct; 22(10): 1172 – 1178.

Van der Weijden F, Dell'Acqua F, Slot DE. Alveolar bone dimensional changes of post-extraction sockets in humans: a systematic review. J Clin Periodontol. **2009** Dec; 36(12): 1048 – 1058.

van Steenberghe D. Outcomes and their measurement in clinical trials of endosseous oral implants. Ann Periodontol. **1997** Mar; 2(1): 291 – 298.

van Steenberghe D. The use of oral implants in compromised patients. Periodontol 2000. **2003**; 33: 9 – 11.

Vela X, Méndez V, Rodríguez X, Segalá M, Tarnow DP. Crestal bone changes on platform-switched implants and adjacent teeth when the tooth-implant distance is less than 1.5 mm. Int J Periodontics Restorative Dent. **2012** Apr; 32(2): 149 – 155.

Velasco-Ortega E, Jos A, Cameán AM, Pato-Mourelo J, Segura-Egea JJ. In vitro evaluation of cytotoxicity and genotoxicity of a commercial titanium alloy for dental implantology. Mutat Res. **2010** Sep 30; 702(1): 17 – 23.

Velvart P, Ebner-Zimmermann U, Ebner JP. Comparison of long-term papilla healing following sulcular full thickness flap and papilla base flap in endodontic surgery. Int Endod J. **2004** Oct; 37(10): 687 – 693.

Vera C, De Kok IJ, Chen W, Reside G, Tyndall D, Cooper LF. Evaluation of post-implant buccal bone resorption using cone beam computed tomography: a clinical pilot study. Int J Oral Maxillofac Implants. **2012** Sep – Oct; 27(5): 1249 – 1257.

Vercellotti T. Piezoelectric surgery in implantology: a case report--a new piezoelectric ridge expansion technique. Int J Periodontics Restorative Dent. **2000** Aug; 20(4): 358 – 365.

Vercruyssen M, Laleman I, Jacobs R, Quirynen M. Computer-supported implant planning and guided surgery: a narrative review. Clin Oral Implants Res. **2015** Sep; 26 (Suppl 11): 69 – 76.

Vervaeke S, Dierens M, Besseler J, De Bruyn H. The influence of initial soft tissue thickness on peri-implant bone remodeling. Clin Implant Dent Relat Res. **2014** Apr; 16(2): 238–247.

Vignoletti F, Johansson C, Albrektsson T, De Sanctis M, San Roman F, Sanz M. Early healing of implants placed into fresh extraction sockets: an experimental study in the beagle dog. De novo bone formation. J Clin Periodontol. **2009** Mar; 36(3): 265–277.

Vignoletti F, Matesanz P, Rodrigo D, Figuero E, Martin C, Sanz M. Surgical protocols for ridge preservation after tooth extraction. A systematic review. Clin Oral Implants Res. **2012** Feb; 23 (Suppl 5): 22–38.

Vignoletti F, Sanz M. Immediate implants at fresh extraction sockets: from myth to reality. Periodontol 2000. **2014** Oct; 66(1): 132–152.

Villa R, Rangert B. Immediate and early function of implants placed in extraction sockets of maxillary infected teeth: a pilot study. J Prosthet Dent. **2007** Jun; 97 (6 Suppl): S96-S108.

Vo TN, Kasper FK, Mikos AG. Strategies for controlled delivery of growth factors and cells for bone regeneration. Adv Drug Deliv Rev. **2012** Sep; 64(12): 1292–1309.

von Arx T, Cochran DL, Hermann JS, Schenk RK, Higginbottom FL, Buser D. Lateral ridge augmentation and implant placement: an experimental study evaluating implant osseointegration in different augmentation materials in the canine mandible. Int J Oral Maxillofac Implants. **2001** May–Jun; 16(3): 343–354.

von Arx T, Broggini N, Jensen SS, Bornstein MM, Schenk RK, Buser D. Membrane durability and tissue response of different bioresorbable barrier membranes: a histologic study in the rabbit calvarium. Int J Oral Maxillofac Implants. **2005** Nov–Dec; 20(6): 843–853.

von Arx T, Buser D. Horizontal ridge augmentation using autogenous block grafts and the guided bone regeneration technique with collagen membranes: a clinical study with 42 patients. Clin Oral Implants Res. **2006** Aug; 17(4): 359–366.

von Arx T, Salvi GE. Incision techniques and flap designs for apical surgery in the anterior maxilla. Eur J Esthet Dent. **2008** Summer; 3(2): 110–126.

Waasdorp JA, Evian CI, Mandracchia M. Immediate placement of implants into infected sites: a systematic review of the literature. J Periodontol. **2010** Jun; 81(6): 801–808.

Waasdorp J, Reynolds MA. Allogeneic bone onlay grafts for alveolar ridge augmentation: a systematic review. Int J Oral Maxillofac Implants. **2010** May–Jun; 25(3): 525–531. (**b**)

Wadhwani, C. Piñeyro, A. Technique for controlling the cement for an implant crown. J Prosthet Dent. **2009** Jul; 102(1); 57–58.

Wadhwani C, Piñeyro A, Hess T, Zhang H, Chung KH. Effect of implant abutment modification on the extrusion of excess cement at the crown abutment margin for cement-retained implant restorations. Int J Oral Maxillofac Implants. **2011** Nov–Dec; 26(6): 1241–1246.

Wadhwani CP, Piñeyro A, Akimoto K. An introduction to the implant crown with an esthetic adhesive margin (ICEAM). J Esthet Restor Dent. **2012** Aug; 24(4): 246–254. (**a**)

Wadhwani C, Rapoport D, La Rosa S, Hess T, Kretschmar S. Radiographic detection and characteristic patterns of residual excess cement associated with cement-retained implant restorations: a clinical report. J Prosthet Dent. **2012** Mar; 107(3): 151–157. (**b**)

Wadhwani C, Chung KH. Effect of modifying the screw access channels of zirconia implant abutment on the cement flow pattern and retention of zirconia restorations. J Prosthet Dent. **2014** Jul; 112(1): 45–50.

Wadhwani C, Goodwin S, Chung KH. Cementing an implant crown: a novel measurement system using computational fluid dynamics approach. Clin Implant Dent Relat Res. **2016** Feb; 18(1): 97–106.

Wallace DG, Cruise GM, Rhee WM, Schroeder JA, Prior JJ, Ju J, Maroney M, Duronio J, Ngo MH, Estridge T, Coker GC. A tissue sealant based on reactive multifunctional polyethylene glycol. J Biomed Mater Res. **2001**; 58(5): 545–555.

Wang F, Zhang Z, Monje A, Huang W, Wu Y, Wang G. Intermediate long-term clinical performance of dental implants placed in sites with a previous early implant failure: a retrospective analysis. Clin Oral Implants Res. **2015** Dec; 26(12): 1443–1449.

Weber HP, Kim FM, Ng MW, Hwang JW, Fiorellini JP. Peri-implant soft-tissue health surrounding cement- and screw-retained implant restorations: a multicenter, 3-year prospective study. Clin Oral Implants Res. **2006** Aug; 17(4): 375–379.

Weber HP, Morton D, Gallucci GO, Roccuzzo M, Cordaro L, Grutter L. Consensus statements and recommended clinical procedures regarding loading protocols. Int J Oral Maxillofac Implants. **2009**; 24 (Suppl): 180–183.

Wechsler S, Fehr D, Molenberg A, Raeber G, Schense JC, Weber FE. A novel, tissue occlusive poly(ethylene glycol) hydrogel material. J Biomed Mater Res A. **2008** May; 85(2): 285–292.

Weisgold AS. Contours of the full crown restoration. Alpha Omegan. **1977** Dec; 70(3): 77–89.

Wennerberg A, Albrektsson T. Effects of titanium surface topography on bone integration: a systematic review. Clin Oral Implants Res. **2009** Sep; 20 (Suppl 4): 172–184.

Wennström JL, Bengazi F, Lekholm U. The influence of the masticatory mucosa on the peri-implant soft tissue condition. Clin Oral Implants Res. **1994** Mar; 5(1): 1–8.

Wennström JL, Ekestubbe A, Gröndahl K, Karlsson S, Lindhe J. Implant-supported single-tooth restorations: a 5-year prospective study. J Clin Periodontol. **2005** Jun; 32(6): 567–574.

Wennström JL, Derks J. Is there a need for keratinized mucosa around implants to maintain health and tissue stability? Clin Oral Implants Res. **2012** Oct; 23 (Suppl 6): 136–146.

Weston JF, Haupt E. Creating aesthetic success through proper clinician and laboratory technical communication. Dent Clin North Am. **2011** Apr; 55(2): 371–382.

Widmann G, Stoffner R, Schullian P, Widmann R, Keiler M, Zangerl A, Puelacher W, Bale RJ. Comparison of the accuracy of invasive and noninvasive registration methods for image-guided oral implant surgery. Int J Oral Maxillofac Implants. **2010** May–Jun; 25(3): 491–498.

Widmark G, Andersson B, Ivanoff CJ. Mandibular bone graft in the anterior maxilla for single-tooth implants. Presentation of surgical method. Int J Oral Maxillofac Surg. **1997** Apr; 26(2): 106–109.

Wiesner G, Esposito M, Worthington H, Schlee M. Connective tissue grafts for thickening peri-implant tissues at implant placement. One-year results from an explanatory split-mouth randomised controlled clinical trial. Eur J Oral Implantol. **2010** Spring; 3(1): 27–35.

Williams D. The golden anniversary of titanium biomaterials. Med Device Technol. **2001** Sep; 12(7): 8–11.

Williams DF. On the mechanisms of biocompatibility. Biomaterials. **2008** Jul; 29(20): 2941–2953.

Wilson TG Jr. positive relationship between excess cement and peri-implant disease: a prospective clinical endoscopic study. J Periodontol. **2009** Sep; 80(9): 1388–1392.

Winkler S. Ring K, Ring JD, Boberick KG. Implant screw mechanics and the settling effect: overview. J Oral Implantol. **2003**; 29(5): 242–245.

Wittneben JG, Buser D, Belser UC, Brägger U. Peri-implant soft tissue conditioning with provisional restorations in the esthetic zone: the dynamic compression technique. Int J Periodontics Restorative Dent. **2013** Jul–Aug; 33(4): 447–455.

Wittneben JG, Millen C, Brägger U. Clinical performance of screw- versus cement-retained fixed implant-supported reconstructions—a systematic review. Int J Oral Maxillofac Implants. **2014**; 29 (Suppl): 84–98.

Wood DL, Hoag PM, Donnenfeld OW, Rosenfeld LD. Alveolar crest reduction following full and partial thickness flaps. J Periodontol. **1972** Mar; 43(3): 141–144.

Yan JJ, Tsai AY, Wong MY, Hou LT. Comparison of acellular dermal graft and palatal autograft in the reconstruction of keratinized gingiva around dental implants: a case report. Int J Periodontics Restorative Dent. **2006** Jun; 26(3): 287–292.

Yilmaz B. Gilbert AB, Seidt JD, McGlumphy EA, Clelland NL Displacement of implant abutments following initial and repeated torqueing. Int J Oral Maxillofac Implants. **2015** Sep–Oct; 30(5): 1011–1018.

Young MP, Carter DH, Worthington H, Korachi M, Drucker DB. Microbial analysis of bone collected during implant surgery: a clinical and laboratory study. Clin Oral Implants Res. **2001** Apr; 12(2): 95 – 103.

Zadik Y, Abu-Tair J, Yarom N, Zaharia B, Elad S. The importance of a thorough medical and pharmacological history before dental implant placement. Aust Dent J. **2012** Sep; 57(3): 388 – 392.

Zalkind M, Hochman N. Alternative method of conservative esthetic treatment for gingival recession. J Prosthet Dent. **1997** Jun; 77(6): 561 – 563.

Zembic A, Sailer I, Jung RE, Hämmerle CH. Randomized-controlled clinical trial of customized zirconia and titanium implant abutments for single-tooth implants in canine and posterior regions: 3-year results. Clin Oral Implants Res. **2009** Aug; 20(8): 802 – 808.

Zembic A, Bösch A, Jung RE, Hämmerle CH, Sailer I. Five-year results of a randomized controlled clinical trial comparing zirconia and titanium abutments supporting single-implant crowns in canine and posterior regions. Clin Oral Implants Res. **2013** Apr; 24(4): 384 – 390.

Zembic A, Kim S, Zwahlen M, Kelly JR. Systematic review of the survival rate and incidence of biologic, technical, and esthetic complications of single implant abutments supporting fixed porstheses. Int J Oral Maxillofac Implants. **2014**; 29 (Suppl): 99 – 116.

Zembic A, Philipp AO, Hämmerle CH, Wohlwend A, Sailer I. Eleven-year follow-up of a prospective study of zirconia implant abutments supporting single all-ceramic crowns in anterior and premolar regions. Clin Implant Dent Relat Res. **2015** Oct; 17 (Suppl 2): e417 – e426.

Zinsli B, Sägesser T, Mericske E, Mericske-Stern R. Int J Oral Maxillofac Implants. **2004** Jan – Feb; 19(1): 92 – 99.

Zitzmann NU, Schärer P, Marinello CP. Factors influencing the success of GBR. Smoking, timing of implant placement, implant location, bone quality and provisional restoration. J Clin Periodontol. **1999** Oct; 26(10): 673 – 682.

Zitzmann NU, Arnold D, Ball J, Brusco D, Triaca A, Verna C. Treatment strategies for infraoccluded dental implants. J Prosthet Dent. **2015** Mar; 113(3): 169 – 174.

Zouras CS, Winkler S. The custom implant impression coping: technical note. Implant Dent. **1995** Fall; 4(3): 178 – 180.

Zucchelli G, Mazzotti C, Mounssif I, Mele M, Stefanini M, Montebugnoli L. A novel surgical-prosthetic approach for soft tissue dehiscence coverage around single implants. Clin Oral Implants Res. **2013** Sep; 24(9): 957 – 962.

Zwahlen RA, Cheung LK, Zheng LW, Chow RL, Li T, Schuknecht B, Grätz KW, Weber FE. Comparison of two resorbable membrane systems in bone regeneration after removal of wisdom teeth: a randomized-controlled clinical pilot study. Clin Oral Implants Res. **2009** Oct; 20(10): 1084 – 1091.